D1574041

Peptide Drug Discovery and Development

Edited by
Miguel Castanho and Nuno C. Santos

Related Titles

Jameel, F., Hershenson, S. (eds.)

Formulation and Process Development Strategies for Manufacturing Biopharmaceuticals

976 pages
Hardcover
ISBN: 978-0-470-11812-2

Jorgenson, L., Nielson, H. M. (eds.)

Delivery Technologies for Biopharmaceuticals

Peptides, Proteins, Nucleic Acids and Vaccines

442 pages
Hardcover
ISBN: 978-0-470-72338-8

Jensen, K. (ed.)

Peptide and Protein Design for Biopharmaceutical Applications

306 pages
Hardcover
ISBN: 978-0-470-31961-1

Rathore, A. S., Mhatre, R. (eds.)

Quality by Design for Biopharmaceuticals

Principles and Case Studies

288 pages
Hardcover
ISBN: 978-0-470-28233-5

Groner, B. (ed.)

Peptides as Drugs

Discovery and Development

242 pages with approx. 38 figures and approx. 8 tables
2009
Hardcover
ISBN: 978-3-527-32205-3

Cavagnaro, J. A. (ed.)

Preclinical Safety Evaluation of Biopharmaceuticals

A Science-Based Approach to Facilitating Clinical Trials

approx. 1064 pages
Hardcover
ISBN: 978-0-470-10884-0

Edited by Miguel Castanho and Nuno C. Santos

Peptide Drug Discovery and Development

Translational Research in Academia and Industry

WILEY-VCH

WILEY-VCH Verlag GmbH & Co. KGaA

The Editors

Prof. Dr. Miguel Castanho
University of Lisbon
Institute of Biochemistry
Av. Egas Moniz
1649-028 Lisboa
Portugal

Prof. Dr. Nuno C. Santos
University of Lisbon
Institute of Biochemistry
Av. Egas Moniz
1649-028 Lisboa
Portugal

■ All books published by **Wiley-VCH** are carefully produced. Nevertheless, authors, editors, and publisher do not warrant the information contained in these books, including this book, to be free of errors. Readers are advised to keep in mind that statements, data, illustrations, procedural details or other items may inadvertently be inaccurate.

Library of Congress Card No.: applied for

British Library Cataloguing-in-Publication Data
A catalogue record for this book is available from the British Library.

Bibliographic information published by the Deutsche Nationalbibliothek
The Deutsche Nationalbibliothek lists this publication in the Deutsche Nationalbibliografie; detailed bibliographic data are available on the Internet at <http://dnb.d-nb.de>.

© 2011 Wiley-VCH Verlag & Co. KGaA, Boschstr. 12, 69469 Weinheim, Germany

All rights reserved (including those of translation into other languages). No part of this book may be reproduced in any form – by photoprinting, microfilm, or any other means – nor transmitted or translated into a machine language without written permission from the publishers. Registered names, trademarks, etc. used in this book, even when not specifically marked as such, are not to be considered unprotected by law.

Cover Design   Adam Design, Weinheim
Typesetting   MPS Limited, a Macmillan Company, Chennai
Printing and Binding   Fabulous Printers Pte Ltd, Singapore

Printed in Singapore
Printed on acid-free paper

Print ISBN: 978-3-527-32891-8
ePDF ISBN: 978-3-527-63675-4
oBook ISBN: 978-3-527-63673-0
ePub ISBN: 978-3-527-63674-7
Mobi ISBN: 978-3-527-63676-1

Contents

Peptide Drug Discovery and Development: Translational Research in Academia and Industry, First Edition.
Edited by Miguel Castanho and Nuno C. Santos.
© 2011 WILEY-VCH Verlag GmbH & Co. KGaA, Weinheim.
Published 2011 by WILEY-VCH Verlag GmbH & Co. KGaA

Preface

The Timeliness of Peptide Drugs

Peptides make good drugs in challenging situations. They may be more expensive and time-consuming to produce than traditional small molecules, have low oral bioavailability, fast clearance in the body, and even, in some cases, be immunogenic. Yet, their ability to be very active, very specific, present very low toxicity, and often to be developed from natural endogenous scaffolds with known biological activity, makes them a desirable solution for unmet complex medical problems. This is not wishful thinking for the future, only. There are examples of very successful peptide drugs in clinical use. The key to this success is very much related to the mutual co-development of peptide biochemistry/biophysics, peptide synthetic chemistry, peptide pharmacology, and peptide biotechnology. This is the basic principle that underlies this book. Peptides have been the passion of many scientists and the investment of many entrepreneurs. Together they made a fantastic world with a very positive contribution to medicine. This book lets the reader know about this world, where peptides bounce between the bench and the bedside.

The numbers that reveal the achievements of peptide drugs are impressive. In 2008 six peptide drugs had attained global sales of US $750 million. Reichert and colleagues say this figure is a consequence of the widespread acceptance of protein therapeutics by both physicians and patients, together with improvements in tackling problems such as a short half-life and challenges with the delivery of these molecules [1]. In the same study, these authors state that the number of peptide drugs entering clinical trials per year was 1.7 in the 1970s, 4.6 in the 1980s, 9.7 in the 1990s and 16.9 in the 2000s up to 2009. Until now, at least 55 therapeutic peptides have been approved for human clinical use by at least one regulatory agency, although 6 of them were withdrawn from their markets afterwards. The approval success rates for peptides that entered clinical trials from 1984 to 2000 were 21–24%. More than 15 peptide candidates were in phase III trials or under regulatory review in 2009; thus, it is expected the field of peptide drugs will continue its positive trend of progress during the years to come. Given the effort of both academic and industrial R&D to overcome the pitfalls of peptide drug candidates [2, 3] and the "scalability challenges" of peptide production [4], it is

Peptide Drug Discovery and Development: Translational Research in Academia and Industry, First Edition.
Edited by Miguel Castanho and Nuno C. Santos.
© 2011 WILEY-VCH Verlag GmbH & Co. KGaA, Weinheim.
Published 2011 by WILEY-VCH Verlag GmbH & Co. KGaA

predictable that peptide drug discovery and development will continue to prosper. We are not alone in our enthusiasm and optimism [5, 6].

From 2000 to 2007, peptides entering trials were most frequently treatments for metabolic disorders (26%). During the 1990s this fraction was less than 10% [1]. This variation shows how fast peptide drugs are evolving and their range of application being broadened. Areas which are today among the less frequent, such as infection and central nervous system, are being intensively researched and have a large potential to grow [4, 7–9]. They may be the future trend in peptide drug pipelines.

Despite all the peptide R&D figures above, the most important numbers are yet to be clearly ascertained: the number of lives saved by peptide drugs and the improvement in the patients' quality of life. These are the figures truly worth working for and we hope this book will transmit knowledge, power and enthusiasm to the readers so that this endeavour is reinforced.

Finally, we wish to thank all contributors to the book. We are proud of their collaboration and engagement to turn this book into something different: a book about academic research translated into pharma industrial development, written by people directly involved and/or privileged inside witnesses. The mission of authors and editors has been to involve the reader in this world. Be welcome!

Miguel Castanho
Nuno C. Santos
Lisbon, March 14, 2011

References

1 Saladin, P.M., Zhang, B.D., and Reichert, J.M. (2009) Current trends in the clinical development of peptide therapeutics. *Idrugs*, **12** (12), 779–784.

2 Sato, A.K., Viswanathan, M., Kent, R.B., and Wood, C.R. (2006) Therapeutic peptides: technological advances driving peptides into development. *Curr. Opin. Biotechnol.*, **17** (6), 638–642.

3 Lien, S. and Lowman, H.B. (2003) Therapeutic peptides. *Trends Biotechnol.*, **21** (12), 556–562.

4 Marx, V. (2005) Watching peptide drugs grow up. *Chem. Eng. News*, **83** (11), 17–24.

5 Ayoub, M. and Scheidegger, D. (2006) Peptide drugs, overcoming the challenges, a growing business. *Chim. Oggi – Chem. Today*, **24** (4), 46–48.

6 Pichereau, C. and Allary, C. (2005) Therapeutic peptides under the spotlight. *Eur. Biopharm. Rev.*, winter issue.

7 Naider, F. and Anglister, J. (2009) Peptides in the treatment of AIDS. *Curr. Opin. Struct. Biol.*, **19** (4), 473–482.

8 Schwarze, S.R., Ho, A., Vocero-Akbani, A., and Dowdy, S.F. (1999) *In vivo* protein transduction: delivery of a biologically active protein into the mouse. *Science*, **285** (5433), 1569–1572.

9 Davis, T.P., Abbruscato, T.J., Brownson, E., and Hruby, V.J. (1995) Conformationally constrained peptide drugs targeted at the blood-brain barrier. in *Membranes and Barriers: Targeted Drug Delivery* (ed. R.S. Rapaka), NIDA Research Monograph 154, NIH, Rockville, MD, pp. 47–59.

List of Contributors

Rina Aharoni
Weizmann Institute of Science
Department of Immunology
PO Box 26
76100 Rehovot
Israel

Frederico Aires da Silva,
Technophage, SA
IMM
Rua Prof. Egas Moniz
Edifício Egas Moniz, Piso 2
1649–028 Lisboa
Portugal

Muharrem Akcan
The University of Queensland
Division of Chemistry and Structural
Biology
Institute for Molecular Bioscience
QLD 4072 Brisbane
Australia

David H Alpers
Washington University School of
Medicine
Department of Internal Medicine
Box 8031, 660 S Euclid Ave
MO 63110 St Louis
USA

Ruth Arnon
Weizmann Institute of Science
Department of Immunology
PO Box 26
76100 Rehovot
Israel

Eduard Bardají
Universitat de Girona, Campus
Montilivi
Laboratori d'Innovació en Processos i
Productes de Síntesi Orgànica
(LIPPSO), Chemistry Department
17071 Girona
Spain

John Broad
Queen Mary, University of London
Barts & The London School of
Medicine and Dentistry, Wingate
Institute of Neurogastroenterology
26 Ashfield Street
E1 2AJ London
UK

Sofia Côrte-Real
Technophage
IMM
Rua Prof. Egas Moniz
Edifício Egas Moniz, Piso 2
1649–028 Lisboa
Portugal

Peptide Drug Discovery and Development: Translational Research in Academia and Industry, First Edition.
Edited by Miguel Castanho and Nuno C. Santos.
© 2011 WILEY-VCH Verlag GmbH & Co. KGaA, Weinheim.
Published 2011 by WILEY-VCH Verlag GmbH & Co. KGaA

David J. Craik
The University of Queensland
Institute for Molecular Bioscience
QLD 4072 Brisbane
Australia

Simoni C. Dias
Universidade Católica de Brasília
Centro de Análises Proteômicas e
Bioquímicas, Programa de Pós-
Graduação em Ciências Genômicas e
Biotecnologia, SGAN Quadra 916,
Modulo B
Av. W5
70790-160 Brasília-DF
Brazil

Dominique Dugourd
BioWest Therapeutics Inc.
Suite 1320–885 West Georgia
Vancouver, BC, V6C 2G2
Canada

Paul J. Edwards
Boehringer Ingelheim (Canada) Ltd,
Research & Development
2100 Rue Cunard
Laval, QC, H7S 3G5
Canada

Octavio L. Franco
Universidade Católica de Brasília
Centro de Análises Proteômicas e
Bioquímicas, Programa de Pós-
Graduação em Ciências Genômicas e
Biotecnologia
SGAN Quadra 916, Modulo B
Av. W5
70790-160 Brasília-DF
Brazil

Henri G. Franquelim
Universidade de Lisboa
Instituto de Medicina Molecular
Faculdade de Medicina
Av. Prof. Egas Moniz
1649-028 Lisboa
Portugal

João Gonçalves
Universidade de Lisboa
Instituto de Medicina Molecular
Faculdade de Farmácia
Av. Prof. Egas Moniz
1649-028 Lisboa
Portugal

Josias H. Hamman
Tshwane University of Technology
Department of Pharmaceutical
Sciences
Private Bag X680, Arcadia Campus,
0001 Pretoria
South Africa

and

North-West University
Unit for Drug Research and
Development
Private Bag X6001
2520 Potchefstroom
South Africa

Wendy J. Hartsock
University of Colorado
School of Medicine, Department of
Biochemistry & Molecular Genetics
CO 80045 Aurora
USA

Robert S. Hodges
University of Colorado
School of Medicine, Department of
Biochemistry & Molecular Genetics
CO 80045 Aurora
USA

Steven R. LaPlante
Boehringer Ingelheim (Canada) Ltd,
Research & Development
2100 Rue Cunard
Laval, QC, H7S 2G5
Canada

Ning Lee
Bristol Myers Squibb
Dep AQ4 ent of Metabolic Diseases
NJ 08534 Hopewell
USA

Christine M. Mack
Amylin Pharmaceuticals Inc.
9360 Towne
Centre Drive
CA 92121 San Diego
USA

Pedro M. Matos
Universidade de Lisboa
Instituto de Medicina Molecular
Faculdade de Medicina
Av. Prof. Egas Moniz
1649-028 Lisboa
Portugal

Graham Molineux
Amgen Inc
Hematology and Oncology Discovery
Research
One Amgen Center Drive, Mailstop
15-2-A, Thousand Oaks,
CA 91320
USA

David G. Parkes
Amylin Pharmaceuticals Inc.
9360 Towne
Centre Drive
CA 92121 San Diego
USA

Mary Ann Pelleymounter
Bristol Myers Squibb
Department of Metabolic Diseases
NJ 08534 Hopewell
USA

Suzana M. Ribeiro
Universidade Católica de Brasília
Centro de Análises Proteômicas e
Bioquímicas, Programa de Pós-
Graduação em Ciências Genômicas e
Biotecnologia, SGAN Quadra 916,
Modulo B
Av. W5
70790-160 Brasília-DF
Brazil

Marta M.B. Ribeiro
Universidade Lisboa,
Instituto de Medicina Molecular,
Faculdade de Medicina
Av. Prof. Egas Moniz
1649-028 Lisboa
Portugal

Jonathan D. Roth
Amylin Pharmaceuticals Inc.
9360 Towne Centre Drive
CA 92121 San Diego
USA

Evelina Rubinchik
BioWest Therapeutics Inc.
Suite 1320–885 West Georgia
Vancouver, BC, V6C 2G2
Canada

Gareth J. Sanger
Queen Mary, University of London
Barts & The London School of
Medicine and Dentistry, Wingate
Institute of Neurogastroenterology
26 Ashfield Street
E1 2AJ London
UK

Sónia Sá Santos
Universidade Lisboa,
Instituto de Medicina Molecular,
Faculdade de Medicina
Av. Prof. Egas Moniz
1649-028 Lisboa
Portugal

Michael Sela
Weizmann Institute of Science
Department of Immunology
PO Box 26,
76100 Rehovot
Israel

Isa D. Serrano
Universidade Lisboa,
Instituto de Medicina Molecular,
Faculdade de Medicina
Av. Prof. Egas Moniz
1649-028 Lisboa
Portugal

Jan H. Steenekamp
North-West University
Department of Pharmaceutics, School
of Pharmacy
Private Bag X6001
Potchefstroom Campus,
2520 Potchefstroom
South Africa

James L. Trevaskis
Amylin Pharmaceuticals Inc.
9360 Towne Centre Drive
CA 92121 San Diego
USA

A. Salomé Veiga
National Cancer Institute
Chemical Biology Laboratory
376 Boyles Street,
MD 21702 Frederick
USA
and
Universidade Lisboa,
Instituto de Medicina Molecular,
Faculdade de Medicina
Av. Prof. Egas Moniz
1649-028 Lisboa
Portugal

Fengshan Wang
Shandong University
Institute of Biochemical and
Biotechnological Drug, School of
Pharmaceutical Sciences
Jinan
250012 Shandong
P. R. China

Yuren Wang
Bristol Myers Squibb
Department of Metabolic Diseases
NJ 08534 Hopewell
USA

Ping Wei
Amgen Inc
Hematology and Oncology Discovery
Research
One Amgen Center Drive, Mailstop
15-2-A
CA 91320 Thousand Oaks
USA

Hao Wu
Beijing You'an Hospital, Capital
Medical University
Department of Infectious Diseases
100069 Beijing
P. R. China

Xiaobin Zhang
FusoGen Pharmaceuticals, Inc.
Ping'an Building B19-A
59 Machang Road
Hexi District,
300203 Tianjin
P. R. China

Part I
The Academia – Market Bouncing of Peptide Drugs – Challenges and Strategies in Translational Research with Peptide Drugs

Peptide Drug Discovery and Development: Translational Research in Academia and Industry, First Edition.
Edited by Miguel Castanho and Nuno C. Santos.
© 2011 WILEY-VCH Verlag GmbH & Co. KGaA, Weinheim.
Published 2011 by WILEY-VCH Verlag GmbH & Co. KGaA

1
Peptides as Leads for Drug Discovery

Paul J. Edwards and Steven R. LaPlante

1.1
Introduction

Peptides have long been used as a source of active material for drug discovery but their use as marketed medicaments is often limited to intravenous administration. The received opinion for peptide drugs delivered via the oral route is that this is a highly challenging endeavor due to the peptides propensity for proteolytic degradation, high clearance, and resulting problems with its delivery, such as low oral bioavailability; all arising from the inclusion of a number of peptide bonds. Scientists have, therefore, sought peptide mimics (peptidomimetics) [1] where degradation of the peptide bonds is hindered (through, for example, N-methylation of the amide nitrogen) and de-peptidization through morphing of the amide (peptide) bonds into peptoids, for example, or through making the molecule more like a small molecule than a peptide. The peptidomimetic would have similar secondary structure as well as other structural features analogous to that of the original peptide, which allows it to displace the original peptide, or protein, from receptors or enzymes [2]. It is in the context of peptidomimics that this work will focus, on peptide-based discovery that has led to advanced (pre-)clinical candidates which are delivered by the oral route of administration.

Fortunately, advances in technologies such as phage-display screening, have enabled the high-throughput discovery of peptides that can inhibit a desired biological reaction for drug discovery purposes [3]. It is now also possible to enable the rapid optimization of peptide mimics to satisfy the many hurdles of drug development. This review intends to expose the fascinating properties and handles that peptides offer and how, through "sensemaking" – that is, the process of gathering and interpreting a body of information relevant to a problem [4] – leading to knowledge building within the project, coupled to synthetic and analytical strategies, successful processes may be adopted that can deliver peptide mimetic (pre-) clinical candidates. We will emphasize our experience from in-house programs where peptide leads were successfully advanced to pre-clinical and clinical candidates (see Figure 1.1). Critical lessons, novel strategies, and examples will be explored at various stages of this process, ranging from the discovery of peptide

Peptide Drug Discovery and Development: Translational Research in Academia and Industry, First Edition.
Edited by Miguel Castanho and Nuno C. Santos.
© 2011 WILEY-VCH Verlag GmbH & Co. KGaA, Weinheim.
Published 2011 by WILEY-VCH Verlag GmbH & Co. KGaA

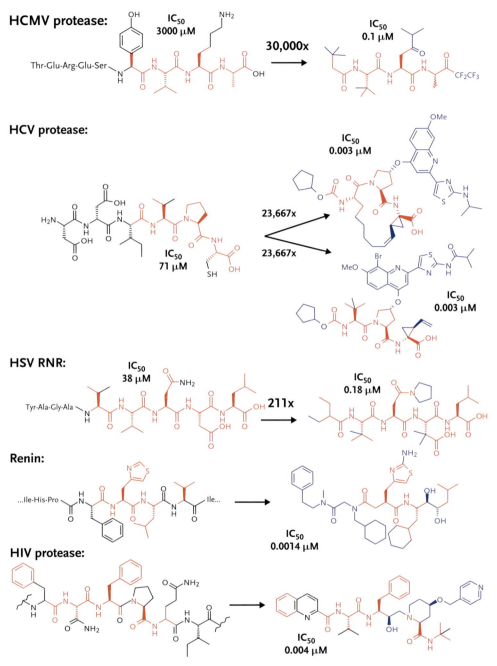

Figure 1.1 Structures of peptide starting points (leads) and their advanced peptide mimics (drugs). The conserved bonds/atoms in both the lead and drug are colored red, whereas the blue and black represent new and modified or deleted sections, respectively.

leads to those that have entered clinical trials. Particularly, we propose that our strategy and work flow (see Schemes 1.1 and 1.2) can represent an expeditious way to render peptides to drugs. This review will be based on exposing major findings/ lessons that have commonality among systems and that can advance drug discovery rapidly, if used appropriately. Central for this purpose, it is demonstrated in Figure 1.1 that there can be a significant degree of similarity between the original peptide hit and the advanced analog. Figure 1.1 shows that one can conserve major segments and structural features of relatively weak lead peptides that are required for achieving potency in drugs (colored as red in Figure 1.1). Also critical are truncations and alterations (colored black) and the addition of new features (colored in blue). In summary, we believe that if one can exploit the latent structural functionality on the peptide starting points effectively, then delivery of orally bioavailable drugs derived from a peptide lead becomes possible.

1.2
Overview of Process for Transforming Peptides to Peptidomimetics

The pharmaceutical industry has developed complex and fascinating processes for discovering and optimizing leads that become drugs. Scheme 1.1 depicts an overview of how one might progress a peptide to peptidomimetic drug project, indicating the various stages (bold text) that will be exemplified in the projects that follow. Of central importance is the "sensemaking" phase (Scheme 1.2), supported by knowledge building, including mapping of the critical binding parts of the peptide with model creation and peptide truncation, and matching of the free state of the peptide to the bioactive conformation through, for example, rigidification, and de-peptidization.

This chapter will consider a number of case studies against different targets where, after hit identification, the minimal peptide fragments were elucidated and then subjected to conformational rigidification. It is well understood that the binding of a ligand to a macromolecule involves numerous recognition events that are strongly influenced by forces such as van der Waal contacts, electrostatic interactions, solvation effects, and also by ligand to macromolecule shape complementarity. Less well appreciated, but no less important and as critical to these recognition events, are the necessary structural and flexibility adaptations of the ligand and receptor to attain the bioactive complex. Therefore, when considering utilizing a peptide hit as a starting point for drug discovery, the tactics utilized should move beyond the classical "lock-and-key" model to a more holistic approach that incorporates the effects of dynamics and conformational changes. In doing so, rational drug design efforts could be accelerated from the knowledge of these adaptive processes. However, to date, few reports of the application of dynamics and conformational changes have appeared in the literature. In part this is due to the paucity of experimental methods that can provide the type of atomic-level information required. Thus, their importance and impact in drug design have not yet been fully realized.

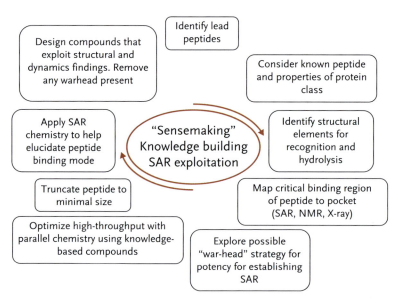

Ideas *Peptide-derived small-molecule drug discovery* Drug

- **Synthesize many compounds (medicinal parallel chemistry)**

- Develop assays

- **Exploit knowledge building and sensemaking strategies**

- Launch from publicly available sources

- **Satisfy assays (binding potency, specificity, cell culture)**

- **Protect discoveries (patents)**

- Identify
  - toxicity limits
  - metabolite liabilities
- Ensure
  - Large scale synthesis
  - Formulation

Identify **essential** biological target	Find inhibitor hits	Optimize lead(s) (multiple criteria)	Candidates for preclinical trials	Clinical trials Phases I,II,III

- **Mimic natural peptide substrates**

- **Screen for peptide leads**

- **Attempt war-head and classical strategies**

- **Exploit literature and patent information**

- Pass disease models

- ADMET, **Metabolism**

- CMC

- Fill pipeline with backup compounds

Scheme 1.1 An overview of the peptide-derived, small-molecule drug discovery. Highlighted in bold text are discovery periods where "sensemaking" and knowledge building cycles can be employed during peptide optimization.

Identify lead peptides

Design compounds that exploit structural and dynamics findings. Remove any warhead present

Consider known peptide and properties of protein class

Apply SAR chemistry to help elucidate peptide binding mode

"Sensemaking" Knowledge building SAR exploitation

Identify structural elements for recognition and hydrolysis

Truncate peptide to minimal size

Map critical binding region of peptide to pocket (SAR, NMR, X-ray)

Optimize high-throughput with parallel chemistry using knowledge-based compounds

Explore possible "war-head" strategy for potency for establishing SAR

Scheme 1.2 An overview of the drug discovery periods that impact and fuel the "sensemaking," knowledge building, and SAR exploitation cycles.

The process we propose may be summarized (Scheme 1.2) as follows:

- Identify lead peptides.
- Understand properties of the protein.
- Map critical binding elements of substrate peptide.
- Understand (by X-ray/NMR) protein–ligand interactions.
- Increase potency, for example, by using a warhead if necessary, to provide meaningful structure–activity relationships (SAR).
- Truncation to minimally active peptide (allowing for initial losses in potency as needed).
- Elucidate free versus bound conformations and ensure SAR designs produce compounds with free conformations matching the bioactive one.
- In parallel, de-peptidize molecule (e.g., by including bulky side-chains or altering the backbone) and remove any warhead present.

This process will be exemplified through the following examples.

1.3
HCMV Protease

1.3.1
HCMV Protease: Identification and Characterization of Antiviral Inhibitors Targeting the Serine Protease Domain of the Human Cytomegalovirus (HCMV Protease)

Human Cytomegalovirus (HCMV) is a pathogen and member of the herpesvirus family that is highly prevalent in the human population [5]. This virus poses a significant risk to immunocompromized individuals, organ transplant recipients and neonates who acquire the infection congenitally [6, 7]. HCMV encodes a unique protease involved in capsid assembly and this protease enzyme is responsible for processing the assembly protein; the latter protein's function is analogous to that of the "scaffolding" protein of bacteriophages [8] and its activity is essential to the production of infectious virions [9–12].

The full-length HCMV protease precursor contains 708 amino acids encoded by the UL80 gene. It was discovered that the enzyme can process its own C-terminus and that the protease can also undergo self-processing at the release site near its amino terminus. This cleavage liberates the 256 amino acid catalytic domain, or HCMV protease. Although this enzyme belongs to the serine protease family, differences between familial members exist, as evidenced through X-ray crystallographic analyses [13–16]. These analyses have shown that it possesses a unique protein fold and an unusual catalytic triad (a histidine replacing the more common aspartate). Additionally its activity arises exclusively from its dimer form [17, 18]. Spectroscopic studies [19] have demonstrated that the binding of substrate-based competitive inhibitors results in a conformational change in the enzyme and that catalysis by HCMV protease is performed through an "induced fit" model [20, 21]. Faced with a need to develop a potent HCMV protease inhibitor, the following research process was undertaken.

1.3.2
Mapping Essential Elements of the Substrate Peptides and Determining Structures of Ligands Bound to HCMV

As substrate hydrolysis by HCMV protease was essential for viral capsid assembly, the first task was to decipher the minimal structural elements of the substrates that were required for recognition and hydrolysis. Enzymological studies revealed that peptides which corresponded to 17 amino acids of the release- and matura-tion-sites (R-site and M-site peptides) were sufficient to induce hydrolysis by HCMV protease (Figure 1.2) [21]. Substitutions of amino acids of the P' residues (using standard nomenclature [22]) had less of an effect on oligopeptide substrate hydrolysis rates than those of P-side residues [23].

Differential line-broadening (DLB) NMR was then valuable for understanding which residues were playing a direct role in the binding of the substrate and product recognition by the enzyme [21]. The DLB method [24] provides atomic-resolution data and was used as a tool within the project to assess ligand binding. As Figure 1.3a shows, using the N-terminal product peptide (R-product) of the release-site, albeit a weak inhibitor (IC$_{50}$ ~ 3000 µM), it nevertheless bound to the protease, as indicated by the selective resonance perturbations observed when the hydrogen resonances of the peptide were compared in the absence versus presence of HCMV protease (Figure 1.3a). The changes in the peak shape and intensity resulted from fast-exchange averaging between the free and bound states (Figure 1.3b). The broadened resonance of the methyl group of Ala 1 (comparing

	...P9 P8 P7 P6 P5 P4 P3 P2 P1 ↑ P1' P2' P3' P4'...P8'	k_{cat}/K_M $(M^{-1}s^{-1})$
R-site	Thr-Glu-Arg-Glu-Ser-Tyr-Val-Lys-Ala - Ser-Val-Ser-Pro...	42
R-mutant	... Asn ...	282
M-site	Arg-Ala-Gln-Ala-Gly-Val-Val-Asn-Ala - Ser-Cys-Arg-Leu...	657
M-mutant	... Lys ...	54
		IC$_{50}$ (µM)
R-product	Thr-Glu-Arg-Glu-Ser-Tyr-Val-Lys-Ala	~3000
M-product	Arg-Ala-Gln-Ala-Gly-Val-Val-Asn-Ala	>1000
1	Gly-Val-Val-Asn-Ala-CF$_3$	1.8

Figure 1.2 Amino acid sequences of peptides/inhibitors with enzymological (k_{cat}/K_M) and inhibitory activity (IC$_{50}$) data [21]. The nomenclature used to denote amino acid positions is given above (i.e., P9 to P4') [22]. The peptides labeled as R-site, R-mutant, M-site, and M-mutant are 17 amino acids in length, but only the sequence to P4' is provided for space-saving. The full sequence can be found elsewhere [21]. Reproduced with kind permission from Springer Science + Business Media: *Top. Curr. Chem.*, Exploiting Ligand and Receptor Adaptability in Rational Drug Design Using Dynamics and Structure-Based Strategies, 272, 2007, 264, Steven R. LaPlante, Figure 2.

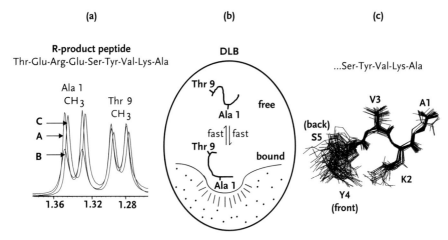

Figure 1.3 DLB mapping that distinguished between residues that were solvent exposed versus those that directly contact the receptor. Shown is the methyl region of the ^{1}H NMR spectrum of R-product showing the P1 and P9 CH$_3$ side-chain doublets [21]. (a) A, free R-product; B, R-product after the addition of HCMV protease at a ratio of 7 : 1; and C, R-product after the addition of HCMV protease and the more potent inhibitor **6** for displacement purposes at a 7 : 1 : 2 ratio. For the sake of clarity, the P1 methyl signals have been skewed slightly. (b) Demonstrates that the DLB method requires fast-exchange binding (averaging) between the free and bound states (on the NMR timescale). (c) The 3D structure of the P5–P1 sequence of R-product when bound to HCMV protease. The 32 overlapped structures determined were derived using transferred NOESY restraints and simulated annealing calculations. Reproduced with kind permission from Springer Science + Business Media: *Top. Curr. Chem.*, Exploiting Ligand and Receptor Adaptability in Rational Drug Design Using Dynamics and Structure-Based Strategies, 272, 2007, 265, Steven R. LaPlante, Figure 3.

"A" with "B" in Figure 1.3a) was due to this group becoming pocket exposed upon binding to HCMV (see the illustration in Figure 1.3b). In contrast, the ^{1}H resonance of the methyl group of Thr 9 changed little, as expected for a group that was predominantly solvent exposed in the free and bound states. Using this method, the ensembles of DLB patterns were monitored for the R-product and M-product peptides, and it was discovered that the P4 to P1 residues directly contacted the protease whereas the P9 to P5 residues were solvent exposed [21].

This was also consistent with enzymology findings that peptides spanning the P4–P1′ M-site core were capable of competitively inhibiting catalysis with binding affinity only fivefold less than that of the P4–P4′ substrate [25]. Overall, the ensemble of data indicated that the structural elements of the substrate which were N-terminal to the scissile bond were clearly crucial for complexation to the enzyme. Thus, the first step in the process of identifying the critical binding parts of the substrate peptides has been completed (i.e., P4–P1).

There was also enzymology effort applied to identifying the (peptide) source of the different processing rates observed between the R-site and M-site peptides (Figure 1.2). Enzymology studies followed that mutated the R-site and M-site peptide substrates (i.e., P5 and P4 residues were separately exchanged), as well as through substitution of the P2 residue of the R-site peptide to that of the M-site (Lys to Asn, and called R-mutant in Figure 1.2). It was discovered that the P2 side-chain played a major role in the observed variation in cleavage rates, suggesting that this P2 side-chain influenced the catalytic triad reactivity and so was integral to modulating the catalytic machinery (i.e., shielding the catalytic triad from solvent effects). It was also envisioned that a better understanding of this phenomenon could be exploited for inhibitor potency improvements. Although the promise of this phenomenon was not sufficiently explored in our HCMV protease program, it was successfully exploited in our efforts at optimizing the P2 position in our HCV protease peptidomimetic program, as described later in this chapter.

1.3.3
Improving Peptide Activity to Allow SAR Studies

Serine proteases are a well-studied class of enzyme [26–28]. Despite significant differences in global protein architecture, they possess similar catalytic machinery (triad), which is thought to arise from convergent structural evolution at the enzyme level. The frequently considered "warhead" strategy was, therefore, employed to create substrate-based activated carbonyl inhibitors [29] to boost potency (i.e., compound 1 in Figure 1.2). The improvement in activity also allowed the generation of meaningful SAR. Warheads involved the synthesis of electrophilic ketones which replaced the C-terminus acid of the N-terminal cleavage products [30]. By allowing attack upon the active-site serine, covalent hemiketal adducts were formed that mimic the transition state of the tetrahedral intermediate formed during the catalytic reaction. In this way, a boost in potency was observed with compound 1 (HCMV protease IC_{50} 1.8 µM) [19, 30], compared to the corresponding M-product peptide containing a C-terminal carboxylate ($IC_{50} > 1000$ µM; Figure 1.2).

With this improved potency, meaningful SAR then became possible. N-terminal truncation of P5 gave an inhibitor with similar potency (e.g., compare compound 1 versus 2 in Figure 1.4), but losses in potency were observed upon further truncation of the P4 and P3 residues (e.g., compare compound 2 with 3 and 4 in Figure 1.4) [30]. Thus, the P4 to P1 peptidyl segment, as suggested by the NMR experiments described above, played a critical role in ligand binding to the active-site of HCMV protease. Further chemistry efforts focussed on optimizing each of the P1–P4 substituents in turn; once one position had been improved significantly, this moiety was incorporated into optimization of the next position along in the sequence. In this way, the best P2 group was as indicated in compound 2 (IC_{50} 3 µM) and the best P3 was found to be the *tert*-butyl group (compound 5; IC_{50} 1.1 µM).

1.3.4
Elucidation of the Binding Mode of the Optimized Peptidyl Segment

Contemporaneous with medicinal chemistry efforts to determine which substituents controlled binding and activity, structural research efforts focussed on

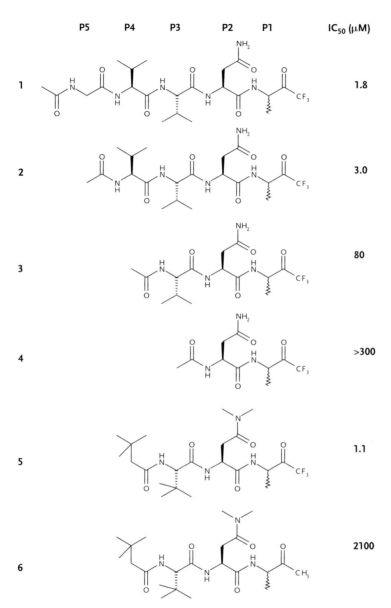

Figure 1.4 Inhibitors **1–6** with inhibition constants. The amino-acid positions are designated on top as P5–P1.

determining the binding mode of these compounds when bound to HCMV protease. It did not prove possible to use the technique of transferred NOESY (nuclear Overhauser spectroscopy) to determine bound conformation, so ligands were designed that as closely as possible resembled the peptidyl portion of the inhibitors without providing the slow exchange phenomenon arising from inactivation of the

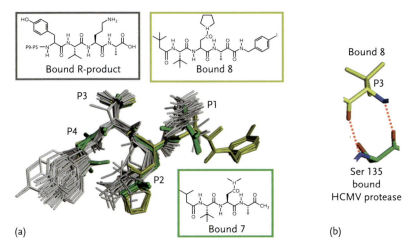

Figure 1.5 (a) Overlap of NMR-derived bound conformations of compound **7** (colored green; 29 conformations), R-product peptide (gray; 32 structures), and the X-ray crystallographic conformations of bound compound **8** (yellow; 4 conformations). (b) Zoomed view of the P3–S3 interaction of compound **8** bound to HCMV protease. Reproduced with kind permission from Springer Science + Business Media: *Top. Curr. Chem.*, Exploiting Ligand and Receptor Adaptability in Rational Drug Design Using Dynamics and Structure-Based Strategies, 272, 2007, 269, Steven R. LaPlante, Figure 7.

enzyme caused by highly electrophilic warhead groups. Thus, methyl ketones **6** [31] and **7** (Figures 1.4 and 1.5, respectively) were designed as NMR-friendly structural probes that could not form covalent complexes when bound to the enzyme, and exhibited fast exchanging binding attributes. In contrast, fluoroketone **5** (Figure 1.4) formed a slow-exchange covalent complex, as determined by ^{13}C NMR experiments [19].

Thus, replacing the C-terminal CF_3 with a CH_3 provided compounds unreactive toward attack by the active-site serine and so provided a useful structural probe of the bioactive conformation. Transferred NOESY data on compound **7** (*vide infra*, Figure 1.5a) and the derived distance restraints were applied to determine the family of bound structures shown in green in Figure 1.5a [31]. These studies indicated that they all bound in the extended conformation with a zigzagged backbone, with the P1 and P3 side-chains lying close to one another, and similarly for the P2 and P4 side-chains. The commonality of this structural feature for all three compounds suggested that this bioactive conformation played an important role for binding and activity. The dramatic losses in potency observed upon N-terminal truncation of P4 and P3 was consistent with this observation.

1.3.5
Ligand Adaptations upon Binding

There followed a stage in the project where compounds were designed that preferentially adopted the bioactive conformation in the free-state. Dramatic

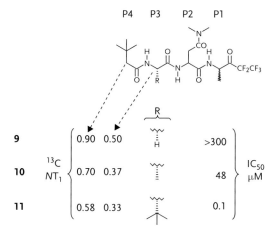

Figure 1.6 Inhibitors **9–11** with inhibition constants. ^{13}C T_1 relaxation data are given for the P3 Cα carbon. For the methylene carbon which has two covalently attached hydrogens, NT_1 values are provided, where N is the number of attached hydrogens, to help in interpreting the relative flexibility between different carbon types. Reproduced with kind permission from Springer Science + Business Media: *Top. Curr. Chem.*, Exploiting Ligand and Receptor Adaptability in Rational Drug Design Using Dynamics and Structure-Based Strategies, 272, 2007, 270, Steven R. LaPlante, Figure 8.

improvements in potency were attained (Figure 1.6) when a glycine at P3 (compound **9**, IC$_{50}$ > 300 μM) was replaced with an alanine (compound **10**, IC$_{50}$ 48 μM) or a *tert*-butyl group (compound **11**, IC$_{50}$ 0.1 μM) [30]. These increases in potency could not be explained by direct contacts with the protease pocket alone. The more overwhelming source for the improvements in potency was a result of the incorporation of the bulkier side-chains which helped to rigidify the compounds to resemble the bioactive conformation.

The relative rigidity (or flexibility) of these compounds was monitored by the NMR technique ^{13}C spin–lattice relaxation measurements (^{13}C T_1) [20]. Overall, shorter relaxation times are indicative of less flexibility. These experiments indicated that the conformational restriction induced by the bulkier P3 side-chain resulted in a minimization of the overall entropic cost of binding. The bulky group forced the critical P3 backbone into the bioactive, extended conformation in the free state which aided in the formation of two hydrogen bonds that were required upon complexation with HCMV protease (see Figure 1.5b) [20, 32].

In considering the ensemble of mounting information and given the highly related findings in our HSV RNR, HCV protease, and HIV protease programs, as described below, the principle of an easily synthesizable, Val or *tert*-butyl side-chain group, certainly proved to be a valuable medicinal chemistry tool, allowing significant improvements in inhibitor potency, where its incorporation is appropriate.

Later in the HCMV program, a peculiar observation was noted where a significant adaptation of the receptor was seen upon substrate or peptidomimetic

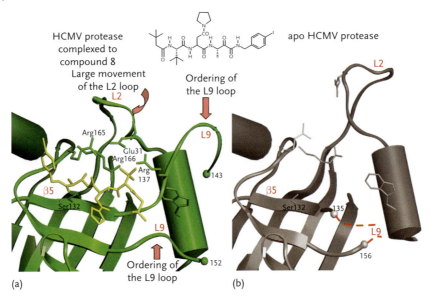

Figure 1.7 Peptidyl ligand-induced conformational changes of HCMV protease. Views of the active site region of (a) the inhibited enzyme (in green) covalently bound with ketoamide **8** shown in yellow and (b) the apoenzyme (in gray). Spheres indicate the points at which there was no electron density further along the L9-loop. Reproduced with kind permission from Springer Science + Business Media: *Top. Curr. Chem.*, Exploiting Ligand and Receptor Adaptability in Rational Drug Design Using Dynamics and Structure-Based Strategies, 272, 2007, 273, Steven R. LaPlante, Figure 11.

binding, as supported by X-ray structure and fluorescence methods (Figure 1.7). In this respect, the process bears elements of protein conformer selection [33]; the peptide guiding the reorganization of the protein around it after association. At this stage of the project, the "sensemaking" indications were that a prerequisite rigidification of the pocket upon peptidyl ligand binding could represent a minimal ceiling in terms of the entropic cost of binding. Thus, this intrinsic feature may ultimately limit any further potency improvements.

In fact, many of our further efforts, and those of competing companies, failed to improve the potency of the peptidyl-activated carbonyl inhibitors. This failure was consistent with the concept of an energetic penalty for protein reorganization on ligand binding. Thus, in this case, many companies aborted efforts at discovering peptidomimetics targeted at this protease (virus). We believe that we went one step further by reasoning that a promising path would be to screen for inhibitors favoring the flexible apo receptor, as we found for beta-lactam inhibitors [5, 20].

1.3.6
Strategic Summary for HCMV Peptide Mimic Design Process

Inhibition of HCMV protease by the peptidyl compounds described above involved the binding of the peptidyl portion to morph the transition state to a catalytically active or activated form of the enzyme. With HCMV protease, an induced-fit catalysis results in binding energy that is expended to compensate for the energy required to convert the enzyme to a thermodynamically less favorable state.

This then explains our strategy of identifying the first lead inhibitor, whereby a C-terminal warhead was incorporated onto N-terminal product peptides. The warhead induced a reversible, covalent mode of binding that mimicked the transition state of substrate cleavage and was utilized to facilitate meaningful SAR studies. However, due to toxicity concerns of deleterious interactions between warheads and proteins, the removal of the warhead from inhibitors was sought, once a level of inhibitor potency had been obtained that allowed the generation of meaningful SAR within the program.

First, the core scaffold of the ligand involved in direct binding to the protease was discovered, followed by utilization of NMR methods to monitor the bioactive conformation of these inhibitors, including the dependence of potency on the free-state flexibility. More potent compounds exhibited similar free and bound (bioactive) conformations, resulting in a reduction in the entropic cost of binding.

Another important finding was that the active-site underwent conformational adaptations upon binding the peptidomimetic ligands and substrates, characterizing HCMV protease as an induced-fit enzyme. The resultant entropic cost required to induce the "activated" state meant there was an intrinsic cost involving the receptor due to changes upon binding. Consistent with this, we and others could not improve inhibitor potencies. In the end, potent ligands were successfully obtained, but the necessity for protein rearrangement precluded further progression of this series of compounds. Throughout this campaign, novel strategies were developed to monitor the bioactive conformation and changes in flexibility of the ligands and receptor. Fortunately, the general nature of these strategies was later applied with success to a highly related campaign that targeted the HCV protease.

1.4
HCV Protease

1.4.1
HCV Protease as an Antiviral Target

Up to 200 million people around the world are infected with the hepatitis C virus [34]. The majority of individuals with persistent HCV infection will develop chronic hepatitis C, a progressive liver disease that can lead to cirrhosis and hepatocellular carcinoma [35–38]. HCV is an enveloped RNA virus belonging to the Flaviviridae family and Hepacivirus genus. As is typical for this family, its positive-sense RNA genome (9.5 kb) encodes a single precursor polyprotein which undergoes proteolytic maturation by enzymes that include host signalases and the viral NS2/3 protease and NS3 protease. NS3 protease (also referred to as HCV protease) is responsible for cleaving four of its non-structural (NS) proteins.

1.4.2
NS3 Serine Protease Possesses a Chymotrypsin-Like Fold

The cleavage sequences have little homology, with the following exceptions: three of four sites have a serine at P1′ and a cysteine at P1, and all four sites have an acidic amino acid at P6 (colored blue, Figure 1.8). Given this permissivity, we employed a peptide substrate having the sequence DDIVPC-SMSYTW [39] for *in vitro* enzymology studies/assays (colored orange, Figure 1.8).

1.4.3
Discovery of the Peptide DDIVPC as an Inhibitor of NS3 Protease

Initial efforts focussed on the approach of designing substrate-based activated carbonyl inhibitors which involved the synthesis of N-terminal cleavage products in which the acid of the C-terminus is replaced with an electrophilic ketone. Upon attack by the active-site serine, a stable covalent hemiketal adduct is formed that mimics the transition state of the tetrahedral intermediate formed during the

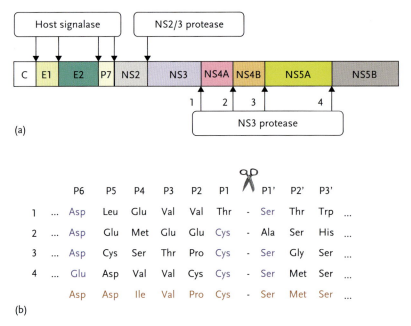

(a)

(b)

		P6	P5	P4	P3	P2	P1		P1′	P2′	P3′	
1	...	Asp	Leu	Glu	Val	Val	Thr	-	Ser	Thr	Trp	...
2	...	Asp	Glu	Met	Glu	Glu	Cys	-	Ala	Ser	His	...
3	...	Asp	Cys	Ser	Thr	Pro	Cys	-	Ser	Gly	Ser	...
4	...	Glu	Asp	Val	Val	Cys	Cys	-	Ser	Met	Ser	...
		Asp	Asp	Ile	Val	Pro	Cys	-	Ser	Met	Ser	...

Figure 1.8 (a) An illustration of the polyprotein encoded by the HCV genome, together with the processing cleavage sites. (b) Sites and sequences cleaved by NS3 protease. The amino-acid positions are designated on top as P6–P3′. The numbers to the left correspond to the numbered sites in (a). Also shown is a model sequence used for enzymology studies and assays (colored orange). Consensus residues are colored blue. Reproduced with kind permission from Bentham Science Publishers Ltd.: Curr. Med. Chem. – Anti-Infective Agents, Dynamics and Structure-based Design of Drugs Targeting the Critical Serine Protease of the Hepatitis C Virus – From a Peptidic Substrate to BILN 2061, 4, 2005, 113, Steven R. LaPlante and Montse Llinàs -Brunet, Figure 2(A).

catalytic reaction [26–28]. Concurrent to this work, we sought to determine the bioactive conformation of bound peptidyl ligands through transferred NOESY NMR methods. Since slow binding ligands, such as activated carbonyl inhibitors, are not suitable for such studies [31], our efforts were directed to the synthesis of N-terminal cleavage peptides having an acid C-terminus. Surprisingly, the activity of the N-terminal product peptide DDIVPC of NS3 protease was more active than expected (IC$_{50}$ 71 µM), thus this became the initial inhibitor lead for further SAR efforts [40]. The next efforts were to replace the reactive cysteine at P1 of DDIVPC with a chemically more stable residue and norvaline was found to be a stable replacement with only a fivefold loss in potency [41]. This loss was then recovered by the replacement of P5 by D-Asp and the addition of a P6 acetyl, resulting in compound **12** having an IC$_{50}$ value of 17 µM. Efforts were then refocussed on replacing the C-terminal acid with an activated-carbonyl warhead to provide an expected boost in activity. However, the C-terminal acid and trifluoromethylketone analogs exhibited comparable activity (compounds **12** and **13** in Figure 1.9) [41].

Unlike the case of HCMV protease, where only compounds with an activated carbonyl were active enough to be considered as a lead for optimization (compound **15** is much more active than **14**, as shown in Figure 1.9) [20, 30], both product

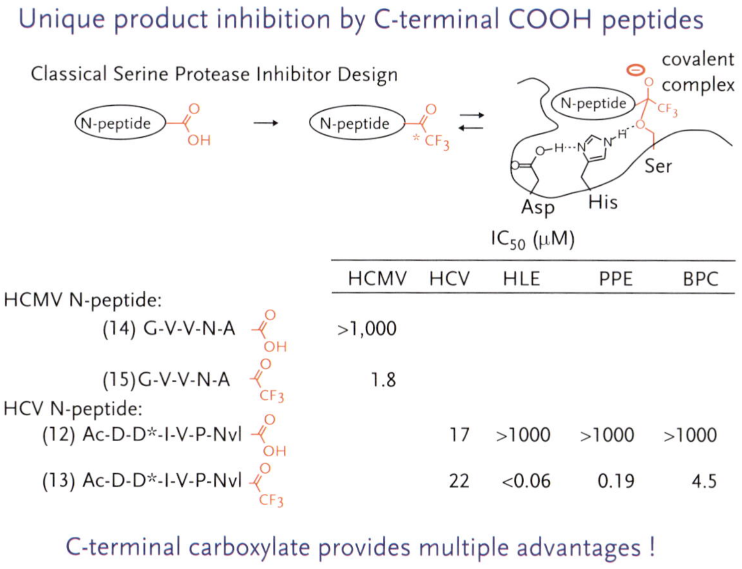

Unique product inhibition by C-terminal COOH peptides

	HCMV	HCV	HLE	PPE	BPC
HCMV N-peptide:					
(14) G-V-V-N-A	>1,000				
(15) G-V-V-N-A	1.8				
HCV N-peptide:					
(12) Ac-D-D*-I-V-P-Nvl		17	>1000	>1000	>1000
(13) Ac-D-D*-I-V-P-Nvl		22	<0.06	0.19	4.5

C-terminal carboxylate provides multiple advantages !

Figure 1.9 Inhibitors of HCMV and HCV are shown with inhibition constants determined using various enzymes. The amino acid positions are designated on top as P6–P1. The inhibition constants involving HCV were determined using the NS3 protease domain and an NS4A peptide [41]. The other binding constants were determined as described elsewhere [30, 40]. The abbreviations for the proteases are defined as follows: HCV, hepatitis C virus; HLE, human leukocyte elastase; PPE, porcine pancreatic elastase; BPC, bovine pancreatic chymotrypsin; HCMV, human cytomegalovirus protease. Selectivity targets were chosen because they represented closely-related chymotrypsin-like serine proteases, when compared to HCV protease.

peptide and activated carbonyl inhibitors of NS3 protease (compounds **12** and **13**) [40–42] had similar potency and were viable starting points as leads. However, the C-terminal acid (compound **12**) had superior attributes to the trifluoromethylketone N-peptide (compound **13**). For example, compound **12** had a superior selectivity profile, as compared to other serine proteases shown in Figure 1.9. Figure 1.9 shows that compound **13** inhibits human leukocyte elastase (HLE) with an $IC_{50} < 0.06$ μM. In contrast, the C-terminal carboxylate inhibitor (compound **12**) provides high specificity for NS3 protease with an IC_{50} 17 μM versus $IC_{50} > 1000$ μM for other typical serine proteases (e.g., human leukocyte elastase, porcine pancreatic elastase, and bovine pancreatic chymotrypsin) [41]. Warheads would be expected to show reduced selectivity toward other proteins and, hence, would be expected to contribute to greater inhibitor toxicity than the carboxylic acid group. The C-terminal carboxyl derivatives also exhibit other favorable qualities, such as chemical stability and aqueous solubility at neutral pH. For all of the above reasons, the carboxylic acid group was preferred over a warhead for inclusion in inhibitor design for this project.

1.4.4
"Sensemaking" and Knowledge Building: Mapping of the Critical Binding Residues of the Peptide and Creation of an Inhibitor-Protease Model

In trying to improve inhibitor potency by modifying the side-chains and reducing the peptidic nature of our early peptides, medicinal chemists undertook a synthetic study in which single amino acid changes (natural and unnatural) were incorporated into hexapeptides, and the effect on potency was monitored. This exercise led to the finding that a benzylmethoxy proline at P2 (compound **16**, Figure 1.10) resulted in a 21-fold improvement in potency (compound **17** versus **18**, Figure 1.11) [43, 44].

To help guide medicinal chemistry efforts, a ligand-focussed NMR strategy was undertaken to determine which sites of the peptides contacted the protease and which were solvent exposed in the bound state [43, 45]. The differential line-broadening (DLB) NMR experiment [24, 45] was used and, in general, ligand sites that contacted the protease could be identified by specific broadening of the corresponding NMR resonances upon addition of small amounts of protease. When applied to DDIVPC and longer sequences spanning P10–P1, it was found that only specific resonances of P4–P1 experienced broadening (Figure 1.10a and b). No broadening was observed for peptides corresponding to the P′ sequences. This suggested that smaller compounds spanning only P4–P1 should retain a reasonable binding affinity [43].

1.4.5
Knowledge Building: Monitoring Ligand Flexibility in the Free-State and Changes Upon Binding – P3 Rigidification

Next we sought to identify any differences that may exist for compound **16** between the free and bound states. Distance information from the bound state was monitored by the transferred NOESY experiment (Figure 1.10c), and the free state

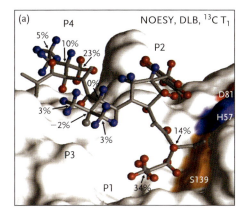

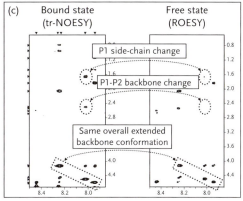

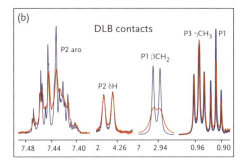

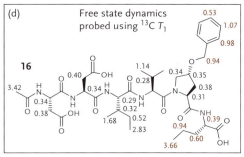

Figure 1.10 "Sensemaking" using NMR-based knowledge building that probed both structure and dynamics information. (a) The first model of the complex between compound **16** and NS3 protease, with a summary of DLB perturbation mapping data, and transferred ^{13}C T_1 data. The complex was determined by docking the bound structure of compound **16** (experimentally determined by transferred NOESY NMR data) to an *apo* X-ray structure of NS3 protease. For the DLB mapping data, hydrogens of compound **16** are colored blue for resonances in which no broadening perturbations were observed upon binding protease, and hydrogens are colored red when significant resonance broadening was observed upon binding. P5 and P6 were determined to be relatively flexible in the bound state and are not shown above. A summary of the transferred ^{13}C T_1 data (placed next to each carbon) is also displayed as the percentage change in ^{13}C T_1 before and after the addition of NS3 protease. (b) DLB perturbation data. Selected ^{1}H NMR resonances of compound **16** are shown (with the exception that P1 CH_2 is of DDIVPC) when free (colored blue) and after adding small amounts of NS3 protease (colored red). (c) A comparison of free-state (ROESY NMR) versus bound-state (tr-NOESY) conformation and dynamics. Note the similarities of the backbone and differences of the side-chains. (d) Inhibitor **16** is shown with its inhibition constant and free-state ^{13}C T_1 relaxation times (next to each carbon). The amino acid positions are designated on top as P6–P1. The inhibition constant was determined using an assay involving the NS3 protease domain and an NS4A peptide [44]. ^{13}C T_1 relaxation data are given next to each protonated carbon. In cases where a carbon has more than one covalently attached hydrogen, NT_1 values are provided, where N is the number of attached protons and NT_1 is the product to help in interpreting the relative flexibility between different carbon types. Reproduced with kind permission from Springer Science + Business Media: *Top. Curr. Chem.*, Exploiting Ligand and Receptor Adaptability in Rational Drug Design Using Dynamics and Structure-Based Strategies, 272, 2007, 287, Steven R. LaPlante, Figure 20.

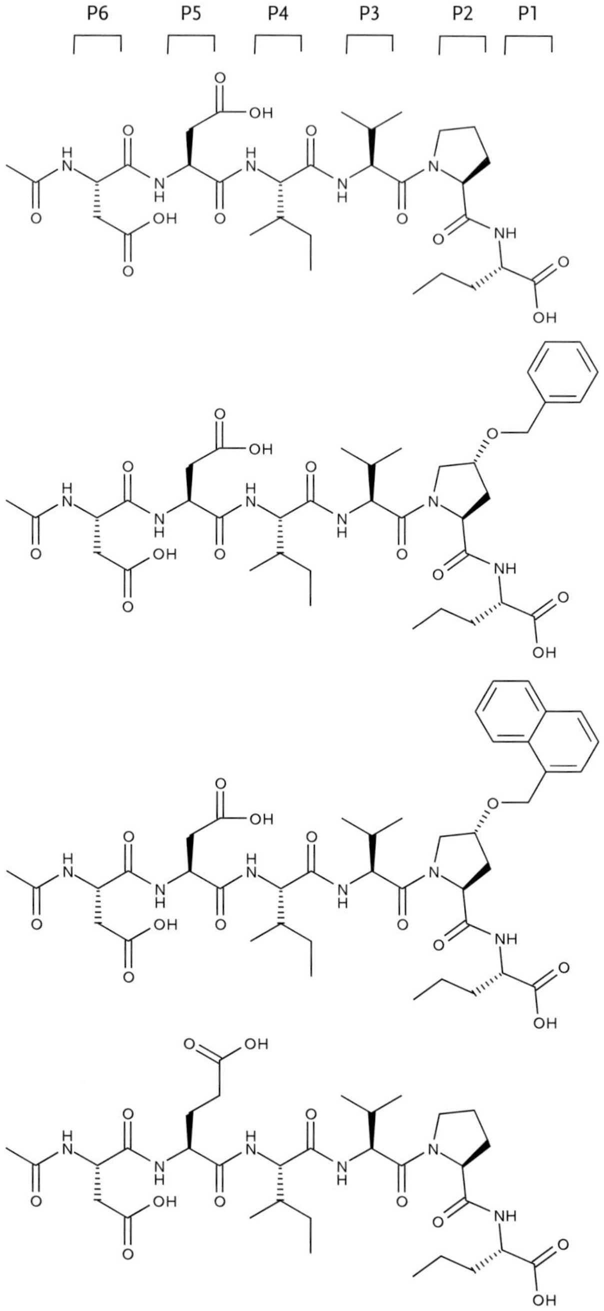

18
$IC_{50} = 150\ \mu M$

17
$IC_{50} = 7\ \mu M$

19
$IC_{50} = 0.39\ \mu M$

20
$IC_{50} = 7.5\ \mu M$

Figure 1.11 Inhibitors **17–21** with inhibition constants determined using an assay that included the NS3 protease domain and an NS4A peptide [44]. The amino acid positions are designated on top as P6–P1.

21
$IC_{50} = 54\ \mu M$

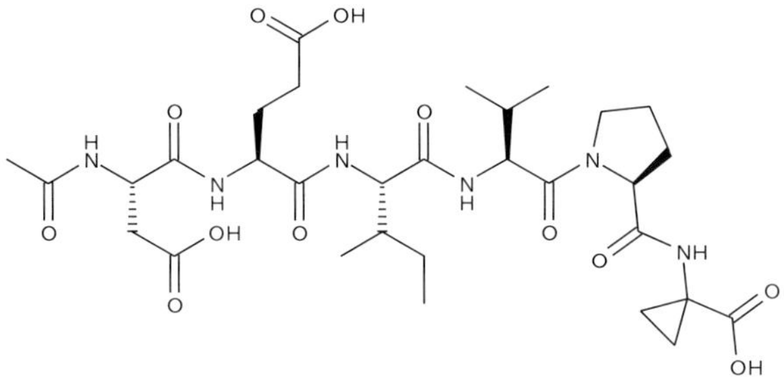

Figure 1.11 *(Continued)*

was probed using an NMR ROESY experiment (Figure 1.10c) [43]. This comparison of the distance-related cross-peaks indicated that compound **16** adopts an extended backbone conformation in both states, with important differences observed for the side-chains.

A better means of monitoring dynamic attributes was sought and led the researchers to consider ^{13}C NMR spin–lattice relaxation experiments ($^{13}C\ T_1$) [43]. $^{13}C\ T_1$ relaxation is sensitive to segmental flexibility in the picosecond to nanosecond timescales, and the internal flexibility of drug-like ligands in the free state, which influences the binding affinity to macromolecules via entropic costs, typically occurs within these timescales. The direct correlation of $^{13}C\ T_1$ relaxation data with molecular flexibility can be made qualitatively for protonated carbons of free ligands where longer relaxation times are generally indicative of increased segmental flexibility [20, 43].

This work indicated that segmental fluctuations of the norvaline group in the free state was evident given the long and incremental increases of $^{13}C\ T_1$ times for the α to δ-carbons (Figure 1.10d, α 0.39, β 0.60, γ 0.94, and δ 3.66 s). Thus, it was reasoned that P1 replacements, which chemically rigidify this side-chain to resemble the bound conformation shown in Figure 1.10a, would likely be more potent owing to a lower entropic cost of binding.

The P2 substituent of **17** also exhibited significant flexibility in the free state, indicating that this aromatic ring underwent fast rotation or spinning along the benzylic/para-carbon axis. Replacement of the phenyl group with a larger naphthyl resulted in an 18-fold improvement in potency (compare compounds **17** and **19**, Figure 1.11) [44], which is likely due, in part, to a reduction in rotational rate and the associated entropic cost of binding (*vide infra*).

The ensemble of data in Figure 1.10 revealed features relevant to the role of P3 for potency. The P3 side-chain played an indirect role in the binding affinity by sterically rigidifying the P3 backbone in the free state to resemble that of the bound extended conformation [20, 43, 45], as was found for the HCMV protease inhibitors. The P3 side-chain had no DLB (Figure 1.10b, and blue-colored hydrogens in Figure 1.10a) indicating that it had no direct binding to the pocket, despite the fact that its removal resulted in significant loss in potency. Thus, given the similarities, and as exploited in the HCMV program, it was suggested to again replace the P3 side-chain with a bulky *tert*-butyl side-chain (*vide infra*).

1.4.6
N-Terminal Truncation and Improved P1, P2 and P5 Substituents

DLB and transferred NOESY mapping suggested that the principle binding residues spanned P4–P1. At first, this appeared to contradict earlier attempts to reduce the size of non-optimized hexapeptides by the removal of N-terminal residues. This resulted in shorter peptides with no significant activity. However, a similar exercise was successful by first improving the potency of the hexapeptide series, to better anchor the inhibitor, using beneficial P1, P2, and P5 replacements [44]. For example, 21- and 384-fold improvements were observed when the P2 proline was substituted with a benzyl-methoxyproline (compound **17** versus **18**, Figure 1.11) and a naphthyl-methoxyproline (compound **19** versus **18**, Figure 1.11), respectively. A further threefold improvement in potency was observed when the P1 norvaline was replaced with a 1-aminocyclopropyl carboxylic (ACCA) (compound **21** versus **20**, Figure 1.11). Replacement of the P5 L-aspartic acid with a D-glutamic acid resulted in a 20-fold gain in affinity (compound **20** versus **18**, Figure 1.11) [44]. Combining these substitutions simultaneously into a single hexapeptide, resulted in an inhibitor with an IC_{50} of 0.013 μM (compound **22**, Figure 1.12) [44].

This potent compound then served as the starting compound for a renewed effort at N-terminal truncation. Removal of the P6 residue and the P5 amide resulted in a 69-fold loss in potency (compound **23** versus **22**, Figure 1.12) and a tetrapeptide having a simple acetyl capping group resulted in a loss in affinity by 269-fold (compound **24** versus **22**, Figure 1.12) [44]. As a result, N-terminal truncation successfully resulted in tetrapeptides that had measurable activity, and that were also more drug-like. The affinity imparted by the P2 naphthyl methoxy and P1 ACCA likely also helped to "anchor" the C-terminal end in the bound state.

Further improvements in potency were sought. It was found that an ethyl appendage on the P1 ACCA provided beneficial contributions to potency (compound **26** is twofold more potent than compound **24**, Figure 1.13) and further improvements could be gained by a vinyl appendage (compound **27** is 12-fold more potent than compound **24**) [46]. The requirement for a specific stereochemistry of the appendage was observed, given that a fourfold loss in affinity was measured for compound **25** as compared to **24** (Figure 1.13). Overall, it is noteworthy that the P1 ACCA group both improved potency and had a more rigidified, bioactive conformation in the free state as compared to the more flexible P1 Nvl (Figure 1.10d). Like P2, the P1 position played multiple roles in the bimolecular interaction. Due to these multiple roles, "sensemaking" exercises were required to qualitatively deconvolute the roles as much as possible, allowing further exploitation.

A combinatorial chemistry approach was also undertaken to identify alternative P2 substituents [48]. A large variety of aromatic groups was appended to the oxy-prolyl group at P2, resulting in two promising lead compounds **28** and **29** (Figure 1.14). The bound structure of each compound was then determined by transferred NOESY and conformational search methods [49]. These structures are

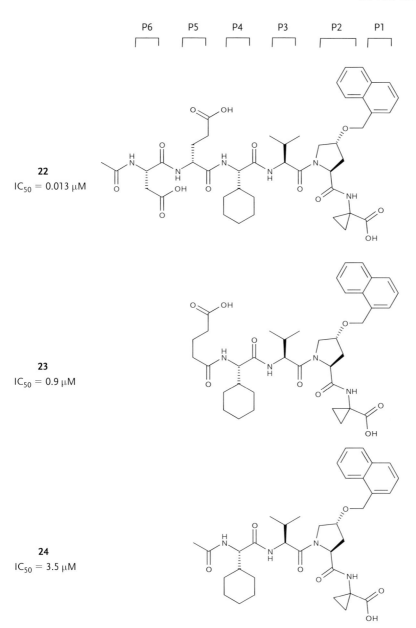

Figure 1.12 Inhibitors **22–24** with inhibition constants determined using an assay that included the NS3 protease domain and an NS4A peptide [44]. The amino acid positions are designated on top as P6–P1. Reproduced with kind permission from Bentham Science Publishers Ltd.: Curr. Med. Chem. – Anti-Infective Agents, Dynamics and Structure-based Design of Drugs Targeting the Critical Serine Protease of the Hepatitis C Virus – From a Peptidic Substrate to BILN 2061, 4, 2005, 119, Steven R. LaPlante and Montse Llinàs -Brunet, Figure 7.

24
$IC_{50} = 7.5\ \mu M$

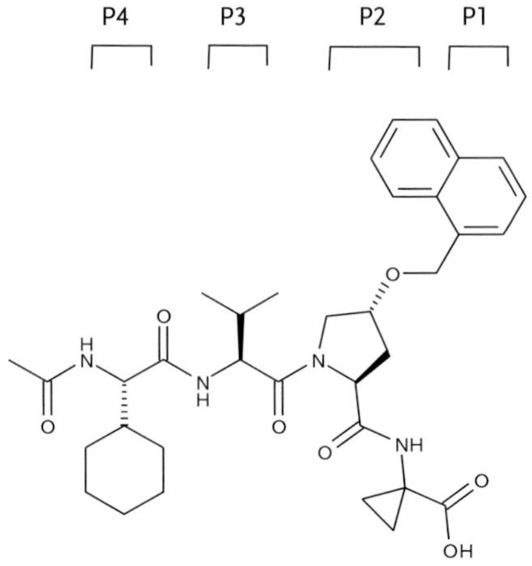

25
$IC_{50} = 32\ \mu M$

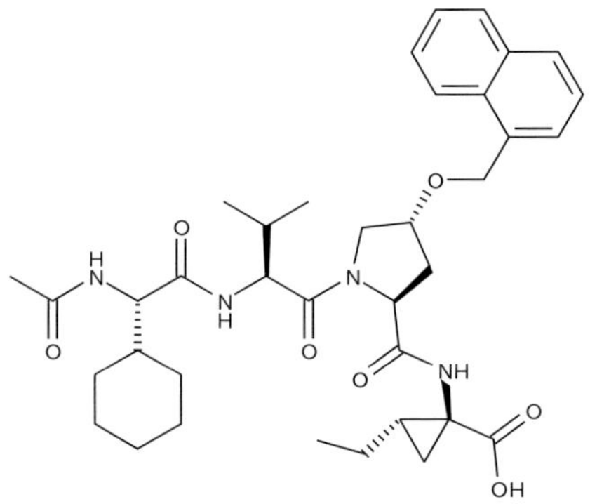

26
$IC_{50} = 4.8\ \mu M$

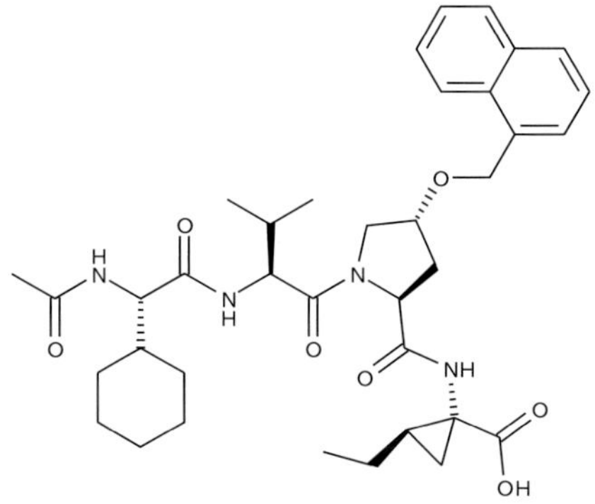

Figure 1.13 Inhibitors **24–27** with inhibition constants determined using an assay that included the full-length NS3–NS4A protein [46, 47]. The amino acid positions are designated on top as P4–P1.

27

$IC_{50} = 0.6 \, \mu M$

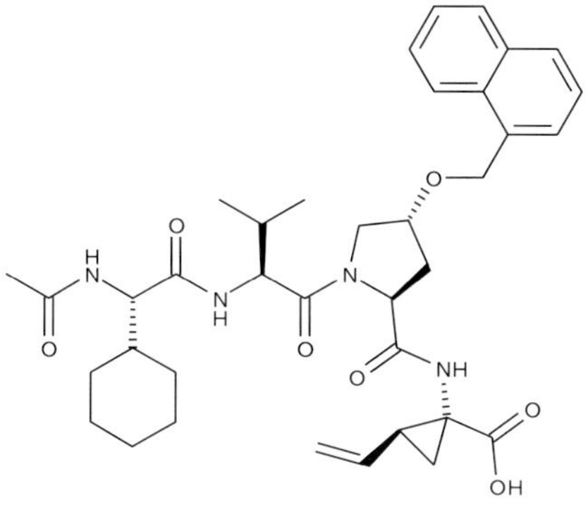

Figure 1.13 (Continued)

shown on the right in Figure 1.14. Given that the biphenyl group of compound **29** and the quinoline ring of compound **28** occupy different physical space when bound to NS3 protease, it was hypothesized that a compound having three rings would better span both regions of space and could result in an improved affinity (see the theoretical superposition of compounds **28** and **29** on the right of compound **30**). A >10-fold improvement in potency was observed (compound **30**), but transferred NOESY data for a compound related to **30** showed that the tricyclic group actually bound in the opposite orientation from that predicted. This was understood when considering the multiple roles played by the P2 substituent (*vide infra*), including its effect on free-state rigidification, solvent shielding of the catalytic triad and electrostatic interactions.

1.4.7
Macrocyclization: Linking the Flexible P1 Side-Chain to P3

At this stage of the project, the following considerations were given to improving the properties of the series. The transferred NOESY model of the complex involving compound **16** (Figure 1.10a) revealed that the P3 side-chain lies on the solvent-exposed surface of the protease and in close proximity to the P1 norvaline side-chain [43, 50]. Transferred ^{13}C T_1 data (Figure 1.10a) indicated that the P1 side-chain underwent rigidification upon binding the protease [51]. It was speculated that intramolecular linking of the P1 side-chain to the P3 side-chain with a hydrocarbon bridge would lead to a macrocyclic inhibitor which would, in the free state, preferentially adopt the bound conformation observed for compound **16** in Figure 1.10a. A rigid macrocyclic scaffold would also ensure that the P2–P3 amide bond would adopt exclusively the trans-geometry observed in the bound conformation, unlike linear peptides which exist as a mixture of cis- and trans-rotamers.

As an example of the impact that macrocyclization can have on potency [50] and free-state flexibility, the macrocyclic compound **32** in Figure 1.15 (15-membered

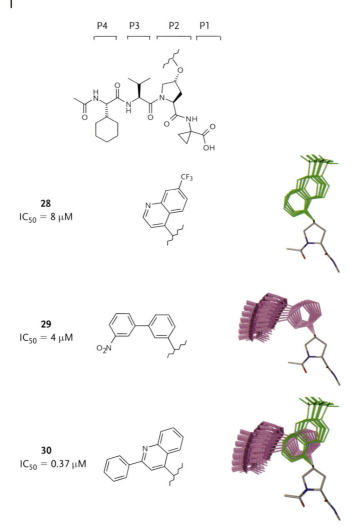

Figure 1.14 Inhibitors **28–30** with inhibition constants determined using an assay that included the NS3 protease domain and an NS4A peptide [40, 49]. The amino acid positions are designated on top as P4–P1. The protease-bound structures of inhibitors **28** and **29** are provide on the right and were determined using transferred NOESY data and a conformational search protocol. Both are overlaid on the right of inhibitor **30** to illustrate the design concept. Reproduced with kind permission from Bentham Science Publishers Ltd.: *Curr. Med. Chem. –* Anti-Infective Agents, Dynamics and Structure-based Design of Drugs Targeting the Critical Serine Protease of the Hepatitis C Virus – From a Peptidic Substrate to BILN 2061, 4, 2005, 122, Steven R. LaPlante and Montse Llinàs-Brunet, Figure 10.

ring) is 10-fold more potent than the acyclic compound **31**. ^{13}C T_1 data are shown for both compounds in Figure 1.15, indicating that a reduction in the flexibility of the P1 side-chain (cyclopropyl and vinyl) was achieved by macrocyclization, as shown by the shorter ^{13}C T_1 relaxation times for this residue in compound **32**

P3   P2   P1

31
$K_i = 0.35\ \mu M$

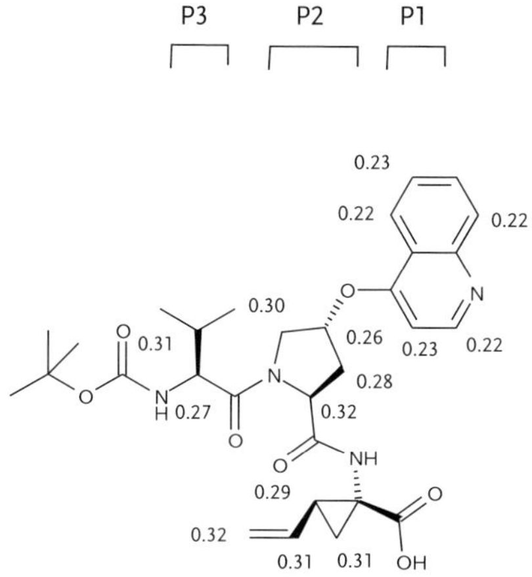

32
$K_i = 0.035\ \mu M$

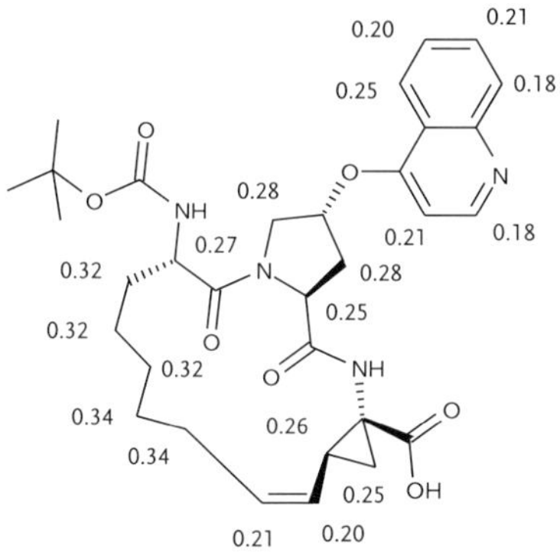

Figure 1.15 Inhibitors **31** and **32** with inhibition constants determined using an assay that included the full-length NS3–NS4A protein. The amino acid positions are designated on top as P3–P1. The free-state ^{13}C NT_1 relaxation times are also provided next to each carbon position (see also the legend of Figure 1.10). Reproduced with kind permission from Bentham Science Publishers Ltd.: *Curr. Med. Chem.* – Anti-Infective Agents, Dynamics and Structure-based Design of Drugs Targeting the Critical Serine Protease of the Hepatitis C Virus – From a Peptidic Substrate to BILN 2061, 4, 2005, 123, Steven R. LaPlante and Montse Llinàs-Brunet, Figure 12.

(Figure 1.15, 0.21–0.26 s) as compared to the acyclic compound **31** (Figure 1.15, 0.29–0.32 s).

The employed strategies described above [40–57] included an early "sensemak-ing" and knowledge building phase in which structural and dynamics data were acquired to, (i) understand the bioactive conformation of lead peptides when bound to HCV protease, (ii) identify the important substituents that directly contact the protease pocket, and (iii) determine the differences in conformational flexibility between the free and bound states of ligands. With the rational use of this information, medicinal chemists identified potent hexapeptide compounds

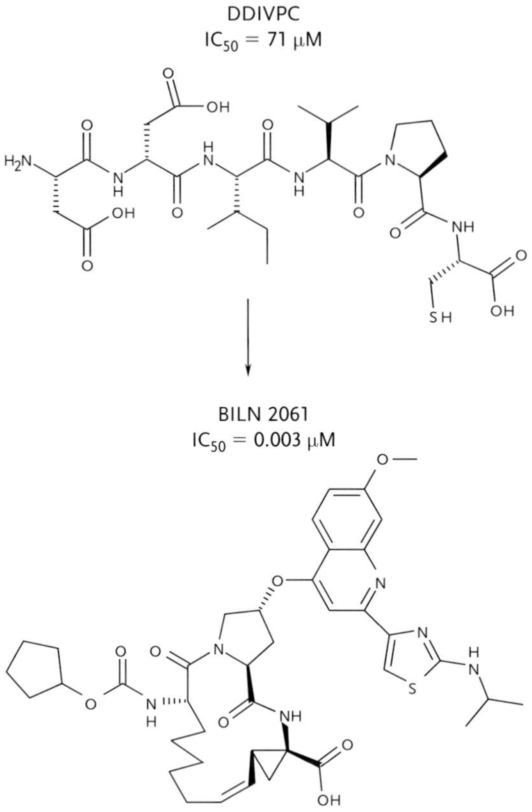

Figure 1.16 Structures of the lead peptide DDIVPC and the clinical compound BILN 2061. Reproduced with kind permission from Springer Science + Business Media: *Top. Curr. Chem.*, Exploiting Ligand and Receptor Adaptability in Rational Drug Design Using Dynamics and Structure-Based Strategies, 272, 2007, 278, Steven R. LaPlante, Figure 14.

with improved P1, P2, and P5 substituents. Efforts to reduce the size and peptidic character resulted in N-terminal truncation to tetra- and tri-peptidic compounds that had novel P1 and P2 substituents. The macrocyclic scaffold was then designed to chemically rigidify the free-state conformation to further resemble the bound-like state, which resulted in a reduction in entropic costs of binding. Having extensive information regarding the binding mode of compounds, medicinal chemists exploited this knowledge in their campaign that eventually led to the BILN 2061 family of compounds. Further SAR efforts at P2 and P4 delivered the first clinical candidate **BILN 2061** (ciluprevir) [58, 59] which was the first compound to show proof of concept in humans for a direct acting anti-HCV protease inhibitor, see Figure 1.16. However, the further development of this compound was discontinued due to the observation of cardiotoxicity in high-dose monkey toxicology studies.

1.4.8
HCV Protease Inhibitor BI00201335

With the discovery of cardiotoxicity and subsequent discontinuation of development of the HCV NS3 protease inhibitor **BILN 2061** [55], this caused a re-evaluation of active material within the project in an effort to discover novel, non-covalent NS3 protease inhibitors [60].

Work continued on the C-terminal carboxylic acid, (1*R*,2*S*)-1-amino-2-vinyl-cyclopropyl carboxylic acid (vinyl-ACCA)-containing inhibitors [46] , as these features provided good potency, excellent selectivity, as well as better solubility than seen with other classes of inhibitors. An advantage of a related linear series of inhibitors [52] lies in the fact that the synthetic complexity and costs associated with drug production are significantly reduced. These points taken together, the project then focussed on merging the SAR of both linear and macrocyclic series of inhibitors [61]. First, the quinoline moiety of **BILN 2061** was cross-fertilized with the linear derivative **33**, providing compound **34** (Figure 1.17) which displayed more than a 10-fold improvement in potency in the replicon assay [61]. This provided the first linear tripeptide inhibitor in our program with cellular activity below 100 nM [61].

Cell-based activity of this linear series needed to be improved whilst concomitantly evaluating and improving its ADME/PK profile. Compound **34** was used as the starting point for further evaluation. From this point in the project, the peptide backbone was retained, as this makes optimal interactions with the enzyme which mimic the canonical substrate binding mode, with both the NH and CO groups of the P3 residue and the NH group of the P1 moiety being involved in key hydrogen bonds with the protein [52]. Additionally, both the vinyl-ACCA derivative at P1 and the *tert*-butyl glycine moiety at P3 were retained as they were found to be optimal. The C-terminal carboxylic acid makes key interactions with the catalytic triad and the oxyanion hole [50], providing good potency and specificity towards NS3 *versus* human and other serine proteases [41]. In addition, one clear advantage over the other classes of reported NS3 protease inhibitors is the observed increase in solubility for this series. The *tert*-butyl found at P3 was also maintained as this was found to rigidify the peptidic backbone and to favor the overall extended conformation, found in the bound state, for the inhibitor in solution [52]. Thus, the SAR focussed on optimizing both the capping group and the P2 aminothiazol-quinoline moiety. SAR at P2 indicated the acetyl group, as in compound **35**, was well tolerated and increasing the size resulted in a loss of potency (Table 1.1). Further substitution on the quinoline core provided compounds **36** and **37** (Table 1.1), both displaying EC_{50} values <20 nM in the replicon assay and these compounds were further improved to compounds **38–40**, Table 1.1. Combining double quinoline-core substitutions with variation of the aminothiazole-acyl group led to **BI00201335**, Table 1.1, which contains a highly optimized peptide backbone, as well as a C-terminal carboxylic acid and large P2 substituent. **BI00201335** has low nM activity in enzymatic and cellular assays, see Table 1.1.

This compound possessed favorable properties, as exemplified by pharmacokinetic parameters in rats, see Table 1.2, is selective in a large panel of human

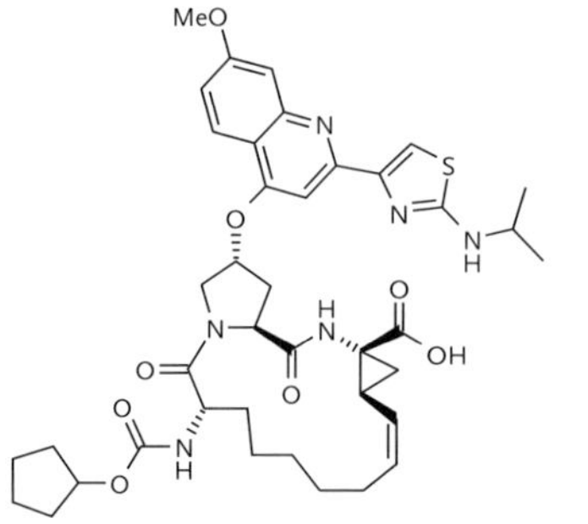

BILN 2061
$IC_{50} = 0.003 \ \mu M$
$EC_{50} = 0.002 \ \mu M$

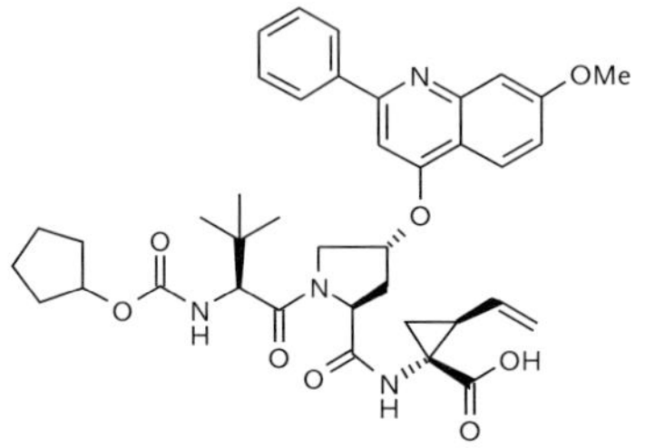

33
$IC_{50} = 0.014 \ \mu M$
$EC_{50} = 0.55 \ \mu M$

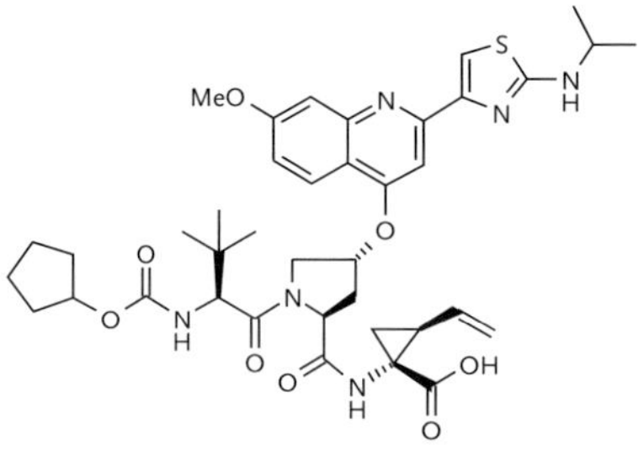

34
$IC_{50} = 0.014 \ \mu M$
$EC_{50} = 0.045 \ \mu M$

Figure 1.17 Linear tripeptide HCV NS3 protease inhibitors. Reprinted with permission from *J. Med. Chem.*, 2010, 53, 6466-6476 (Table 1) Discovery of a potent and selective noncovalent linear inhibitor of the hepatitis C virus NS3 protease (BI 201335). Llinàs-Brunet, M., Bailey, M.D., Goudreau, N., Bhardwaj, P.K., Bordeleau, J., Bös, M., Bousquet, Y., Cordingley, M.G., Duan, J., Forgione, P., Garneau, M., Ghiro, E., Gorys, V., Goulet, S., Halmos, T., Kawai, S.H., Naud, J., Poupart, M.-A., White, P.W. Copyright 2010 Americal Chemical Society.

proteases and is currently in phase III clinical trials. The genesis of this compound owes its existence to the careful inhibitor design of progenitor macrocyclic and linear series, along with the transfer of "sensemaking" lessons from the earlier HCMV program, *vide supra*, and illustrates that peptides can be de-peptized and turned successfully into clinical candidates.

In HCV-infected patients, an impressive (average) viral load decrease of -5.3 $\log_{10}$ has been seen with a 240 mg qd dose of **BI00201335** in combination with pegylated Interferon-α and ribavirin over 28 days of treatment, see Figure 1.18 [62]. No viral breakthroughs were observed for the six patients treated under this regime.

In conclusion for these two targets, this work has the distinction of systematically monitoring the structure and dynamics features of ligands using

Table 1.1 Optimization of linear tripeptide NS3 HCV protease inhibitors.

Compound	R1	R2	IC$_{50}$ (nM)	EC$_{50}$ (nM)
35	H		5	34
36	Me		8	19
37	Me		10	17
38	F		7	36
39	Cl		7	11
40	Br		7	5
BI00201335	Br		3	3

Table 1.2 Pharmacokinetic parameters of BI00201335 in rats following oral and intravenous administration.

Compound	Oral 5 mg/kg		i.v 2 mg/kg			
	C$_{max}$ (μM)	AUC$_{0-\infty}$ (μM h)	T$_{1/2}$ (h)	V$_{ss}$ (L/kg)	Cl (mL/min/kg)	F%
BI00201335	0.6	1.7	1.2	1.9	20	40

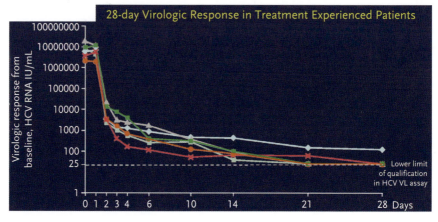

Figure 1.18 Structure of BI00201335 and viral load decline in patients.

multidisciplinary strategies. It is certain that the well-characterized systems described here are not unique and that most bi-molecular interactions involve a range of adaptive processes. The simplistic "lock-and-key" and "induced-fit" views of ligand binding must evolve to a better understanding of intermediate events and properties. The work described here can serve as an example for monitoring and exploiting adaptive features.

1.5
Herpes Simplex Virus

1.5.1
Herpes Simplex Virus-Encoded Ribonucleotide Reductase Inhibitors

Herpes simplex viruses (HSV-1 and HSV-1) are responsible for a number of human diseases, such as genital and oral lesions, ocular disease, and encephalitis. HSV encoded the enzyme ribonucleotide reductase (RR) which is responsible for the conversion of ribonucleoside diphosphates into the corresponding 2'-deoxyribonucleotides. As RR is an essential viral pathogen, a selective RR inhibitor is an attractive target for drug development. HSV RR is composed of two distinct homodimeric subunits [63, 64]. Association of these two subunits is essential for catalytic activity, and the C-terminus of the smaller of the two sub-units is critical for association [65]. When this small subunit lacks seven amino acids at the C-terminus, it does not bind to the larger subunit [66] and catalytic activity is lost. Peptides and peptide mimetic inhibitors of this region have been investigated as a route to new drug design [66–70].

NMR studies found that the last 32 amino acid residues of the C-terminus of R2 are disordered [71]: A published X-ray structure of *E.coli* RR R2 [72] was consistent with this, and also suggested that this region was disordered (no electron density was observed). It is important to determine this to understand whether con-formationally-constrained inhibitor design would work. Researchers found that the last six amino acids are more mobile that the rest of the protein, that these amino acids are conformationally similar to the corresponding amino acids of the 15-amino acid analogous peptide and that this corresponds to the critical binding region of the C-terminus responsible for subunit recognition. Critically, the researchers found that it was not necessary to study the small subunit C-terminus further and that conformational analysis of C-terminal peptides and their deriva-tives could be sufficient to gain insight into the bioactive conformation.

Knowledge of the bound conformation of peptides to the large subunit was then sought [70]. It was know that the nonapeptide H-Tyr-Ala-Gly-Ala-Val-Val-Asn-Asp-Leu-OH **41** corresponds to the nine- C-terminal amino acids of the HSV RR small subunit and that this inhibits HSV RR with an IC_{50} of 38 µM by preventing subunit association, see Table 1.3. It was desired to used **41** as a starting point to further improve inhibitor potency and reduce its size. The first tactic undertaken was to truncate the peptide at the N-terminus by up to four amino acids in **41** and this still provided inhibitors with some level of activity: compound **42** has an IC_{50} of 760 µM against HSV RR [65, 73]. It was deduced that peptapeptide **42** contained the minimum structural requirements for binding to the large subunit. SAR continued on analogs of this peptide **42**.

Earlier SAR had established that replacement of the asparagine side-chain NH_2 with a pyrrolidine provided a 50-fold boost in potency (**43**; IC_{50} 13 µM), see Table 1.4 [72]. This potency boost was necessary to undertake meaningful SAR studies and **43** was used as the basis for SAR investigations.

Table 1.3 Truncation of nonapeptide to minimum active fragment.

	Compound	IC_{50} (μM)
41	H-Tyr-Ala-Gly-Ala-Val-Val-Asn-Asp-Leu-OH	38
	H-Ala-Gly-Ala-Val-Val-Asn-Asp-Leu-OH	280
	H-Gly-Ala-Val-Val-Asn-Asp-Leu-OH	220
	H-Ala-Val-Val-Asn-Asp-Leu-OH	190
42	H-Val-Val-Asn-Asp-Leu-OH	760
	H-Val-Asn-Asp-Leu-OH	> 2000
	H-Tyr-Ala-Gly-Ala-Val-Val-Asn-Asp-OH	> 2000

Table 1.4 Modifications at the N-terminus

Compound	X	IC$_{50}$ (μM)
43		13
44		> 1000
45		1.5
46		1.5

Moving from the N-terminus to the C-terminus and optimizing substituents at each position before incorporating this optimized substituent into the optimization of the following round for the next substituent, we see that the capping group for the N-terminus supports lipophilic groups, with the simple acetyl compound being essentially inactive (**44**; IC$_{50}$ > 1000 μM), Table 1.4, whereas the cyclohexylamine (**45**; IC$_{50}$ 1.5 μM) and the diethylacetyl-chain (**46**; IC$_{50}$ 1.5 μM) were equally active. The latter is smaller and less lipophilic and so was taken forward into the next design round. Modifying the Ile-side chain led to compound rigidification by incorporation of a *tert*-butyl group, see Table 1.5 (**47**; IC$_{50}$ 0.6 μM), forcing the inhibitor to access the bioactive conformation. Compare this to the simple methyl **48** and proton compounds **49** that are less active. It is noteworthy that this knowledge inspired the use of similar *tert*-butyl groups in the HCMV and HCV programs (*vide supra*). SAR of the asparagine position failed to improve potency over that achieved with the pyrrolidine substituent, whereas addition of a geminal-dimethyl group to the aspartic acid side chain improved potency further. Finally, modification of the C-terminal position confirmed that a substituted carboxylate at the aspartic acid position was the optimal group for potency, compound **50**.

Table 1.5 Modifications leading to inhibitors accessing the bioactive conformation

Compound	X	IC$_{50}$ (μM)
46		1.5
47		0.6
48	CH$_3$	11
49	H	77

50: IC$_{50}$ 0.18 μM

Compounds were tested for selectivity of HSV ribonucleotide reductase inhibition over human RR. Table 1.6 indicates that selectivity was maintained.

Thus, SAR studies led to the identification of a substituted tetrapeptide **50** with a 200-fold improvement in potency over the nona-peptide (**41** in Table 1.3) and >4000-fold more potent over the peptapeptide (**42** in Table 1.3). Further SAR studies provided **51**, Figure 1.19, [74] which has an (s)-isopropyl side chain on the aspartate group and provides a compound with an IC$_{50}$ of 8 nM. NMR studies confirmed the conformational preference in solution for these inhibitors. The orientation of the carboxylate group was profoundly affected by the beta-alkyl group. Based on these and other conformation preferences deduced from NMR studies, a conformational restriction approach was attempted, with some success. From these efforts, compound **52**, which possessed an IC$_{50}$ of 56 nM, was synthesized.

Further optimization of the aspartic acid side chain, this time to a cyclopentyl-side chain and isopropyl to *tert*-butyl side chain modification at the leucine residue and the N-terminal cap to a phenylethylacetyl group, provided **BILD 1257** (Figure 1.20: EC$_{50}$ 35 μM [HSV-1]; 30 μM [HSV-2]). However, compounds in this

Table 1.6 Selectivity of HSV ribonucleotide reductase inhibition over human ribonucleotide reductase

	IC$_{50}$ (μM)	
Compound	HSV-RR	Human-RR
47	0.6	>1000
46	1.5	>1000
50	0.18	>1000

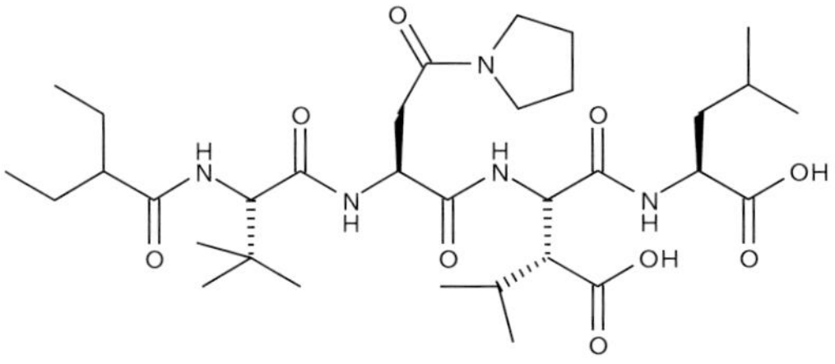

51: IC$_{50}$ 0.008 μM

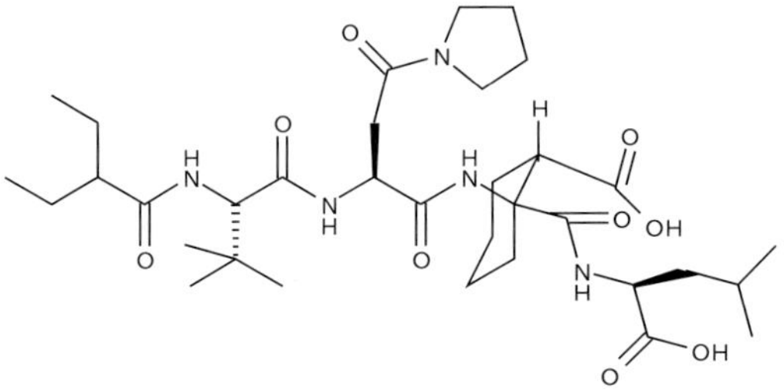

52: IC$_{50}$ 0.056 μM

Figure 1.19 HSV ribonucleotide reductase inhibitors.

series were not cell penetrant. Analogous to strategies in the HIV protease field, neutral or basic compounds showed higher cell penetration. In this HSV series of compounds, the C-terminal carboxylate was changed to a hydroxymethyl group, giving compound **BILD 1263** which possessed reasonable cellular potency (Figure 1.20: EC$_{50}$ 3.1 μM for HSV-1 and 4.2 μM for HSV-2).

These discoveries led to the discovery of **BILD 1263** as a topical treatment that was shown to reduce the severity and incidence of HSV-1-induced stromal keratitis and corneal neovascularization in a murine occular model [75]. A combination of NMR and molecular mechanics models was used to suggest a potential 3D structure for the inhibitors in the bound state as matching that in solution. Figure 1.21 indicates the groups important for binding and orientation into the

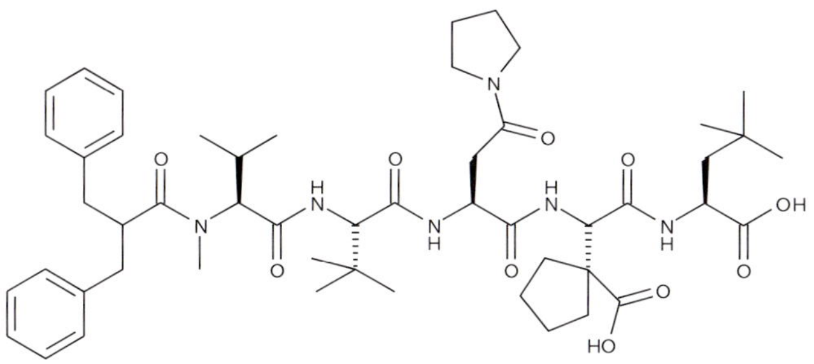

BILD 1257: EC$_{50}$ 35 μM (HSV-1)
EC$_{50}$ 30 μM (HSV-2)

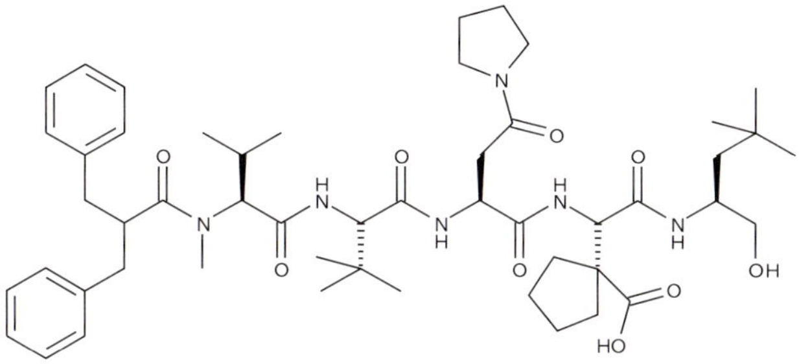

BILD 1263: EC$_{50}$ 3.1 μM (HSV-1)
EC$_{50}$ 4.2 μM (HSV-2)

Figure 1.20   Structures of advanced peptide mimics BILD 1257 and BILD 1263.

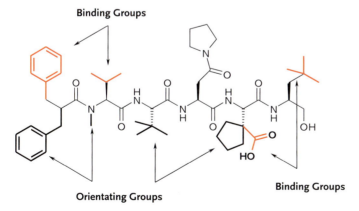

Binding Groups

Orientating Groups

Binding Groups

Figure 1.21   Proposed 3D structure for the inhibitors in the bound state matching that in solution. Reprinted with permission from *J. Med. Chem.*, 1995, 38, 3617-3623 (Figure 2). Peptidomimetic Inhibitors of Herpes Simplex Virus Ribonucleotide Reductase: A New Class of Antiviral Agents. Moss, N., Beaulieu, P., Duceppe, J.S., Ferland, J.M., Gauthier, J., Ghiro, E., Goulet, S., Grenier, L., Llinàs-Brunet, M., Plante, R., Wernic, D., Déziel, R. Copyright 1995 American Chemical Society.

bioactive conformation for peptide inhibitors. In the absence of X-ray information, correlation of potency with the structure of conformationally-restricted inhibitors has been undertaken to provide evidence of the bioactive conformation. Understanding an inhibitor's bioactive conformation and how the molecule binds to its target requires knowledge of what inhibitor functionalities are important for binding potency and why these are so.

A related target varicella zoster virus (VSV) RR is also inhibited by compounds in this series. The C-terminal sequence of VZV RR (YAGTVINDL) is similar to that of HSV RR(YAGAVVNDL) so it was reasoned that the same series of compounds could be active in both [76]. Table 1.7 gives the binding affinities of the nonapeptides corresponding to the C-terminal sequences of VZVRR and HSV RR (**53** and **54**, respectively). The peptides were reduced in size to find the minimum binding sequence to elicit activity, leading to compound **55** (Table 1.7: IC_{50} of 4000 nM for HSV RR and 15000 nM for VZV and compound **56** (Table 1.7: IC_{50} of 24 nM for HSV RR and 588 nM for VZV). Following changes to the side chains to improve activity, compound **57** was obtained, Table 1.7, which possessed an IC_{50} of 1 nM for HSV RR and 37 nM for VZV.

1.6
Renin

1.6.1
Aspartyl Protease Renin as a Target

Renin is an aspartyl protease that catalyzes the first rate-limiting step in the renin-angiotensin cascade [77]. Renin-angiotensin plays an important role in the regulation of blood pressure and the maintenance of sodium and volume homeostasis, where renin cleaves its substrate angiotensinogen (its only natural substrate) generating the decapeptide angiotensin I, which in turn is processed to the octapeptide angiotensin II by the angiotensin converting enzyme (ACE). Angiotensin II is a potent vasoconstrictor, therefore inhibitors of renin have been sought for the treatment of hypertension.

The potential of renin as a target has been recognized for decades but many potent peptides and peptidomimetics active against renin have displayed poor oral efficacy, attributed to poor absorption, a high first-pass clearance and/or proteolytic degradation.

A series of renin inhibitors, which are non-peptide inhibitors possessing a dipeptide replacement for the P2–P3 segment (see Figure 1.22) was designed by researchers, as well as a known diol transition state analog, 4,5- and 3,5-dihydroxyhexanamide [78].

The inhibitors **58** and **59** span the P_3 P_1' to positions and it had been shown that with renin inhibitors, the P_3 carbonyl interacts with the enzyme while the P_2–P_3 amide NH forms a non-critical hydrogen bond [79]. The P_2–P_3 replacements must achieve critical hydrogen bonds with the enzyme and orient the P_3 side chain whilst lacking the P_4 residue.

Table 1.7 Truncation of the nona-peptides corresponding to the C-terminal sequences of VZV RR.

Compound		Binding Assay IC$_{50}$ (nM)	
		HSV	VZV
53		8 000	11 000
54		25 000	42 000
55		4 000	15 000

(Continued)

Table 1.7 (Continued)

Compound	Binding Assay IC$_{50}$ (nM)	
	HSV	VZV
56	24	588
57	1	37

Figure 1.22 Dipeptide replacement for the P2–P3 segment of Renin and inhibitors spanning the P_3 to P'_1 positions of Renin. Reprinted from *Bioorganic & Medicinal Chemistry*, 6, Jung, G.L., Anderson, P.C., Bailey, M., Baillet, M., Bantle, G.W., Berthiaume, S., Lavallée, P., Llinàs-Brunet, M., Thavonekham, B., Thibeault, D., Simoneau, B., Novel Small Renin Inhibitors Containing 4,5- or 3,5-Dihydroxy-2-substituted-6-phenylhexanamide Replacements at the P_2-P_3 Sites, 2317-2336 (Figure 2), Copyright 1998, with permission from Elsevier Science Ltd.

On route to optimizing this series of inhibitors, NMR spectroscopy was used to identify and compare the preferred solution conformations of the inhibitors [80]. Comparisons were also made between the unbound structures determined by NMR, and the renin-bound structures determined by X-ray crystallography [81].

Determination of solution conformations of inhibitors **60** to **62** (Figure 1.23a) in the unbound state indicated a major conformer for these inhibitors. By using NMR-derived restraints, the solution structures of the inhibitors were modeled using a combination of distance geometry, energy minimization, and molecular dynamics. The lowest 25 energy structures that satisfied the NMR data were superimposed (colored in black, Figure 1.23c). These were then compared with the crystal structures of renin complexed with inhibitors **60** to **62** [82], see the red

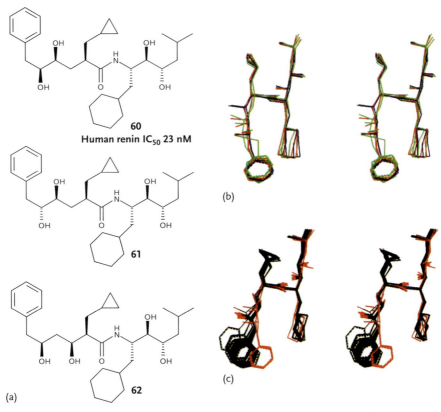

60

Human renin IC$_{50}$ 23 nM

61

62

(a)

(b)

(c)

Figure 1.23 Renin inhibitors. (a) structures of inhibitors **60–62**. (b) Stereoviews of the renin-bound structures of inhibitors **60–62** as determined by X-ray crystallography [82]. Inhibitors **60–62** are colored red, green and blue, respectively. Since there are two independent renin complexes per asymmetric unit, both forms for each inhibitor are shown. (c) Stereoviews of the solution structures of **60** (black) in the unbound state (determined by NMR) are shown superimposed with the renin-bound structures of **60** (red) (determined by X-ray crystallography).

colored structures in Figure 1.23c. As can be seen from Figure 1.23c, the inhibitors adopt similar confirmations in the unbound and renin-bound states. Also, all three inhibitors have a similar overall conformation (Figure 1.23b), with the P$_3$ showing the greatest variability. It was found that, although the inhibitors displayed similar conformations with renin-bound and unbound, the gross conformational changes of the inhibitor are not a prerequisite to binding renin. Differences were observed, for example, between the P$_3$ position between inhibitors themselves and between renin-bound and unbound conformations. These differences were not detrimental to inhibitor potency.

Medicinal chemistry proceeded to attempt to optimize this series of peptidomimetics but this ultimately failed to deliver a series that was optimizable for

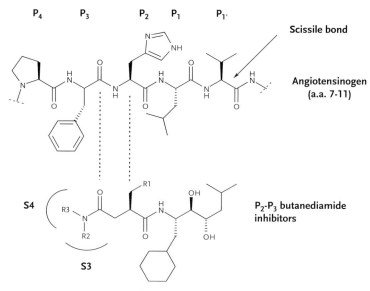

Figure 1.24 Proposed P$_2$–P$_3$ butanediamide inhibitors. Reprinted from *Bioorganic & Medicinal Chemistry*, 7, Simoneau, B., Lavallée, P., Anderson, P.C., Bailey, M., Bantle, G., Berthiaume, S., Chabot, C., Fazal, G., Halmos, T., Ogilvie, W.W., Poupart, M.-A., Thavonekham, B., Xin, Z., Thibeault, D., Bolger, G., Panzenbeck, M., Winquist, R., Jung, G.L., Discovery of non-peptidic P$_2$–P$_3$ butanediamide renin inhibitors with high oral efficacy, 489–508 (Figure 1), Copyright 1999, with permission from Elsevier Science Ltd.

physicochemical properties, such as water solubility. One of the most promising compounds from this series was **60** which possessed an IC$_{50}$ of 23 nM, see Figure 1.23. [78].

Although potent (**60**: human plasma renin IC$_{50}$ 23 nM), inhibitors at this stage of the program lacked water solubility and so this series was abandoned in favor of a series where the focus for design was placed on the P$_2$–P$_3$–P$_4$ segment of the inhibitors [83] while maintaining a known transition state analog at P1–P1′ [84].

Research centered around replacing the P$_2$–P$_3$ peptide moiety with a butanediamide (Figure 1.24) as the NH at P$_2$ is not involved in an essential hydrogen bond it can, therefore, be replaced by a methylene. One stereogenic center is thus eliminated, leading to a decomplexation of overall structure. A medicinal chemistry program then followed to optimize potency and physico-chemical properties, varying substituents at P$_2$–P$_3$–P4. Optimization for potency at P$_1$ led to the introduction of a 2-amino-4-thiazolyl-group **63**, Figure 1.25; at P$_3$ to a cyclohexylmethyl substituent **64** and at P$_4$ to the introduction of an N,N-dimethylacetamide side chain **63**. Compound **63** was evaluated in a conscious sodium deplete cynomologous monkey, given orally at a 10 mg/kg dose and this compound gave a statistically significant decrease in mean arterial blood pressure. Further

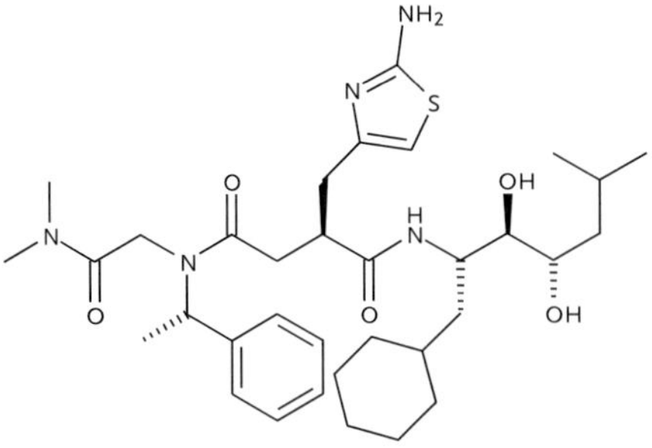

63: Human renin IC$_{50}$ 1.1 nM

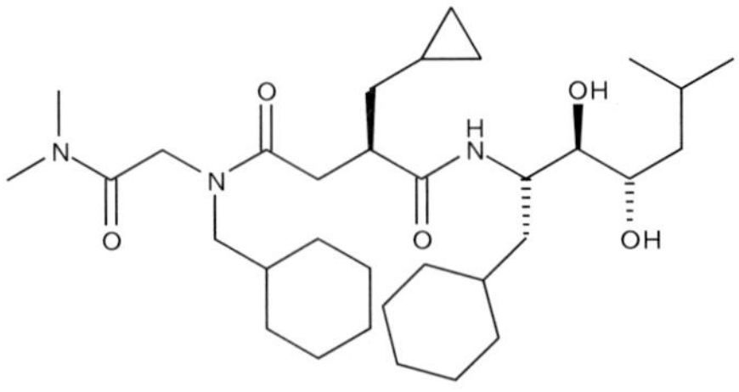

64: Human renin IC$_{50}$ 11 nM

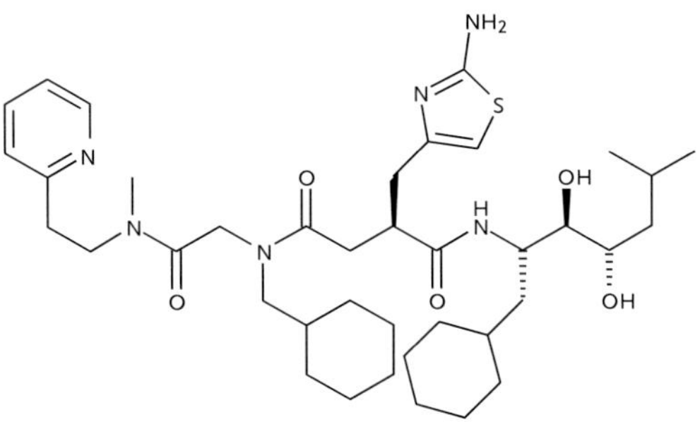

BILA 2157: Human renin IC$_{50}$ 1.4 nM

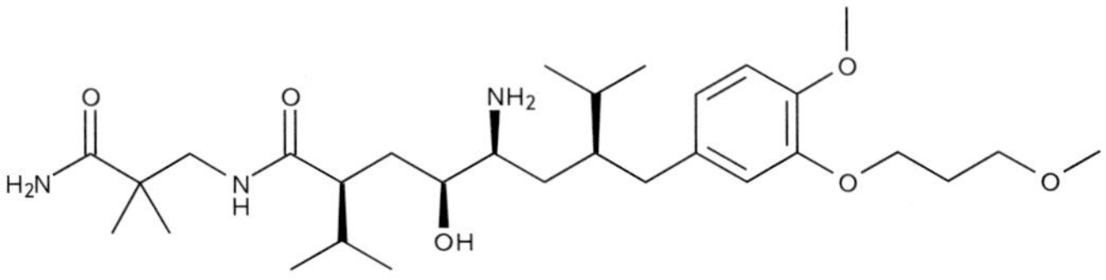

Aliskirin

Figure 1.25 P$_2$–P$_3$ butanediamide Renin inhibitors.

optimization for compound **63** based on *in vivo* activity followed, focussing on the P$_4$ and P$_3$ positions by replacement of the *N,N*-dimethylamide fragment with an *N*-methyl-2-pyridylethyl-substituent. This compound **BILA 2157** was selected as the clinical candidate [85].

BILA 2157 was potent, selective, possessed a simplified chemical structure and displayed a good oral activity of 40% in cynomolgus monkey, as well as displaying a statistically significant lowering of blood pressure in sodium-depleted animals, given at an oral dose of 3 mg/kg [83]. Further clinical development of this compound was stopped due to unforeseen toxicology observed in rats and dogs under chronic administration.

Some years later a related compound (Spp-100; Tekturna; Aliskirin®) was launched onto the market (see Figure 1.25).

1.7
HIV

1.7.1
HIV Protease Inhibitors

The human immunodeficiency virus (HIV) has been identified as the causative agent of acquired immune deficiency syndrome (AIDS). Studies of the virus' life-cycle have revealed a number of potential therapeutic intervention points: One of the most studied being the aspartyl protease enzyme of HIV, which has been shown to be essential for viral replication [86–89]. The enzyme is essential for processing the viral *gag* and *gag-pol* gene products through specific cleavage of peptide bonds [90–93]. The rational design of HIV protease inhibitors has relied upon the transition state mimic concept, applied to the cleavage of an amide bond. In this case, replacing an amide bond by a non-cleavable hydroxyethylamine dipeptide isostere, see Figure 1.26. In this way, a number of potent peptide-mimic viral replication inhibitors of the enzyme have been produced and made it to market [94, 95].

Originally, the highly peptidic nature of these HIV protease inhibitors resulted in limited oral bioavailability, short *in vivo* half-lives and complex structures [96]. From our own work aimed at simplifying the structure of HIV protease inhibitors, reducing the peptidic nature of the inhibitors as well as reducing charge and hydrophobicity, these efforts led to the synthesis of palinavir [97, 98] which contains a (R)-hydroxyethylamine transition state mimic and a novel 4-substituted pipecolic amide (see Figure 1.27). Palinavir is a highly potent and specific inhibitor of HIV-1 (EC$_{50}$ 4 nM) and HIV-2 proteases (EC$_{50}$ 10 nM), see Table 1.8 and Figure 1.27.

The bioavailability of palinavir in rats is 26%, significantly higher than that of Saquinavir (oral bioavailability 3%). Palinavir was nominated as the first clinical candidate against HIV protease (Figure 1.27), but development of this compound

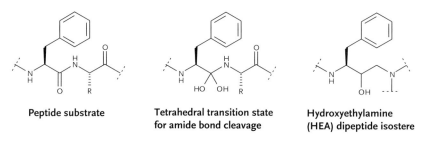

| Peptide substrate | Tetrahedral transition state for amide bond cleavage | Hydroxyethylamine (HEA) dipeptide isostere |

Figure 1.26 Dipeptide isostere. Reprinted with permission from *J. Org. Chem.*, 1996, 61, 3635-3645 (Figure 1). Preparation of Aminoalkyl Chlorohydrin Hydrochlorides: Key Building Blocks for Hydroxyethylamine-Based HIV Protease Inhibitors. Beaulieu, P. and Wernic, D. Copyright 1996 American Chemical Society.

Substrate sequence

Palinavir

- Peptidomimetic
- Stopped just before entering clinical phase

Tipranavir (Aptivus)

- Non-peptidomimetic, potent against resistant mutants
- Approved by FDA in 2005
- On the market

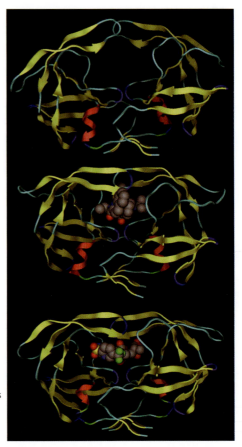

Figure 1.27 Conserved features of relatively weak lead peptide substrates (colored red), with truncations and alterations (colored black) and the addition of new features (colored blue) for Palinavir and Tipranavir, together with bound crystal structures of each.

Table 1.8 Inhibition of HIV-1 and HIV-2 proteases by Palinavir and activity against human aspartyl proteases

Aspartyl Protease	EC$_{50}$ (nM)
HIV-1	4 (0.031[a])
HIV-2	10 (0.134[a])
Renin	> 50 000
Cathepsin D	100 000
Pepsin	33 000
Gastricsin	45 000

[a] K_i was determined by a steady-state velocity method.

was stopped just before entering clinical trials. In a separate program, a non-peptidic drug was rationally discovered and is now marketed as Tipranavir (Figure 1.27). Tipranavir possesses a complimentary resistance profile to that seen with other peptidomimetic drugs in this class [99–101].

1.8
Conclusions

Historically, the process of taking a peptide hit and turning this into a marketed, orally bioavailable drug has been time consuming and prone to failure. Through the process outlined in this chapter (Schemes 1.1 and 1.2), resting on a "sense-making" approach to the creation of knowledge and understanding of the therapeutic target of interest and how the peptide starting point(s) interact with this target, the success rate in taking a peptide and creating an orally bioavailable peptide mimic can be increased. We have exemplified this process in detail for two targets: HCMV protease and HCV protease and have teased out important strategic peptide mimic design considerations for a number of other targets such as herpes simplex virus, renin aspartyl protease, and HIV protease. As a testament to the approach taken to peptide mimic design outlined here, we have delivered a number of clinical candidates, including the HCV protease inhibitors BILN 2061 and BI00201335, which are currently in Phase III clinical trials.

Although a number of important design stage posts will be present in any peptide to peptide mimic program, important points for consideration include mapping of the critical binding elements of the substrate to the protein (determining the bioactive conformation of the inhibitor), increasing peptide potency where necessary in order to generate meaningful SAR, often by incorporating a warhead; remembering to remove the warhead in later medicinal chemistry design iterations when appropriate. Additionally, through truncation of the peptide, to find the minimally active peptide and building back potency (and concurrently de-peptidizing), in part through matching of the inhibitor's free-state conformation to its biologically active bound conformation, resulting in a reduction in the entropic cost of binding.

Systematically monitoring the structure and dynamic features of ligands using multidisciplinary strategies has broad application: most bi-molecular interactions involve a range of adaptive processes. Critical to biomolecular recognition events are the necessary structural and flexibility adaptations of the ligand and receptor to attain the bioactive complex. Therefore, peptide to peptide mimic strategies need to recognize these facts and the tactics used need to move to a more holistic approach that incorporates the effects of dynamics and conformational changes, thus moving beyond the simplistic "lock-and-key" and "induced-fit" views of ligand binding to one where we have a better understanding of intermediate events and properties. We believe that by following this strategy and tactics in their application to rational drug design, the discovery process could be accelerated from the knowledge of these adaptive processes. However, to date, few reports of the application of dynamics and conformational changes have appeared in the literature. The work described here can serve as examples to monitor and exploit adaptive features and will, hopefully, prompt other researchers to incorporate these design strategies into their work.

References

1 Wu, Y.-D. and Gellman, S. (2008) Peptidomimetics. *Acc. Chem. Res.*, **41**, 1231–1232.

2 Gante, J. (1994) Peptide mimics – tailor-made enzyme inhibitors. *Angew. Chem., Int. Ed. Engl.*, **33**, 1699–1720.

3 Ladner, R.C., Sato, A.K., Gorzelany, J., and de Souza, M. (2004) Phage display-derived peptides as therapeutic alternatives to antibodies. *Drug Discov. Today*, **9**, 525–529.

4 Buckingham, S., Quintas, P., and Hopkins, M. (2002) The cost of knowledge, in *B823 Managing Knowledge* (ed. The Open University), Dorset, Henry Ling Ltd., **3**, p. 10.

5 LaPlante, S.R. (2007) Exploiting ligand and receptor adaptability in rational drug design using dynamics and structure-based strategies. *Top. Curr. Chem.*, **272**, 259–296.

6 Mocarski, E.S. Jr (1995) Cytomegaloviruses and their replication, in *Fields Virology*, **2** (eds B.N. Fields, D.M., Knipe, and P.M. Howley), Lippincott-Raven, Philadelphia, PA, pp. 2447–2492.

7 Britt, W.J. and Alford, C.A. (1995) Cytomegalovirus, in *Fields Virology*, **2** (ed. B.N. Fields), Lippincott-Raven, Philadelphia, PA, pp. 2493–2525.

8 Casjens, S. and King, J. (1975) Virus assembly. *Annu. Rev. Biochem.*, **44**, 555–611.

9 Gibson, W., Welch, A.R., and Hall, M.R.T. (1995) Assembling a herpes virus serine maturational proteinase and new molecular target for antivirals. *Perspect. Drug Discov. Des.*, **2**, 413–426.

10 Gao, M., Matusick-Kumar, L., Hurlburt, W., DiTusa, S.F., Newcomb, W.W., Brown, J.C., McCann, P.J. III,

Deckman, I., and Colonno, R.J. (1994) The protease of herpes simplex virus type 1 is essential for functional capsid formation and viral growth. *J. Virol.*, **68**, 3702–3712.

11 Preston, V.G., Coates, J.A.V., and Rixon, F.J. (1983) Identification and characterization of a herpes simplex virus gene product required for encapsidation of virus DNA. *J. Virol.*, **45**, 1056–1064.

12 Matusick-Kumar, L., McCann, P.J. III, Robertson, B.J., Newcomb, W.W., Brown, J.C., and Gao, M. (1995) Release of the catalytic domain N(o) from the herpes simplex virus type 1 protease is required for viral growth. *J. Virol.*, **69**, 7113–7121.

13 Tong, L., Qian, C., Massariol, M.-J., Bonneau, P.R., Cordingley, M.G., and Lagacé, L. (1996) A new serine-protease fold revealed by the crystal structure of human cytomegalovirus protease. *Nature*, **383**, 272–275.

14 Qiu, X., Culp, J.S., DiLella, A.G., Hellmig, B., Hoog, S.S., Janson, C.A., Smith, W.W., and Abdel-Meguid, S.S. (1996) Unique fold and active site in cytomegalovirus protease. *Nature*, **383**, 275–279.

15 Shieh, H.-S., Kurumbail, R.G., Stevens, A.M., Stegeman, R.A., Sturman, E.J., Pak, J.Y., Wittwer, A.J., Palmier, M.O., Wiegand, R.C., Holwerda, B.C., and Stallings, W.C. (1996) Three-dimensional structure of human cytomegalovirus protease. *Nature*, **383**, 279–282.

16 Chen, P., Tsuge, H., Almassy, R.J., Gribskov, C.L., Katoh, S., Vanderpool, D.L., Margosiak, S.A., Pinko, C., Matthews, D.A., and Kan, C.-C. (1996)

Structure of the human cytomegalovirus protease catalytic domain reveals a novel serine protease fold and catalytic triad. *Cell*, **86**, 835–843.

17 Margosiak, S.A., Vanderpool, D.L., Sisson, W., Pinko, C., and Kan, C.-C. (1996) Dimerization of the human cytomegalovirus protease: kinetic and biochemical characterization of the catalytic homodimer. *Biochemistry*, **35**, 5300–5307.

18 Darke, P.L., Cole, J.L., Waxman, L., Hall, D.L., Sardana, M.K., and Kuo, L.C. (1996) Active human cytomegalovirus protease is a dimer. *J. Biol. Chem.*, **271**, 7445–7449.

19 Bonneau, P.R., Grand-Maître, C., Greenwood, D.J., Lagacé, L., LaPlante, S.R., Massariol, M.-J., Ogilvie, W.W., O'Meara, J.A., and Kawai, S.H. (1997) Evidence of a conformational change in the human cytomegalovirus protease upon binding of peptidyl-activated carbonyl inhibitors. *Biochemistry*, **36**, 12644–12652.

20 LaPlante, S.R., Bonneau, P.R., Aubry, N., Cameron, D.R., Déziel, R., Grand-Maître, C., Plouffe, C., Tong, L., and Kawai, S.H. (1999) Characterization of the human cytomegalovirus protease as an induced-fit serine protease and the implications to the design of mechanism-based inhibitors. *J. Am. Chem. Soc.*, **121**, 2974–2986.

21 LaPlante, S.R., Aubry, N., Bonneau, P.R., Cameron, D.R., Lagacé, L., Massariol, M.-J., Montpetit, H., Plouffe, C., Kawai, S.H., Fulton, B.D., Chen, Z.G., and Ni, F. (1998) Human cytomegalovirus protease complexes its substrate recognition sequences in an extended peptide conformation. *Biochemistry*, **37**, 9793–9801.

22 Berger, A. and Schechter, J. (1970) Mapping the active site of papain with the aid of peptide substrates and inhibitors. *Philos. Trans. R. Soc. London, Ser. B.*, **257**, 249–264.

23 Sardana, V.V., Wolfgang, J.A., Veloski, C.A., Long, W.J., Legrow, K., Wolanski, B., Emini, E.A., and LaFemina, R.L. (1994) Peptide substrate cleavage specificity of the human cytomegalovirus protease. *J. Biol. Chem.*, **269**, 14337–14340.

24 Ni, F. (1994) Recent developments in transferred NOE methods. *Prog. NMR Spectrosc.*, **26**, 517–606.

25 LaFemina, R.L., Bakshi, K., Long, W.J., Pramanik, B., Veloski, C.A., Wolanski, B.S., Marcy, A.I., and Hazuda, D.J. (1996) Characterization of a soluble stable human cytomegalovirus protease and inhibition by M-site peptide mimics. *J. Virol.*, **70**, 4819–4824.

26 Fersht, A. (ed.) (1985) *Enzyme Structure and Mechanisms*, 2nd edn, Freeman and Co, New York.

27 Polgár, L. (ed.) (1989) *Mechanisms of Protease Action*, CRC Press Inc, Boca Raton FL, Chapter 3.

28 Hedstrom, L. (2002) Serine protease mechanism and specificity. *Chem. Rev.*, **102**, 4501–4524.

29 Mercer, D.F., Schiller, D.E., Elliott, J.F., Douglas, D.N., Hao, C., Rinfret, A., Addison, W.R., Fischer, K.P., Churchill, T.A., Lakey, J.R.T., Tyrrell, D.L.J., and Kneteman, N.M. (2001) Hepatitis C virus replication in mice with chimeric human livers. *Nature Medicine*, **7**, 927–933.

30 Ogilvie, W.W., Bailey, M., Poupart, M.-A., Abraham, A., Bhavsar, A., Bonneau, P.R., Bordeleau, J., Bousquet, Y., Chabot, C., Duceppe, J.-S., Fazal, G., Goulet, S., Grand- Maître, C., Guse, I., Halmos, T., Lavallée, P., Leach, M., Malenfant, E., O'Meara, J.A., Plante, R., Plouffe, C., Poirier, M., Soucy, F., Yoakim, C., and Déziel, R. (1997) Peptidomimetic inhibitors of the human cytomegalovirus protease. *J. Med. Chem.*, **40**, 4113–4135.

31 LaPlante, S.R., Cameron, D.R., Aubry, N., Bonneau, P.R., Déziel, R., Grand-Maître, C., Ogilvie, W.W., and Kawai, S.H. (1998) The conformation of a peptidyl methyl ketone inhibitor bound to the human cytomegalovirus protease. *Angew. Chem. Int. Ed. Engl.*, **37**, 2729–2732.

32 Tong, L., Qian, C., Massariol, M.-J., Déziel, R., Yoakim, C., and Lagacé, L. (1998) Conserved mode of

peptidomimetic inhibition and substrate recognition of human cytomegalovirus protease. *Nature Struct. Biol.*, **5**, 819–826.

33 Cao, Y., Musah, R.A., Wilcox, S.K., Goodin, D.B., and Mcree, D.E. (1998) Protein conformer selection by ligand binding observed with crystallography. *Protein Sci.*, **7**, 72–78.

34 LaPlante, S.R., Llinàs-Brunet, M. (2005) Dynamics and structure-based design of drugs targeting the critical serine protease of the Hepatitis C Virus – from a peptide substrate to BILN 2061. *Curr. Med. Chem.*, **4**, 111–132.

35 Choo, Q.L., Kuo, G., Weiner, A.J., Overby, L.R., Bradley, D.W., and Houghton, M. (1989) Isolation of a cDNA clone derived from a blood-borne non-A, non-B viral hepatitis genome. *Science*, **244**, 359–362.

36 Kuo, G., Choo, Q.L., Alter, H.J., Gitnick, G.L., Redeker, A.G., Purcell, R.H., Miyamura, T., Dienstag, J.L., Alter, M.J., and Stevens, C.E. (1989) An assay for circulating antibodies to a major etiologic virus of human non-A, non-B hepatitis. *Science*, **244**, 362–364.

37 Di Bisceglie, A.M. (1998) Hepatitis C. *Lancet*, **351**, 351–355.

38 World Health Organization (1999) Global surveillance and control of hepatitis C. Report of a WHO consultation organized in collaboration with the viral hepatitis prevention board, Antwerp, Belgium. *J. Virol. Hepat.*, **6**, 35–47.

39 Kakiuchi, N., Hijikata, M., Komoda, Y., Tanji, Y., Hirowatari, Y., and Shimotohno, K. (1995) Bacterial expression and analysis of cleavage activity of HCV serine proteinase using recombinant and synthetic substrate. *Biochem. Biophys. Res. Comm.*, **210**, 1059–1065.

40 Llinàs-Brunet, M., Bailey, M., Fazal, G., Goulet, S., Halmos, T., LaPlante, S., Maurice, R., Poirier, M., Poupart, M.-A., Thibeault, D., Wernic, D., and Lamarre, D. (1998) Peptide-based inhibitors of the hepatitis C virus serine protease. *Bioorg. Med. Chem., Lett.*, **8**, 1713–1718.

41 Llinàs-Brunet, M., Bailey, M., Déziel, R., Fazal, G., Gorys, V., Goulet, S., Halmos, T., Maurice, R., Poirier, M., Poupart, M.-A., Rancourt, J., Thibeault, D., Wernic, D., and Lamarre, D. (1998) Studies on the C-terminal of hexapeptide inhibitors of the hepatitis C virus serine protease. *Bioorg. Med. Chem. Lett.*, **8**, 2719–2724.

42 Bailey, M., Halmos, T., Goudreau, N., Lescop, E., and Llinàs-Brunet, M. (2004) Novel azapeptide inhibitors of hepatitis C virus serine protease. *J. Med. Chem.*, **47**, 3788–3799.

43 LaPlante, S.R., Cameron, D.R., Aubry, N., Lefebvre, S., Kukolj, G., Maurice, R., Thibeault, D., Lamarre, D., and Llinàs-Brunet, M. (1999) Solution structure of substrate – based ligands when bound to hepatitis C virus NS3 protease domain. *J. Biol. Chem.*, **274**, 18618–18624.

44 Llinàs-Brunet, M., Bailey, M., Fazal, G., Ghiro, E., Gorys, V., Goulet, S., Halmos, T., Maurice, R., Poirier, M., Poupart, M.-A., Rancourt, J., Thibeault, D., Wernic, D., and Lamarre, D. (2000) Highly potent and selective peptide-based inhibitors of the hepatitis C virus serine protease: towards smaller inhibitors. *Bioorg. Med. Chem. Lett.*, **10**, 2267–2270.

45 LaPlante, S.R., Aubry, N., Bonneau, P., Kukolj, G., Lamarre, D., Lefebvre, S., Li, H., Llinàs-Brunet, M., Plouffe, C., and Cameron, D.R. (2000) NMR line-broadening and transferred NOESY as a medicinal chemistry tool for studying inhibitors of the hepatitis c virus NS3 protease domain. *Bioorg. Med. Chem. Lett.*, **10**, 2271–2274.

46 Rancourt J., Cameron, D.R., Gorys, V., Lamarre, D., Poirier, M., Thibeault, D., and Llinàs- Brunet, M. (2004) Peptide-based inhibitors of the hepatitis C virus NS3 protease: structure-activity relationship at the C-terminal position. *J. Med. Chem.*, **47**, 2511–2522.

47 Pause, A., Kukolj, G., Bailey, M., Brault, M., Do, F., Halmos, T., Lagace, L., Maurice, R., Marquis, M., McKercher, G., Pellerin, C., Pilote, L., Thibeault, D., and Lamarre, D. (2003)

An NS3 serine protease inhibitor abrogates replication of subgenomic hepatitis C virus RNA. *J. Biol. Chem.*, **278**, 20374–20380.

48 Poupart, M.-A., Cameron, D.R., Chabot, C., Ghiro, E., Goudreau, N., Goulet, S., Poirier, M., and Tsantrizos, Y. (2001) Solid-phase synthesis of peptidomimetic inhibitors for the hepatitis C virus NS3 protease. *J. Org. Chem.*, **66**, 4743–4751.

49 Goudreau, N., Cameron, D.R., Bonneau, P., Gorys, V., Plouffe, C., Poirier, M., Lamarre, D., and Llinàs-Brunet, M. (2004) NMR structural characterization of peptide inhibitors bound to the hepatitis C virus NS3 protease: design of a new P2 substituent. *J. Med. Chem.*, **47**, 123–132.

50 Tsantrizos, Y., Bolger, G., Bonneau, P., Cameron, D.R., Goudreau, N., Kukolj, G., LaPlante, S.R., Llinàs-Brunet, M., Nar, H., and Lamarre, D. (2003) Macrocyclic inhibitors of the NS3 protease as potential therapeutic agents of hepatitis C virus infection. *Angew. Chem. Int. Ed. Eng.*, **42**, 1356–1360.

51 LaPlante, S.R., Aubry, N., Déziel, R., Ni, F., and Xu, P. (2000) Transferred 13C T1 relaxation at natural isotopic abundance: a practical method for determining site-specific changes in ligand flexibility upon binding to a macromolecule. *J. Am. Chem. Soc.*, **122e**, 12530–12532.

52 Llinàs-Brunet, M., Bailey, M.D., Ghiro, E., Gorys, V., Halmos, T., Poirier, M., Rancourt, J., and Goudreau, N. (2004) A systematic approach to the optimization of substrate-based inhibitors of the hepatitis C virus NS3 protease: discovery of potent and specific tripeptide inhibitors. *J. Med. Chem.*, **47**, 6584–6594.

53 Goudreau, N., Brochu, C., Cameron, D.R., Duceppe, J.-S., Faucher, A.-M., Ferland, J.-M., Grand- Maître, C., Poirier, M., Simoneau, B., and Tsantrizos, Y.S. (2004) Potent inhibitors of the hepatitis C virus NS3 protease: design and synthesis of macrocyclic substrate-based -strand mimics. *J. Org. Chem.*, **69**, 6185–6201.

54 Ali, S., Pellerin, C., Lamarre, D., and Kukolj, G. (2004) Hepatitis C virus subgenomic replicons in the human embryonic kidney 293 cell line. *J. Virol.*, **78**, 491–501.

55 Llinàs-Brunet, M., Bailey, M., Bolger, G., Brochu, C., Faucher, A.M., Ferland, J.-M., Garneau, M., Ghiro, E., Gorys, V., Grand- Maître, C., Halmos, T., Lapayre -Pachette, N., Liard, F., Poirier, M., Rheame, M., Tsantrizos, Y.S., and Lamarre, D. (2004) Structure- activity study on a novel series of macrocyclic inhibitors of the hepatitis C virus NS3 protease leading to the discovery of BILN 2061, *J. Med. Chem.*, **47**, 1605–1608.

56 Thibeault, D., Bousquet, C., Gingras, R., Lagace, L., Maurice, R., White, P., and Lamarre, D. (2004) Sensitivity of NS3 serine proteases from hepatitis C virus genotypes 2 and 3 to the inhibitor BILN 2061. *J. Virol.*, **78**, 7352–7359.

57 Faucher, A.-M., Bailey, M., Beaulieu, P. L., Brochu, C., Duceppe, J.-S., Ferland, J.-M., Ghiro, E., Gorys, V., Halmos, T., Kawai, S.H., Poirier, M., Simoneau, B., Tsantrizos, Y.S., and Llinàs-Brunet, M. (2004) Synthesis of BILN 2061, an HCV NS3 protease inhibitor with proven antiviral effect in humans. *Org. Lett.*, **6**, 2901–2904.

58 Lamarre, D., Anderson, P.C., Bailey, M., Beaulieu, P., Bolger, G., Bonneau, P., Bös, M., Cameron, D.R., Cartier, M., Cordingley, M.G., Faucher, A.-M., Goudreau, N., Kawai, S.H., Kukolj, G., Lagace, L., LaPlante, S.R., Narjes, H., Poupart, M.-A., Rancourt, J., Sentjens, R.E., St George, R., Simoneau, B., Steinmann, G., Thibeault, D., Tsantrizos, Y.S., Weldon, S.M., Yong, C.L., and Llinàs-Brunet, M. (2003) An NS3 protease inhibitor with antiviral effects in humans infected with hepatitis C virus. *Nature*, **426**, 186–189.

59 Hinrichsen, H., Benhamou, Y., Wedemeyer, H., Reiser, M., Sentjens, R.E., Calleja, J.L., Forns, X., Erhardt, A., Cronlein, J., Chaves, R.L., Yong, C.L., Nehmiz, G., and Steinmann, G.G.

(2004) Short-term antiviral efficacy of BILN 2061, a hepatitis C virus serine protease inhibitor, in hepatitis C genotype 1 patients. *Gastroenterology*, **127**, 1347–1355.

60 Venkatraman, S. and Njoroge, F.G. (2009) Macrocyclic inhibitors of HCV NS3 protease. *Expert Opinion on Therapeutic Patents*, **19**, 1277–1303.

61 Llinàs-Brunet, M., Bailey, M.D., Goudreau, N., Bhardwaj, P.K., Bordeleau, J., Bös, M., Bousquet, Y., Cordingley, M.G., Duan, J., Forgione, P., Garneau, M., Ghiro, E., Gorys, V., Goulet, S., Halmos, T., Kawai, S.H., Naud, J., Poupart, M.-A., and White, P.W. (2010) The discovery of BI 201335: a potent and selective non-covalent inhibitor of the hepatitis C Virus NS3 protease. *J. Med. Chem.*, **53**, 6466–6476

62 Manns, M.P., Bourlière, M., Benhamou, Y., Pol, S., Bonacini, M., Trepo, C., Wright, D., Berg, T., Calleja, J.L., White, P.W., Stern, J.O., Steinmann, G., Yong, C.L., Kukolj, G., Scherer, J., and Boecher, W.O. (2010) Potency, safety and pharmacokinetics of the NS3/4A protease inhibitor BI201335 in patients with chronic HCV genotype-1 infection. *J. Hepatol.*, **54**, 1114–1122.

63 Lammers, M. and Follman, H. (1983) The ribonucleotide reductases – a unique group of metalloenzymes essential for cell proliferation. *Struct. Bonding*, **54**, 27–91.

64 Ingemarson, R. and Lankinen, H. (1987) The herpes simplex virus type 1 ribonucleotide reductase is a tight complex of the type $\alpha 2\beta 2$ composed of 40K and 140K proteins, of which the latter shows multiple forms due to proteolysis. *Virology*, **156**, 417–422.

65 Filatov, D., Ingemarson, R., Graslund, A., and Thelander, L. (1992) The role of herpes simplex virus ribonucleotide reductase small subunit carboxyl terminus in subunit interaction and formation of iron-tyrosyl center structure. *J. Biol. Chem.*, **267**, 15816–15822.

66 Krogsrud, R.L., Welchner, E., Scouten, E., and Liuzzi, M. (1993) A solid-phase assay for the binding of peptidic subunit association inhibitors to the herpes simplex virus ribonucleotide reductase large subunit. *Anal. Biochem.*, **213**, 386–394.

67 Chang, L.L., Hannah, J., Ashton, W.T., Rasmusson, G.H., Ikeler, T.J., Patel, G.F., Garsky, V., Uncapher, C., Yamanaka, G., McClements, W.L., and Tolman, R.L. (1992) Substituted penta- and hexapeptides as potent inhibitors of herpes simplex virus type 2 ribonucleotide reductase. *Bioorg. Med. Chem. Lett.*, **2**, 1207–1212.

68 Gaudreau, P., Brazeau, P., Richer, M., Cormier, J., Langlois, D., and Langelier, Y. (1992) Structure–function studies of peptides inhibiting the ribonucleotide reductase activity of herpes simplex virus type I. *J. Med. Chem.*, **35**, 346–350.

69 Liuzzi, M. and Déziel, R. (1993) *The Search for Antiviral Drugs* (eds J. Adams and V.J. Merluzzi), Birkhauser, Boston, pp. 225–238.

70 Moss, N., Déziel, R., Adams, J., Aubry, N., Bailey, M., Baillet, M., Beaulieu, P., DiMaio, J., Duceppe, J.-S., Ferland, J.-M., Gauthier, J., Ghiro, E., Goulet, S., Grenier, L., Lavallée, P., Lépine-Frenette, C., Plante, R., Rakhit, S., Soucy, F., Wernic, D., and Guindon, Y. (1993) Inhibition of herpes simplex virus type 1 ribonucleotide reductase by substituted tetrapeptide derivatives. *J. Med. Chem.*, **36**, 3005–3009.

71 LaPlante, S.R., Aubry, N., Liuzzi, M., Thelander, L., Ingemarson, R., and Moss, N. (1994) The critical C-terminus of the small subunit of herpes simplex virus ribonucleotide reductase is mobile and conformationally similar to C-terminal peptides. *Int. J. Peptide Protein Res.*, **44**, 549–555.

72 Nordlund, P., Sjoberg, B.-M., and Eklund, H. (1990) Three-dimensional structure of the free radical protein of ribonucleotide reductase. *Nature (London)*, **345**, 593–598.

73 Stubbe, J. (1990) Ribonucleotide reductases: amazing and confusing. *J. Biol. Chem.*, **265**, 5329–5332.

74 Moss, N., Déziel, R., Ferland, J.-M., Goulet, S., Jones, P.-J., Leonard, S.F., Pitner, P., and Plante, R. (1994) Herpes Simplex virus ribonucleotide reductase subunit association inhibitors: the effect and conformation of -alkylated aspartic acid derivatives. *Bioorg. Med. Chem.*, **2**, 959–970.

75 Brandt, C.R., Spencer, B., Imesch, P., Garneau, M., and Déziel, R. (1996) Evaluation of a peptidomimetic ribonucleotide reductase inhibitor with a murine model of herpes simplex virus type 1 ocular disease. *Antimicrob. Agents Chemother.*, **40**, 1078–1084.

76 Llinàs-Brunet, M., Moss, N., Scouten, E., Liuzzi, M., and Déziel, R. (1996) Peptidomimetic inhibitors of herpes virus ribonucleotide reductase, correlation between herpes simplex and varicella zoster virus. *Bioorg. Med. Chem. Lett.*, **6**, 2881–2886.

77 Rosenberg, S.H. (1995) Renin inhibitors, in *Progress in Medicinal Chemistry* (eds G.P. Ellis and D.K. Luscombe), Elsevier, New York, pp. 37–114.

78 Jung, G.L., Anderson, P.C., Bailey, M., Baillet, M., Bantle, G.W., Berthiaume, S., Lavallée, P., Llinàs-Brunet, M., Thavonekham, B., Thibeault, D., and Simoneau, B. (1998) Novel small renin inhibitors containing 4,5- or 3,5-Dihydroxy-2-substituted-6-phenylhexanamide replacements at the P2–P3 sites. *Bioorg. Med. Chem.*, **6**, 2317–2336.

79 Hutchins, C. and Greer, J. (1991) Comparative modeling of proteins in the design of novel renin inhibitors. *Crit. Rev. Biochem. Mol. Biol.*, **26**, 77–127.

80 LaPlante, S.R., Tong, L., Aubry, N., Pav, S., Jung, G., and Anderson, P.C. (1996) Several polyhydroxymonamide renin inhibitors assume similar conformations in the unbound and renin-bound states. *Int. J. Peptide Protein Res.*, **48**, 401–410.

81 LaPlante, S.R., Tong, L., Aubry, N., Pav., S., Jung, G., and Anderson, P.C. (1995) *Proceedings of the Fourteenth American Peptide Symposium. Peptides: Chemistry, Structure and Biology*, (eds P. T.P. Kaumaya and S.R. Hodges) Mayflower Scientific Ltd., Kingswinford, UK.

82 Tong, L., Pav, S., Lamarre, D., Pilote, L., LaPlante, S., Anderson, P., and Jung, G. (1995) High resolution crystal structures of recombinant human renin in complex with polyhydroxymonoamide inhibitors. *J. Mol. Biol.*, **250**, 211–222.

83 Simoneau, B., Lavallée, P., Anderson, P. C., Bailey, M., Bantle, G., Berthiaume, S., Chabot, C., Fazal, G., Halmos, T., Ogilvie, W.W., Poupart, M.-A., Thavonekham, B., Xin, Z., Thibeault, D., Bolger, G., Panzenbeck, M., Winquist, R., and Jung, G.L. (1999), Discovery of non-peptidic P2–P3 butanediamide renin inhibitors with high oral efficacy. *Bioorg. Med. Chem.*, **7**, 489–508.

84 Luly, J.R., BaMaung, N., Soderquisat, J., Fung, A.K.L., Stein, H., Kleinert, H.D., Marcotte, P.A., Egan, D.A., Bopp, B., Merits, I., Bolis, G., Greer, J., Perun, T.J., and Plattner, J.J. (1988) Renin inhibitors. Dipeptide analogs of angiotensinogen utilizing a dihydroxyethylene transition-state mimic at the scissile bond to impart greater inhibitory potency. *J. Med. Chem.*, **31**, 2264–2276.

85 Beaulieu, P.L., Gillard, J., Bailey, M., Beaulieu, C., Duceppe, J.-S., Lavallée, P., and Wernic, D. (1999) Practical synthesis of BILA 2157 BS, a potent and orally active renin inhibitor: use of an enzyme-catalyzed hydrolysis for the preparation of homochiral succinic acid derivatives. *J. Org. Chem.*, **64**, 6622–6634.

86 Kohl, N.E., Emini, E.A., Schleif, W.A., Davis, L.J., Heimbach, J.C., Dixon, R.A. F., Scolnick, E.M., and Sigal, I.S. (1988) Active human immunodeficiency virus protease is required for viral infectivity. *Proc. Natl. Acad. Sci. U.S.A.*, **85**, 4686–4690.

87 Gottlinger, H.G., Sodroski, J.G., and Haseltine, W.A. (1989) Role of capsid precursor processing and myristoylation in morphogenesis and infectivity of human immunodeficiency virus type 1. *Proc. Natl. Acad. Sci. U.S.A.*, **86**, 5781–5785.

88 Peng, C., Ho, B.K., Chang, T.W., and Chang, N.T. (1989) Role of human immunodeficiency virus type 1-specific protease in core protein maturation and viral infectivity. *J. Virol.*, **63**, 2550–2556.

89 McQuade, T.J., Tomasselli, A.G., Liu, L., Karacostas, V., Moss, B., Sawyer, T.K., Heinrikson, R.L., and Tarpley, W.G. (1990) A synthetic HIV-1 protease inhibitor with antiviral activity arrests HIV-like particle maturation. *Science*, **247**, 454–456.

90 Ratner, L., Haseltine, W., Patarca, R., Livak, K.J., Starcich, B., Josephs, S.F., Doran, E.R., Rafalski, J.A., Whitehorn, E.A., Baumeister, K., Ivanoff, L., Petteway, S.R. Jr, Pearson, M.L., Lautenberger, J.A., Papas, T.S., Ghrayeb, J., Chang, N.T., Gallo, R.C., and Wong-Staal, F. (1985) Complete nucleotide sequence of the AIDS virus, HTLV-III. *Nature*, **313**, 277–2.

91 Hellen, C.U.T., Kraeusslich, H.V.G., and Wimmer, E. (1989) Proteolytic processing of polyproteins in the replication of RNA viruses. *Biochemistry*, **28**, 9881–9890.

92 Henderson, L.E., Copeland, T.D., Sowder, R.C., Schultz, A.M., and Oroszlan, S. (1988) Analysis of proteins and peptides purified from sucrose gradient banded HTLV-III. UCLA Symposia on Molecular and Cellular Biology, New Series. *Human Retroviruses, Cancer and AIDS: Approaches to Prevention and Therapy*, Liss, New York, pp. 135–147.

93 Copeland, T.D., Wondrak, E.M., Tozser, J., Roberts, M.M., and Oroszlan, S. (1990) Substitution of proline with pipecolic acid at the scissile bond converts a peptide substrate of HIV proteinase into a selective inhibitor. *Biochem. Biophys. Res. Commun.*, **169**, 310–314.

94 Roberts, N.A., Martin, J.A., Kinchington, D., Broadhurst, A.V., Craig, J.C., Duncan, I.B., Galpin, S.A., Handa, B.K., Kay, J., Krohn, A., Lambert, R.W., Merrett, J.H., Mills, J.S., Parkes, K.E.B., Redshaw, S., Ritchie, A.J., Taylor, D.L., Thomas, G.J., and Machin, P.J. (1990) Rational design of peptide-based HIV proteinase inhibitors. *Science*, **248**, 358–361.

95 Tsantrizos, Y.S. (2008) Peptidomimetic therapeutic agents targeting the protease enzyme of the human immunodeficiency virus and hepatitis C virus. *Acc. Chem. Res.*, **41**, 1252–1263.

96 Beaulieu, P.L., Wernic, D., Abraham, A., Anderson, P.C., Bogri, T., Bousquet, Y., Croteau, G., Guse, I., Lamarre, D., Liard, F., Paris, W., Thibeault, D., Pav, S., and Tong, L. (1997) Potent HIV protease inhibitors containing a novel (Hydroxyethyl) amide isostere. *J. Med. Chem.*, **40**, 2164–2176.

97 Beaulieu, P.L., Lavallée, P., Abraham, A., Anderson, P.C., Boucher, C., Bousquet, Y., Duceppe, J.-S., Gillard, J., Gorys, V., Grand- Maître, C., Grenier, L., Guindon, Y., Guse, I., Plamondon, L., Soucy, F., Valois, S., Wernic, D., and Yoakim, C. (1997) Practical, stereoselective synthesis of palinavir, a potent HIV protease inhibitor. *J. Org. Chem.*, **62**, 3440–3448.

98 Lamarre, D., Croteau, G., Wardrop, E., Bourgon, L., Thibeault, D., Clouette, C., Vaillancourt, M., Cohen, E., Pargellis, C., Yoakim, C., and Anderson, P.C. (1997) Antiviral properties of palinavir, a potent inhibitor of the human immunodeficiency Virus Type 1 protease. *Antimicrob. Agents Chemother.*, **41**, 965–971.

99 Baxter, J.D., Schapiro, J.M., Boucher, C.A.B., Kohlbrenner, V.M., Hall, D.B., Scherer, J.R. and Mayers, D.L. (2006) Genotypic changes in human immunodeficiency Virus Type 1 protease associated with reduced susceptibility and virologic response to the protease inhibitor tipranavir. *J. Virol.*, **80**, 10794–10801.

100 Larder, B.A., Hertogs, K., Bloor, S., van den Eynde, C., DeCianc, W., Wang, Y., Freimuth, W.W., and Tarpley, G. (2000) Tipranavir inhibits broadly protease inhibitor-resistant HIV-1 clinical samples. *AIDS*, **14**, 1943–1948.

101 Muzammil, S., Armstrong, A.A., Kang, L.W., Jakalian, A., Bonneau, P.R., Schmelmer, V., Amzel, L.M., and Freire, E. (2007) Unique thermodynamic response of tipranavir to human immunodeficiency Virus Type 1 protease drug resistance mutations. *J. Virol.*, **81**, 5144–5154.

2
Marketing Antimicrobial Peptides: A Critical Academic Point of View

Eduard Bardají

2.1
Introduction

When the editors asked me to contribute a chapter describing my personal experience related to technology transfer activities derived from results generated and accumulated during nearly 10 years of research in the field of antimicrobial peptides at the University of Girona, I agreed, mainly encouraged by the enthusiasm to communicate and share my knowledge and opinions on how to find the most effective way to translate the results of academic research into products or services on the market. I tried to share all the perspectives and problems generated, keeping in mind that at this time many changes are happening, and, more importantly, a large list of latent opportunities are still waiting for a positive or negative resolution. This contribution is essentially a report about the steps taken over the years, from a traditional position working on public funded academic research, and the factors that influenced the steps taken for the adoption of a 'technology push' orientation and to seek adequate strategies to place new antimicrobial peptides in the market.

The decision to direct our research projects to the field of antimicrobial peptides was based on the opportunity to find adequate funding in the agrochemical research field. It was a strategic decision that, with time, turned out to be relevant and positive, because it led to the decision to set up an internal cluster at the University of Girona on this topic. The association of the researchers of the peptide-organic chemistry group (LIPPSO) and the plant pathology group (CIDSAV) started with the aim to set a solid collaboration and to focus our research on antimicrobial peptide discovery. After nearly 10 years, this collaboration has evolved to a full strategic alliance culminating with the setting up of a shared platform for antimicrobial technology discovery at the Scientific Park of the University of Girona, and the creation of AMPbiotech, a new spin-off company [1]. All this had several beneficial effects: sustained access to grants to fund basic and applied research, and also for the acquisition of specific instrumentation; a

Peptide Drug Discovery and Development: Translational Research in Academia and Industry, First Edition.
Edited by Miguel Castanho and Nuno C. Santos.
© 2011 WILEY-VCH Verlag GmbH & Co. KGaA, Weinheim.
Published 2011 by WILEY-VCH Verlag GmbH & Co. KGaA

continued improvement of our processes and growth in knowledge and capabilities. From an initial collaboration based on the synthesis and *in vitro* testing of peptides, we have grown to a multidisciplinary level where these activities are complemented with early toxicity and biodegradability assays, full proof of concept for plant protection products, including expertise about the use of bioproduction for the future synthesis of new antimicrobial peptides.

2.2
Basic Research: Antimicrobial Peptides

Antimicrobial peptides (AMPs) have a wide range of potential market applications and are emerging as a promising solution to overcome problems generated by extensive use of antibiotics and pesticides and to avoid the associated microorganism resistances. AMPs may show broad spectrum antimicrobial activity, mainly against bacteria and fungi, and differ from actual antibiotics or fungicides in their mechanism of action, derived from their cationic and amphipathic structure, responsible for their electrostatic interaction with cytoplasmic membranes of target microorganisms, and resulting in a cell-killing mode of action that makes the selection of resistance in target pathogens very difficult [2–7]. Our research, oriented to the development of new antimicrobial peptides, led us, in a first stage, to the study of two families of products.

The first family of compounds was based on the improvement of existing antimicrobial undecapeptides [8, 9] and ended with the discovery of a new and patentable collection of peptides optimized through a combinatorial approach and called CECMEL11 library [10]. The antimicrobial evaluation of this library has led to the identification of peptides with high activity against Gram-negative bacteria, Gram-positive bacteria, and fungi [11, 12]. One of the most striking results was the finding that the bactericidal peptide KKLFKKILKYL-NH$_2$ (BP100) was effective *in vivo* to prevent infections by *Erwinia amylovora*, the microorganism responsible for the Blight fire of several trees and ornamental plants of economic importance. Apart from BP100, other lead compounds have been identified for Gram-positive bacteria (BP018) or fungi (BP021), and also compounds with antibacterial and antifungal activities, like BP015 (Figure 2.1). All these compounds show very low toxicity and also have suitable biodegradability profiles, making them good candidates for the development of new antimicrobial products for the market. Additionally, due to the fact that all aminoacids are of natural L-configuration, the possibility to produce such compounds using bioproduction approaches makes them even more attractive for the development of new products.

The second family of products is a still underexploited collection of Leu-Lys containing cyclopeptides that were also good antimicrobials [13, 14]. Trying to find good products active against Gram-negative bacteria, we synthesized a collection of linear Leu-Lys-containing peptides of several sizes and we found that they showed poor or no antimicrobial activity. This situation was overcome by making their cyclic counterparts, and ended with a good collection of active compounds based

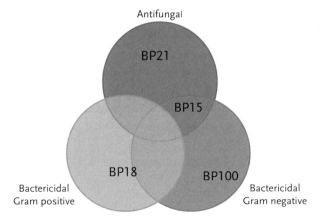

Figure 2.1 Different selectivity profiles of antibacterial and antifungal activities of selected peptides from CECMEL11 antimicrobial peptide library.

X_1-X_2-KLFKKILK-X_3-L-NH2

X_1 = H,Ac,Ts,Bz,Bn,Pam
X_2 = W, F, Y, L, K
X_3 = W, F, Y, V, K

Figure 2.2 General formula for CECMEL11 library.

on a chemical library of cyclic decapeptides [15]. Cyclization not only improved antimicrobial activity, it improved stability against protease degradation and did not affect their hemolytic activity. Cyclic peptides appear then as an important option to improve the properties of linear peptides, and, in our hands, several projects have proved this hypothesis; recently we have reported a family of cyclic peptides with promising anticancer activities and potential applications [16, 17].

One of the main advantages of AMPs for the development of new bactericidal and fungicidal products is the possibility to easily modulate their activity, toxicity, and degradability within an optimized family of compounds. In our case, the series of linear undecapeptides called the CECMEL11 library [5, 9] is based on a sequence where only two amino acid positions and N-terminal substitution change for each compound (Figure 2.2); subtle changes in these positions produce clear and somehow unexpected results on antibacterial and hemolytic activities. The analysis of a set of 25 results obtained during the study of the activity of the CECMEL11 library against the three plant pathogenic Gram-negative bacteria, *Erwinia amylovora* (fire blight), *Xanthomonas vesicatoria* (bacterial spot of tomato and pepper) and *Pseudomonas syringae* (several blight diseases), shows how antimicrobial and hemolytic activity changes are difficult to predict (Figure 2.3). For example, peptides having a K-Y pair of amino acids in position 1 and 10, respectively, include BP100, a good and safe product, but their

N-terminal modifications (benzoylation, BP103, or tosylation, BP102) are less active and more hemolytic. BP76, a K-F peptide, also shifts to a less active and more hemolytic version after acetylation (BP77) or tosylation (BP78). From these results N-terminal modification seems to be an inadequate option but, in contrast, two of the best products are benzoylated (BP126) or tosylated (BP125) at this position, both having two lysines in their sequence on positions 1 and 10. Products with a potential good safety profile, like BP15, BP76, BP100, BP125, and BP126 (indicated with black arrows, Figure 2.3) can be detected; also, we can detect products with bad safety profiles, like BP11, BP19, and BP103, or even being ten times more hemolytic than antibacterial, like BP08, BP10, or BP12. This is an example of how adequate AMPs can be selected from our libraries for the development of a product oriented to a specific application. This technology is patent protected and is the background necessary in our case to start a technology transfer activity with the aim being to find adequate strategies to place new antimicrobial peptides in the market.

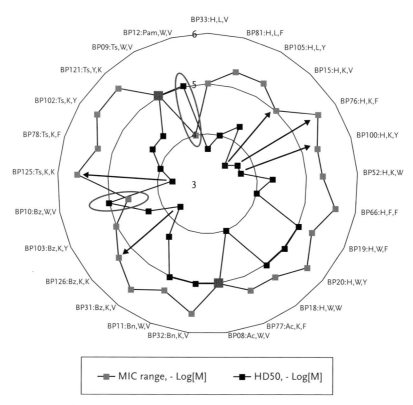

Figure 2.3 Changes on antimicrobial (MIC) and hemolytic activity (HD50) in a sample of 25 peptides from the CECMEL11 library showing different patterns of variation. Labels indicate the code sequence and the type of substitutions at N-terminal and positions 1 and 10.

2.3
Patents

Filing a patent is, from the academic point of view, always a complicated decision. Patents have to be filed without having disclosed any information about the invention, but many academic researchers tend not to want stop the presentation of papers, theses, or research reports in order to protect their academic progress or the career development of their collaborators. If the results obtained from a research program have potential application, and if the invention can be protected by filing a patent, for us this means some restrictions. The first restriction is not to publish anything before filing a patent, and also to delay all publications as long as possible after the date of priority of the filed patent. Because patents remain undisclosed for 6–12 months, it is highly recommended to delay any public communication for at least the first year. This is strictly not necessary, but is an extended strategy that helps to keep the technology secret for as long as possible. Therefore, in EU countries, where we need to delay scientific publication for at least few months, and sometimes for more than one year, we have a clear disadvantage compared to US academics who can make public their innovative technologies and file a patent later. To do so, it is necessary to be diligent and reduce using the invention (performing proof-of-concept tests or developing prototypes) that has been previously disclosed; thus, a previous communication may constitute an evidence of conception of such invention, and, consequently, the first inventor to have conceived an invention will be the inventor entitled to the patent, even if another inventor had filed an earlier patent application. This system, where a patent may be filed after disclosing the innovation and still be granted, offers special advantages for US scientists because the time available for marketing their technology is greater than in the rest of the world (Figure 2.4). Under this legal structure, it is easy to offer and transfer the technology, with the competitive advantage of being able to offer also the property of the patent to the company that adopts the technology, saving time, and costs, for all parties. It is important to remember that filing a first patent gives priority and protection for 12 months, and that, before the end of this period, it is necessary to decide to extend the patent to

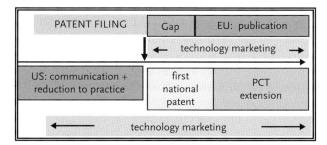

Figure 2.4 Difference in time available for marketing a technology between the United States and the rest of the world before reaching the end of PCT protection.

PCT level (that extends the period of protection for an additional period of 18 months) or to enter directly into national phases.

As a consequence of being non-US members, we have to handle an important drawback from our legal system. The morale and enthusiasm of the researchers involved in a first-to-file process, where filing a patent stops all communication for a period of time, never remain unaltered and, due to the need to publish as much and as soon as possible for evident reasons, the management of research projects and the interests of young researchers are often in conflict. This has a negative impact on their motivation and also helps to develop a latent and disturbing feeling of excessive sacrifice due to the need to keep everything secret and give priority to filing a patent. During our research activities we have been through the process of filing a patent and delaying the papers for at least 3 or 4 months several times, and it is worth saying that this effort is not always well rewarded.

Another important issue to take into account when planning to protect technology is to be aware of the costs of patents (exclusive rights for the commercialization of protected inventions in given countries) and terms from the first moment. Filling a first patent as a national patent may cost between 3000 and 6000€, including a patentability study to assess a high probability to be granted. A PCT patent can also be filed as a first option or as a second stage; its cost is around 10 000€. In Europe it is possible to file a European patent, that costs between 6000 and 9000€, and the only advantage of this procedure is that it is a single process for the approval of a patent for mainly all European countries; after a European patent concession it is necessary to file the extension to national patents in all the desired European countries, and that means that the protection of a technology in Europe is at least 10–20 times more expensive than in the United States and Canada combined. At the end of the PCT protection and/or European patent grant concession, national extensions have to be faced with a cost of between 2000 and 5000€ per country, including all single European countries. In summary, the costs of filing a patent and their extensions may range from 10 000€ (one or two selected countries) up to more than 100 000–200 000€, depending on the number of national extensions and the number of language translations required. It should not be forgotten that from the date of priority it is necessary to pay an annual rate in each country. These fees start at around 200–400€ per year and country, and are incremented every successive year according to the national regulations of each country up to the limit of 20 years. Patent annuities after 5 years may cost around 500–1000€/country and 1200–1600€/country at year 10. Exact values depend on national regulations and the extension of patent claims. Once each one of the national extensions has been filed, a specific and sometimes cumbersome process starts. Each national patent office will proceed to examine the patent, and this may include two or three steps of request and response in order to go forward with the concession of the patent grant or not. All those steps have specific and additional costs that can add an extra charge of 1500–5000€ per country spread over several years (often 3–5 years).

For Universities to take patents far beyond the PCT level is a stage impossible to assume, except for special opportunities or well-funded institutions with a strong

Table 2.1 Costs for patenting a series of linear antimicrobial peptides.

Stage/Year	2006	2007	2008	2009	2010	2011	2012
National patent (Spain)							
Patentability study	4000						
Preparation	3000						
Filing	800						
PCT filing		2500					
Translations (indicated as*)			3200	Annuities and examen costs			
EEUU filing (*)				4000	2000	1000	1000
Canada filing				2200	500	2000	600
Indian filing				2800	850	900	900
Brazil filing (*)				1000	550	750	900
Mexico filing				2300	650	750	900
China filing (*)				2775	800	1000	1000
European filing				7950	750	850	950
Australia filing				2780	1500	1000	1000
	7800	2500	3200	25805	7600	8250	7250

technology transfer organization. Since national patents may be filed at reduced fees for Universities, it is easy to decide to start filing a national patent as a first stage. In our case, involving the antimicrobial peptide technologies generated from basic research, we have filed up to four national patents on antimicrobial peptides. Two of these patents were extended to PCT and only one was selected to be extended to other countries. Table 2.1 summarizes all the steps taken and all the costs incurred during all those years for patenting the series of linear antimicrobial peptides. Altogether, it is evident that still most academic and public research institutions are partially unaware of the whole process that starts after filing a patent and fixing a priority date; thus, more structured and focused technology transfer departments are needed, with specific funds for patents and proof of concept assays, in order to better select and promote their own technologies.

2.4
Potential Applications of AMPs

Antimicrobial peptides (AMPs) have several potential market applications. Human infections produced by Gram-negative or Gram-positive bacteria require new compounds with efficacy similar to actual antibiotics and with better selectivity profiles, in order to develop therapies with less risk of inducing microbial cross resistances [18]. In particular, compounds for treating human infections produced by ESKAPE microorganisms are an important growing need. ESKAPE is the acronym for *Enterococcus faecium* (E), *Staphylococcus aureus* multiresistant (S),

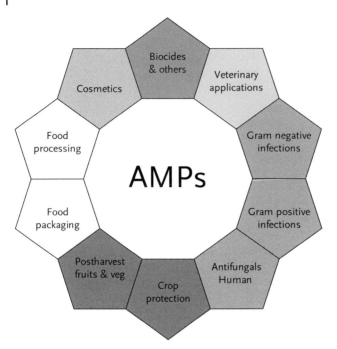

Figure 2.5 Potential market applications for AMPs.

Klebsiella pneumoniae and *Escherichia coli* (K), *Acinetobacter baumannii* (A), *Pseudomonas aeuroginosa* (P), and *Enterobacter* species (E), all related to emerging resistances and increasing mortalities due to the lack of effective compounds to treat such severe infections [19].

In parallel to the pharmaceutical sector, the veterinary or agrochemical sectors also require new products to protect animal health or crops with reduced risk for the environment and consumers; even more so in Europe where a large number of pesticides are being banned in the agrochemical sector. Other sectors of potential application for new AMPs include biocides, food preservatives and food packaging, biomaterials, and materials sciences (Figure 2.5). Any of these potential applications of AMPs has several market opportunities with a range of development costs per project that start at 1 M€ and rise to 30–40 M€ for specific pharmaceutical indications; new product development is becoming more and more expensive due to increasing regulatory requirements based on human, animal, and environmental protection.

2.5
Technology Transfer: Valorization, Licensing, or Spin-Off Creation

Technology transfer has become a central aspect of European public-funded research in the last decade due to the growing concern about the need to generate new products and services based on innovations and leading technologies that can help to transform industrial-based economies into more knowledge-based economies. Therefore, there is an increasing need to detect potential market applications and find adequate strategies to transform scientific findings from research laboratories with potential application into useful products, processes and services in the commercial sector. All this runs in parallel to permanent comparison with the strong and experienced technology transfer system in the United States, and the actual pressure from Asian countries where the number of patents is growing at an exceptional rate. Information extracted from the latest world intellectual property indicators reflects the leading position of the United States, based on the origin of patent filings, followed by Japan, China, and Korea, with some relevant distances between these countries, and with European countries far behind [20]. Interestingly, the US patent filing profile shows 52% of patents filed in house rather than abroad, and with a number of extensions, close to 50%, to their most relevant markets (Mexico, Canada, Hong Kong, and Singapore); the rest of the strong (United Kingdom, Japan, Germany, France, Russia, etc.) and emerging economies (China, Korea) show 75–80% of patent filings originating from their own country and with a low rate (10–15% for Japan or Germany) or very low rate (1–5% for China or Korea) of extensions to foreign countries, when compared to the United States.

When a basic research program delivers results with potential application and innovative enough to be protected, several strategies can be faced: patenting and licensing-out, valorization and commercialization, or spin-off creation. In all cases it is necessary to have a consistent proof-of-concept, demonstration or prototype, to convince potential investors to fund further development or to attract the attention of stakeholders.

Patenting and licensing is becoming a significant market activity, mainly oriented toward earning revenues or sharing technologies between companies; although licensing markets are less developed than they could be, licensing out is a growing activity and many indicators show the relevance of such commercial activity at present. The use of patents for raising funds from venture capital and private equities is recognized as very important by many European firms, and the emergence of patent-related services (technology brokers, internet platforms, patent funds, auction houses, IP consulting companies) offering a variety of commercialization tools (partnering, patent portfolio management, and valorization) is a clear indication of the importance of such activities [21].

Patenting the results of research and licensing out the technology developed from a university is complicated due to all the reasons stated before, especially because the time available for marketing a technology before having to decide on national patent extensions is always too short. Valorization and commercialization are essentially activities that may help to find opportunities and, as in some successful examples, end up with a good license agreement for the university. However, the real experience tells us that this system is mainly growing because an increasing number of technology transfer agents and consultants find a way to develop their business based mostly on database analysis and contact management, activities mainly funded by government departments. Entering this world may represent for academics and scientists a real nightmare and may often be perceived as a major deviation from the essential dedication to science, also adding expenses to the technology transfer process without a clear return for them or their institution. This paradigm has to be inverted and the potential market opportunities for university innovations have to be outlined before applying for public grants in order to get funds for basic and applied research. Universities and public research institutions are essentially innovators, and innovators require the existence of adaptors in order to be able to place technological developments into the market. Regulatory issues play a central role, depending on the sector of application, and due to the level of costs associated with product development, marketing authorization is often very expensive and in most cases represents a real barrier for the new products being developed.

It is necessary then to change the paradigm of funding public research and to clearly differentiate between research grants oriented toward promoting the advancement of science in a wide sense and applied research oriented toward placing innovations in the market. The first has to be managed by public and privately funded academic and science institutions, exploiting networking activities as much as possible in order to promote the advancement of knowledge and science, and will not be considered further now. The second covers essentially all research activities focused on placing new technologies in the market. Applied research programs have to adopt a real open innovation strategy and the contribution of all agents has to be planned from the moment of program design. It is necessary to foster innovation, but without reducing the relevance of brokering research results and increasing the collaboration from the first moment between all agents required to reach the commercialization step. To do this, university spin-off companies are, in my opinion, the real solution, but considered under a revised perspective.

2.6
Spin-Off Creation: An Academic Point of View

The most relevant barrier for an academic becoming an entrepreneur is the considerable difference between a traditional university culture and an entrepreneurial culture based on different decision-making processes. Academics tend to place more emphasis on researching new ideas and, at the same time, believe that their technological ideas have commercial potential on a global scale, and, hence, that somebody else should buy or take those innovations further, mainly because their effort, dedication, and brilliant results are worth it. However, market opinions differ from these thoughts; often industry players have the perception that academic results have not been fully researched for commercial viability. This divergence of opinions is essentially based on the fact that university research has been performed, in most cases, before envisaging the commercialization steps in detail, and a clear market orientation of their potentially marketable results has not been planned. Public researchers and their institutions have to develop a more market-oriented system for planning and developing basic research programs in order to increase their influence in the development of new technologies and improve social impact visibility.

Spin-off companies are considered a specific tool for the promotion to market of the university research results, with the aim to provide part of the benefits back to universities as royalties. Licensing patents or technologies generated from university research programs is their major objective. At an early stage, spin-off companies are normally set up and organized by researchers, with the help of incubator and entrepreneurship programs, and focused to sell their "protected" technology; in a second stage, the need to invest further in their developments to obtain products or services for the market forces the incorporation of capital and management partners that, in most cases, ends with a company configured far away from the initial expectations created when it was born around the academic environment. In such a situation it is normal that researchers involved in the project exit the company and return to essential academic activities, or simply evolve to a consultant position while holding some marginal shares in the company. At this level, the spin-off company has usually suffered an evolution that in most cases need not have happened. It is clear that when a technology is protected and well studied there still remains a large number of proofs or assays to be done; that is why so few university inventions end up with a real marketed application. Instead of planning spin-off creation as a need to make profit from the exploitation of the results from academic research, spin-off companies should be created to provide the market with specific, high level, and competitive know-how for the development of real solutions for the market, introducing an added value at the institution. The process involved in the spin-off creation is generally placed in the middle of a sequence of events that starts with the research program execution and ends with the decision to sell the technology or the associated products (Figure 2.6). A level of improvement can be introduced in such a scheme. The greatest value is the human capital behind results and patents, researchers and their know-how accumulated during years, integrated in facilities that have been improved due to the productivity and sustained funding, and that normally are excluded from spin-off conception and kept in a secondary role, that used to evolve to a non-continued collaboration due to the lack of integration of basic research and participation in the spin-off project.

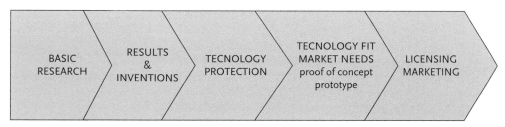

Figure 2.6 Traditional sequence for the development of university technologies and spin-off creation for their commercialization.

From an academic point of view, spin-off companies have to be created with the aim to maintain an effective link with all know-how and expertise accumulated at the university and to establish a clear scheme of collaboration between the new company and the already existing research facilities (persons and technologies) at the university. Additionally, the university will have the benefits of promoting a spin-off venture without weakening their academic and research structure. Not skipping this step will help the new company to start with the lowest rate of investment possible, and this will allow managing the relationships with customers and business partners at a reasonable cost for each stage of development. Applying this vision, we must think of spin-off companies as real and sustainable development departments at universities –autonomous companies that profit from their privileged connexion with the university and that are free to negotiate and set agreements with the optimal marketing partners, and also are a source of reward to the institution of origin. Developing the right product or service for a market application is a matter of meeting at the right time and place several factors and players, and it is difficult to find a place to sell specific technologies with a small margin of adaptation. It is better to apply all efforts to developing the right applications for specific market needs. This means establishing a platform of integration of existing know-how and accumulated expertise with the other players: governments and regulatory agencies, SMEs (small and medium-sized enterprises) and large companies, other specialized high-tech companies, and end users. In this situation, using all human capital and facilities existing at universities, and adapting as much as possible the strategy of the new spin-off company to find key alliances with companies operating in specific sectors, should result in several competitive advantages: the university provides strong scientific background and high level infrastructures, that, combined with the oriented contribution provided by co-developers and strategic partners, will be essential for the development of specific solutions at the lowest reasonable cost (Figure 2.7). This fast development strategy based on synergisms and lower risk assumption for all parties has to be rewarded in terms of royalties and sustained partnerships. This will help to set and manage spin-offs companies in a sustainable way, adopting just the amount of risk needed and contributing to science and social advancement.

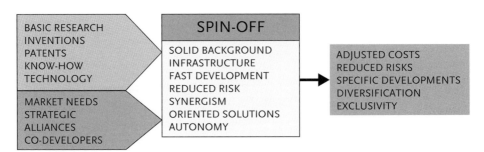

Figure 2.7 Spin-off strategy relying on university and market stakeholders based strategic alliances for the development of adapted solutions for the market.

References

1 LIPPSO: http://web2.udg.edu/lippso; **CIDSAV**: http://www.udg.edu/cidsav; AMPbiotech: http://www.ampbiotech .com

2 Ajesh, K. and Sreejith, K. (2009) Peptide antibiotics: an alternative and effective antimicrobial strategy to circumvent fungal infections. *Peptides*, **30**, 999–1006.

3 Brogden, K.A. (2005) Antimicrobial peptides: pore formers or metabolic inhibitors in bacteria?. *Nat. Rev. Microbiol.*, **3**, 238–250.

4 Bulet, P., Stöcklin, R., and Menin, L. (2004) Antimicrobial peptides: from invertebrates to vertebrates. *Immunol. Rev.*, **198**, 169–184.

5 Jenssen, H., Hamill, P., and Hancock, R.E.W. (2006) Peptide antimicrobial agents. *Clin. Microbiol. Rev.*, **19**, 491–511.

6 Yeaman, M.R. and Yount, N.Y. (2003) Mechanisms of antimicrobial peptide action and resistance. *Pharmacol. Rev.*, **55**, 27–55.

7 Zasloff, M. (2002) Antimicrobial peptides of multicellular organisms. *Nature*, **415**, 389–395.

8 Cavallarin, L., Andreu, D., and San Segundo, B. (1998) Cecropin A-derived peptides are potent inhibitors of fungal plant pathogens. *Mol. Plant-Microbe Interact.*, **11**, 218–227.

9 Ferre, R., Badosa, E., Feliu, L., Planas, M., Montesinos, E., and Bardaji, E. (2006) Inhibition of plant-pathogenic bacteria by short synthetic cecropin A-melittin hybrid peptides. *Appl. Environ. Microbiol.*, **72**, 3302–3308.

10 Bardají, E., Montesinos, E., Badosa, E., Feliu, L., Planas, M., and Ferre, R. (2007) Antimicrobial linear peptides. WO 2007/125142.

11 Badosa, E., Ferre, R., Planas, M., Feliu, L., Besalú, E., Cabrefiga, J., Bardají, E., and Montesinos, E. (2007) A library of linear undecapeptides with bactericidal activity against phytopathogenic bacteria. *Peptides*, **28**, 2276–2285.

12 Badosa, E., Ferre, R., Francés, J., Bardají, E., Feliu, L., Planas, M., and Montesinos, E. (2009) Sporicidal activity of synthetic antifungal undecapeptides and control of penicillium rot of apples. *Appl. Environ. Microbiol.*, **75**, 5563–5569.

13 Monroc, S., Badosa, E., Besalú, E., Planas, M., Bardají, E., Montesinos, E., and Feliu, L. (2006) Improvement of cyclic decapeptides against plant pathogenic bacteria using a combinatorial chemistry approach. *Peptides*, **27**, 2575–2584.

14 Bardají, E., Montesinos, E., Badosa, E., Feliu, L., Planas, M., and Monroc, M. (2007) Antimicrobial cyclic peptides. WO 2007/074185.

15 Monroc, S. (2008) Synthesis and evaluation of cyclic cationic peptides as antimicrobial agents for use in plant protection. PhD Thesis. University of Girona.

16 Feliu, L., Oliveras, G., Cirac, A.D., Besalú, E., Rosés, C., Colomer, R., Bardají, E., Planas, M., and Puig, T. (2010) Antimicrobial cyclic decapeptides with anticancer activity. *Peptides*, **31**, 2017–2026.

17 Bardají, E., Feliu, L., Montesinos, E., Planas, M., and Puig, T. (2010) Péptidos cíclicos inhibidores de crecimiento celular. ES 2010/30239.

18 Livermore, D.M. (2006) The need for new antibiotics. *Clin Microbiol Infect*, **10** (Supp. 4), 1–9.

19 Obritsch, M.D., Fish, D.N., Maclaren, R., and Jung, R. (2005) Nosocomial infections due to multidrug-resistant pseudomonas aeruginosa: epidemiology and treatment options. *Pharmacotherapy*, **25**, 1353–64.

20 WORLD INTELLECTUAL PROPERTY INDICATORS Publication No. 941 (2010) http://www.wipo.int/ freepublications/en/intproperty/941/ wipo_pub_941.pdf, accessed October 2010.

21 Pluvia Zuniga, M., and Guellec, D. (2009) Who licenses out patents and why?: lessons from a business survey, OECD Science, Technology and Industry Working Papers, 2009/5, OECD Publishing.

3
Oral Peptide Drug Delivery: Strategies to Overcome Challenges

Hamman, Josias H. and Steenekamp, Jan H.

3.1
Introduction

A variety of protein and peptide drugs have been established as important therapeutics for the treatment of different types of diseases, such as certain cancers and autoimmune diseases, hormone deficiencies, diabetes and hepatitis [1]. The oral route of drug administration is preferred due to certain advantages above many other routes of drug administration. A specific example where oral delivery of a peptide drug would be highly beneficial to the patient is that of insulin because it is naturally released from the pancreas into the portal vein, then it moves to the liver, followed by the peripheral circulation. The oral route delivers insulin directly to the liver, while other routes of administration cause peripheral hyperinsulinemia, which predisposes hypoglycemia that is linked to weight gain or metabolic abnormalities over the long term [2]. Unfortunately, poor oral bioavailability of protein and peptide drugs constitutes a major drawback for the development of orally administered medicinal products that are more acceptable to patients than injections. Furthermore, low bioavailability leads to high intersubject variability and poor control over plasma concentrations as well as pharmacological effects. By optimizing the pharmacokinetic profile of peptide drugs, their pharmacological efficacy will also be maximized [3, 4].

Designing a dosage form for effective oral peptide drug delivery requires several features such as stabilizing the drug to obtain a reasonable shelf-life, protecting the drug against acidity in the stomach and the enzymes in the gastrointestinal lumen, and facilitating membrane permeation [4]. Effective delivery of therapeutic polypeptides not only involves overcoming the low bioavailability of these drugs, caused by their instability and poor membrane permeation, but also needs to consider issues such as their short biological half-lives, immunogenicity, conformational stability (e.g., secondary, tertiary, or quaternary structures), site of absorption, dose requirements, aggregation, and precipitation [5, 6].

Peptide Drug Discovery and Development: Translational Research in Academia and Industry, First Edition.
Edited by Miguel Castanho and Nuno C. Santos.
© 2011 WILEY-VCH Verlag GmbH & Co. KGaA, Weinheim.
Published 2011 by WILEY-VCH Verlag GmbH & Co. KGaA

3.2
Challenges Associated with Oral Peptide Delivery

3.2.1
Transport Pathways Across the Intestinal Epithelium

There are two main routes by which a molecule can move across the intestinal epithelium, namely between adjacent cells (paracellular transport) and through cells (transcellular transport) [7] (see Figure 3.1). The mechanisms of transcellular transport include passive diffusion, carrier-mediated (active or facilitated) and endocytocis [7, 8]. The major pathway for absorption of a drug depends on its physicochemical characteristics as well as the membrane features. In general, lipophilic drug molecules cross the intestinal epithelium transcellularly, whereas hydrophilic drug molecules cross the epithelium paracellularly [9]. In terms of peptides, it is believed that the intestinal absorption of di- and tri-peptides is carrier mediated. Certain drugs such as cephalexin and other β-lactam antibiotics are also transported by carriers [10, 11]. Proteins like IgG and epidermal growth factor are believed to be absorbed by endocytosis [12]. All other proteins are assumed to be absorbed by passive diffusion, if at all [13].

The gastrointestinal tract is designed to impede the entry of pathogens, toxins, and undigested macromolecules, while simultaneously digesting and absorbing nutrients such as peptides, proteins, vitamins, and cofactors. For this purpose, the intestinal mucosa uses biochemical as well as physiological mechanisms to complement its physical barrier [7]. The oral bioavailability of many peptide drugs typically ranges between 1 and 2% [14]. The low bioavailability of these drugs can be attributed to various causes, such as poor membrane permeability of the intestinal membrane, susceptibility to the strong acidic environment of the stomach and proteolytic enzymes, as well as first-pass metabolism. Furthermore, the large

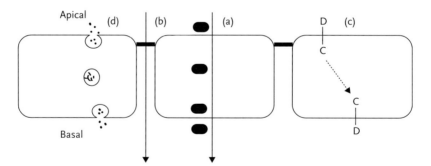

Figure 3.1 A schematic representation of transcellular and paracellular transport pathways across intestinal epithelial cells (a) passive transcellular diffusion; (b) paracellular transport, dependent on opening of the tight junctions; (c) carrier-mediated transcellular transport (active or facilitated; C, the carrier and D, the drug); and (d) transcellular endocytosis followed by exocytosis.

molecular size and hydrophilic nature of peptide and protein drugs aggravate the bioavailability problems [15, 16].

3.2.2
Unfavorable Physicochemical Properties of Peptide Drugs

3.2.2.1 Molecular Size, Hydrophilicity, and Physical Stability

The transcellular transport of drugs is the most common means for drug transport and depends on the physicochemical properties of the drugs [17]. Peptide drugs often have molecular weights in excess of 500 Da, exhibit low lipophilicity, have charged groups and tend to associate with water by hydrogen bonds. These features are generally associated with poor diffusion across the intestinal membrane [18]. Beside these properties, peptide drugs are prone to non-enzymatic as well as enzymatic degradation. Non-enzymatic degradation of peptides can be classified into two major types, namely chemical and physical changes. Physical changes include aggregation and precipitation. Aggregation can be caused by various factors such as general environmental factors that include exposure to light and temperature; solution factors that include pH, ionic strength and protein or peptide concentration; and processing factors which include freezing, thawing and shearing. Aggregation is a common mode of potein instability and can occur via various pathways [19]. Both precipitation and aggregation may lead to a loss in conformation and, as a consequence, poor absorption as well as loss of activity. Chemical changes include β-elimination, deamidation, disulfide exchange, and oxidation [16].

In addition to these unfavorable physicochemical properties of peptide drugs, intestinal absorption is also hampered by physical and biochemical barriers, as well as efflux systems.

3.2.3
Physical Barriers of the Gastrointestinal Tract

3.2.3.1 Transcellular Pathway

As mentioned before, the transcellular pathway is the mechanism through which most drugs are absorbed after oral administration. However, because of the physicochemical properties of peptide drugs, such as molecular size and low lipophilicity, the transcellular pathway is restricted for most peptide drugs. The major components of the physical barrier to the transcellular pathway will each be discussed separately in the following sections.

Unstirred Water Layer The epithelial cells of the intestine are covered by a stagnant aqueous layer consisting of water, glycoproteins, electrolytes, proteins, and nucleic acids. This aqueous layer is bound to the apical cell surface by the glycocalyx [20]. The glycocalyx is a 500 nm thick glycoprotein structure which is covalently linked to the brush border membrane and is part of the unstirred water layer. The unstirred water layer is the result of incomplete mixing of the luminal contents [21]. The unstirred water layer protects the underlying membrane from the corrosive elements in the luminal contents [22, 23].

The mucus layer hinders the diffusion of compounds and this effect is dependent on the size of the diffusing molecules [24]. It was demonstrated that the unstirred water layer is neglible compared to the intestinal cell membrane as the rate-limiting barrier to the intestinal uptake of highly permeable solutes like glucose and antipyrine [21]. However, the absorption of fluorescein isothiocyanate labeled dextran (FD-4), a poorly absorbed hydrophilic compound, was markedly improved when the drug was co-administered with certain penetration enhancers and N-acetylcysteine, a mucolytic agent. The results of this study supported the hypothesis that the unstirred water layer might be a significant barrier to the intestinal absorption of hydrophilic compounds like peptide and protein drugs. Furthermore, the results of different studies indicated that the mucus barrier might be an important barrier to the absorption of hydrophilic drugs [25, 26].

Apical Epithelial Cell Membrane The most important intestinal epithelial cells in terms of nutrient and drug absorption are the absorptive cells, also known as enterocytes. The apical surface of the absorptive cells is characterized by a striated border. This striated border consists of many closely packed microvilli approximately 0.5–1.5 µm in length and 0.1 µm in width, depending on the mamalian species [27]. The presence of villi and microvilli increases the surface area of the small intestine to 200 m^2 in humans. The glycocalyx, as described in the previous section, extends 0.1 µm from the tips of the microvilli [28]. The apical cell membrane is composed of a phospholipid double layer. The major lipid components are phosphatidylcholine, phosphatedylethanolamine, phosphatedylserine, phosphatedylinositol, phosphatidic acid, cholesterol, and glycolipids [20, 29].

Generally, the transport of molecules across the phospholipid bilayer has been correlated with their lipophilicity. Molecules need a certain degree of lipophilicity to cross the phospholipid bilayer and also have a low molecular size [30]. From this it is evident that the phospholipid bilayer of the apical membrane acts as an absorption barrier to hydrophilic molecules like peptides and proteins. Certain hydrophilic molecules like water, ions, and di- and tri-peptides cross the plasma membrane by other means, for example, pores or carrier-mediated transport. Overall, to take advantage of the transcellular transport pathway, drugs need to possess the necessary lipophilicity and size characteristics to support passive diffusion or they need to be recognized by the appropriate carrier if carrier-mediated transport is to be used [28].

Basal Epithelial Cell Membrane The basal membrane of absorptive cells is approximately 7 nm thick. The lipid composition of the basal membrane differs substantially from that of the apical microvillus membrane. This difference in composition is most probably the cause of the higher fluidity of the basal cell membrane compared to the apical membrane [27]. The higher fluidity might cause a less pronounced barrier function compared to the apical membrane [20].

3.2.3.2 Paracellular Pathway

When a molecule moves across the intestinal epithelium by passing through the intercellular space between adjacent cells, it is called paracellular transport [7]. Translocation through the paracellular pathway is primarily passive [14]. Hydrophilic molecules that are not recognized by a carrier cannot partition into the hydrophobic membrane and have to traverse the epithelial barrier via the paracellular pathway [31]. This transport of hydrophilic molecules via the paracellular pathway is, however, restricted by the presence of tight junctions (zonula occludens) [14]. The controlled and reversible opening of the tight junction represents an attractive approach to increasing the absorption of hydrophilic drugs, like peptide and protein drugs, especially in view of the fact that degradation by intracellular enzymes is avoided [9, 14, 31].

The fact that the paracellular route is devoid of proteolytic activity, it is an aqueous-filled channel and has an estimated surface area of about 200–2000 cm^2, should not be underestimated for peptide and protein delivery [32].

3.2.4
Biochemical Barriers of the Gastrointestinal Tract

Protein and peptide drugs are susceptible to the strong acidic environment of the stomach and the proteolytic enzymes of the gastrointestinal tract [15]. Digestion by the intestinal proteases starts in the stomach with pepsin and is continued throughout the gastrointestinal tract by various enzymes located in the intestinal lumen as well as at subcellular fractions of the enterocytes. Examples of peptides and the enzymes responsible for their degradation are listed in Table 3.1. The enzymes located in the enterocytes are mainly located in three subcellular fractions, namely the brush border membrane, the cytoplasm, and the lysosomes [33, 34].

As a consequence of the high susceptibility of peptide and protein drugs to the acid environment of the stomach and the proteolytic enzymes located at various sites within the gastrointestinal tract, the biochemical barrier is one of the most important barriers to protein and peptide drug absorption [36, 37]. To illustrate

Table 3.1 Examples of enzymes that cause degradation of protein and peptide drugs [35].

Peptide/protein	Enzyme
Leucin encephalin	Aminopeptidase
	Endopeptidase
Morphiceptin	Dipeptidylpeptidase
Renin inhibitor	Brush border aspartyl- or zinc protease
L-arginine vasopressin	Trypsin
	Carboxypeptidase
Insulin	Chymotrypsin, trypsin

the ubiquitiousness of the proteolytic barrier, it will be discussed in the following sections according to the location of the enzymes, namely luminal, brush border (membrane bound), and intracellular.

3.2.4.1 Luminal Enzymes

The luminal enzymes include those from the pancreatic secretions. This mixture of enzymes includes the endopeptidases trypsin, chymotrypsin, and elastase, as well as exopeptidases of which carboxypeptidase A and carboxypeptidase B are examples. The products of these enzymes include amino acids and peptides with two to six amino acid residues. The endopeptidases work in concert to hydrolyze internal peptide bonds, whereas the exopeptidases, like carboxypeptidase, preferentially hydrolyze peptide bonds at the carboxy-terminus [33, 38, 39].

3.2.4.2 Brush Border Membrane Bound Enzymes and Intracellular Enzymes

Degradation by luminal enzymes accounts for 5–20% of the total degradation in a given intestinal segment. The rest of the degradation and final degradation of peptides occur upon contact with the brush border or following entry into the cell [38]. Whether degradation occurs at the brush border or in the cytoplasm depends on the resistance of a given peptide to the peptidases at the brush border [40]. Among the exopeptidases of the brush border membrane are peptidases that hydrolyze peptides from the amino-terminal end. Important aminopeptidases of the brush border include aminopeptidase A, P, and W. Other important brush border enzymes include endopeptidases and carboxy-exopeptidases P and M [33].

Intracellular peptide degradation can also occur in the lysosomes following endocytosis. Proteolytic degradation in the lysosomes is mainly catalyzed by the catephsins and may involve endo- and exo-peptidase activity. Proteolytic activity at the brush border seems to be more important than the proteolytic activity in the lysosomes [33].

3.2.5
Efflux Transport Systems

The barrier function of the intestinal mucosa cannot be described by the physical or metabolic (enzymatic) barriers alone [14]. The intestinal epithelium possesses efflux pathways, which have a secretory function to actively move solutes out of tissues, thus limiting the absorption of drugs [41, 42]. These efflux systems are located at the apical membrane and include P-glycoprotein (P-gp), the focus of intense study, as well as other efflux transporter proteins [42, 43].

P-glycoprotein-like mechanisms have been implicated in the intestinal secretion of certain drugs, including peptides like cyclosporin and, as a consequence, may contribute significantly to the poor bioavailability of these drugs [42, 44]. The effect of these efflux transporters on the bioavailability of drugs might be augmented by intracellular enzymes, which not only modify compounds but can also produce metabolites that are themselves substrates for these transport proteins [43].

3.2.6
Gastrointestinal Transit Time and Site-Specific Absorption

Besides the enzymatic degradation of peptides that might be site-dependent, it should also be kept in mind that the absorption of peptides might be site-dependent. Both site-dependent degradation and site-specific degradation have been suggested for leuprolide [45]. It was found that the absorption of leuprolide is significantly higher from the ileum and colon than from the jejunum. It was concluded that targeting the lower intestine might be advantageous for oral leuprolide delivery. In another study [46] investigating the site-specific delivery with regard to insulin it was found that the optimal site for insulin absorption after oral administration to rats was the lower intestine.

3.3
Strategies to Overcome the Barriers of the Gastrointestinal Tract

The increasing demand for protein and peptide drugs, together with the advantages of the oral route of administration, stimulated research efforts to find ways of overcoming the many obstacles associated with their effective oral delivery [47]. It is important to mention that many peptide drugs are very potent hormones, which means that only relatively small amounts need to be absorbed to provide the desired pharmacological effect. This makes the oral route of administration a realistic option for effective delivery of peptide and protein drugs [48].

Several strategies have been suggested for the development of needle-free delivery systems for polypeptides and, although good progress has been made in this area, technologies to deliver these drugs have not kept pace with the advancements in methods to manufacture them on a large scale. The most commonly investigated strategies or approaches to improve the systemic availability of polypeptide drugs after oral administration include co-administration of absorption enhancers, chemical or physical modification of the peptide drug molecules, particulate carrier systems, the use of enzyme inhibitors, and mucoadhesion [47].

Since more than one factor is often responsible for the low bioavailability of peptide drugs, a combination of absorption-enhancing strategies may provide a more successful approach. For example, it was shown that overcoming the enzymatic barrier as a strategy to improve peptide stability resulted in only limited success, while including both a permeation enhancer and an enzyme inhibitor improved the bioavailability of insulin to a greater extent than either of the strategies alone [49–51].

3.3.1
Absorption Enhancing Agents

Absorption or permeation enhancers are defined as compounds that temporarily disrupt the physical barrier of the gastrointestinal tract to improve the permeation of drug molecules across the epithelium into the blood and/or lymph circulation. The action of the ideal absorption enhancer should be quick and should occur at the same time that the drug is present at the site of absorption, but should not cause any damage to the epithelial tissue. Furthermore, permeation enhancers that are not absorbed themselves and/or that are not pharmacologically active would avoid systemic toxicity [3, 4, 52].

Absorption enhancers can improve macromolecular drug permeation across the physical epithelial cellular barrier through one of two distinct mechanisms or through a combination of both these mechanisms. The first mechanism involves alteration of the structure of the epithelial cell membranes to enhance transcellular passive diffusion, while the other mechanism involves opening of the tight junctions to allow paracellular diffusion through the intercellular spaces [53].

The obvious disadvantage of absorption enhancers is their potential to cause toxicity, such as completely destroying the epithelial cell membranes and, thereby, causing inflammation and also, potentially, allowing entrance of unwanted xenobiotics or pathogens [47, 51, 54]. In this regard, the most promising permeability enhancers seem to function by means of a transient, reversible opening of the tight junctions to increase paracellular transport [55].

Compounds with chemically diverse structures have been identified as absorption enhancers that showed varied levels of increased macromolecular permeation. A summary of different categories of absorption enhancers and their proposed mechanisms of action is shown in Table 3.2.

Although transcellular absorption enhancement is often associated with damage to the intestinal epithelial cell layer, the rapid reversibility of this effect was shown in some cases, such as the permeation enhancing effects of the bile salt taurodeoxycholate and the non-ionic surfactant nonylphenoxypolyoxyethylene [3, 77]. The effects of tight junction modulators that allow paracellular transport of macromolecules are often fully reversible such as zonula occludens toxin (ZOT) [70, 78], *Aloe vera* gel [75], and sinomenine [76]. Polymeric absorption enhancers also showed potential reversibility, but the complete reversibility of the effect of the cationic polymer chitosan and its trimethylated derivative on the transepithelial electrical resistance of Caco-2 cell monolayers was difficult to prove with *in vitro* tests due to their mucoadhesive properties that prevented complete removal of the material from the cell layer without damaging the cells [79].

3.3.2
Chemical and Physical Modifications

The main structural features that determine the passive diffusion of peptide drugs across cell membranes are size, charge, and hydrophilicity. The concept of optimized physicochemical properties by means of chemical modification has been shown to be very successful in improving the bioavailability of certain peptide drugs. For example, the oral bioavailability of peptidic renin inhibitors has been substantially increased by derivitization (i.e., up to 50% from 2% for the parent compound). A common structural modification that is used to increase the

Table 3.2 Categories of absorption enhancing agents and their mechanisms of action.

Category and example(s) of absorption enhancers	Mechanism of action	Reference
Bile salts: Sodium cholate, sodium deoxycholate, sodium taurocholate	Facilitation of drug diffusion through the cell membrane by means of the formation of reverse micelles or other mechanisms, reduction of mucous viscosity on the epithelial surface, opening of tight junctions and, thereby, increasing paracellular transport.	[56]
Surfactants: Sodium dodecylsulfate, nonylphenoxypoly-oxyethylene, polysorbate 80, cremophore EL	Changes in the lipid order, orientation and fluidity, thereby, altering the structure of the bilayer membrane. Inhibition of efflux transport.	[55, 57–59]
Polymers: Cationic polymers such as chitosan and its derivatives	Combination of mucoadhesion and tight junction opening through ionic interactions with the cell membrane.	[60–62]
Anionic such as carbopol and poly(acrylic acid) derivatives	Combination of enzyme inhibition and tight junction opening through extracellular calcium removal.	[63, 64]
Efflux inhibitors: Verapamil, cyclosporine A, cremophor EL	Competitive or allosteric blocking of efflux transporter binding sites, interfering with ATP hydrolysis and altering integrity of cell membrane lipids.	[65]
Fatty acids: Sodium caprylate, sodium caprate and sodium laurate	Paracellular: increased intracellular calcium levels by activating phospholipase C in the membrane, contractions of actin microfilaments and opening of tight junctions. Transcellular: potential inhibition of efflux transporters.	[66, 67]
Acylcarnitines and alkanoylcholines: Palmitoyl-DL-carnitine chloride	Opening of tight junctions with a calcium-independent mechanism, changes in lipid order of membranes.	[3]
Chelating agents: ethylene glycol-bis(2-aminoethylether)-N,N,N',N'-tetraacetic acid (EGTA)	Extracellular calcium removal by chelation with disruption of intracellular junctions resulting in a decrease in transepithelial electrical resistance and an increase in paracellular permeability.	[68]

(Continued)

Table 3.2 (Continued)

Category and example(s) of absorption enhancers	Mechanism of action	Reference
Toxins, venoms, and microorganisms:		
Zonula occludens toxin (ZOT), hemagglutinin (HA)	ZOT binds to a putative receptor on the apical surface of enterocytes resulting in a cascade of events such as protein kinase C-mediated polymerization of soluble G-actin followed by opening of tight junction. HA affects distribution of occludin, ZO-1, E-cadherin, and β-catenin leading to increased tight junction permeability.	[69, 70–72]
Melittin	Transcellular membrane perturbation through both toroidal pore and carpet mechanisms and paracellular drug absorption enhancement via inhibition of calmodulin.	[67, 73]
Baker's yeast such as *Saccharomyces cerevisiae*	Opening of tight junctions by translocation of ZO-1 and occludin from the membrane to cytoskeletal cell areas, which could involve protein kinase C activation.	[74]
Phytoconstituents:		
Aloe vera gel and whole leaf	Reversible opening of tight junctions as indicated by reduction in transepithelial electrical resistance of Caco-2 cell monolayers.	[75]
Sinomenine	Opening of tight junctions and/or efflux inhibition.	[76]

stability of peptides towards proteolysis is substitution of the L-amino acid with a D-amino acid at either or both termini, while cyclization substantially increases metabolic stability [14].

Prodrug strategies involve reversible chemical modifications of the peptide drug to improve bioavailability while retaining optimum pharmacological activity. Once the absorption barrier has been circumvented, the prodrug is converted to the parent drug by means of enzymatic or non-enzymatic catalyzed reactions [80]. In general, prodrug strategies for peptide drugs include modification of a single functional group, the formation of cyclic prodrugs by using chemical linkers, or conjugation with a polymer to form a polymeric prodrug. The advantages of the formation of prodrugs, especially polymeric prodrugs, include an increase in the water solubility, protection against degradation and deactivation, improved pharmacokinetics, reduced antigenicity and immunogenicity, passive or active targeting of the drug to the site of action, and the potential to produce a novel complex drug delivery system [4, 81, 82].

It was shown that conjugation of fatty acids to peptides can enhance their membrane permeability, while stabilizing the peptide–receptor interaction through additional hydrophobic interactions. In contrast, such a modification may, in some cases, reduce the affinity of the protein for the receptor due to conformation changes. Linking agents such as tris (2-amino-2-hydroxy-methyl-1,3-propanediol) have been used to attach fatty acyl groups to peptides. One example where this technique was applied includes the conjugation of core peptide with tris-glycine-tripalmitate, which showed therapeutic activity against inflammation in acute adjuvant induced arthritis. Reversible aqueous lipidization technology has been used to improve the pharmacological effect and half-lives of proteins such as octreotide, somatostatin, desmopressin, and salmon calcitonin [47, 83].

PEGylation is the term describing a process whereby one or more molecules of activated polyethylene glycol (PEG) reacts chemically with a biomolecule, usually a protein or peptide, resulting in a recognized new molecular entity with improved pharmacokinetic properties that is more effective compared to the predecessor parent molecule. So far, nine PEGylated products have been approved by the FDA, of which eight involve proteins like cytokines, hormones, and growth factors. The most commonly used functional group on proteins and peptides to link the PEG molecule via a linker is the primary amino group ($-NH_2$), such as those from the N-terminus or from the lysine residues, but the sulfhydryl ($-SH$) group is another potential functional group for linking PEG molecules [84]. A conjugated insulin product, developed by Nobex® Corporation, that consists of hexyl insulin mono-conjugate 2 (HIM2) showed high potential to decrease glucose levels after oral administration. This strategy involves the covalent attachment of an amphiphilic PEG oligomer via an amide bond to the free amino group of the lysine residue in position 29 of the β-chain of recombinant human insulin. Besides improved oral bioavailability (to about 5%), the conjugate also provides improved stability and is currently one of the most promising products for effective oral delivery of insulin [1, 85, 86].

Cell penetrating proteins (also referred to as protein transduction domains, membrane translocating sequences, Trojan peptides or membrane transduction peptides) are short chain peptides capable of crossing cell membranes in an apparent energy-independent manner [87]. When conjugated to cargo, which may vary from small molecular weight drugs to macromolecules, and even liposomes and nanoparticles, they facilitate their systemic delivery by acting as vectors to carry them through cell membranes. They have been investigated to translocate their cargo across membranes of different mammalian cells to reach the cytoplasm and nucleus, but surprisingly few studies have looked into the possibility to deliver drugs across epithelial cell monolayers when linked to cell penetrating proteins. However, some reports have indicated higher permeability of the cargo after conjugation with these cell penetrating peptides. For example, insulin conjugated to one such cell penetration peptide (i.e., Tat peptide) showed a sixfold increase in transport across Caco-2 cell monolayers compared to insulin alone [88–90].

3.3.3
Targeting Strategies

3.3.3.1 Targeting Specific Regions of the Gastrointestinal Tract
The absorption of some drugs administered by the oral route is region-specific, due to pH dependent solubility, poor stability due to the secretion of enzymes in

specific regions of the gastrointestinal tract, region-selective occurrence of active and efflux transporters and pre-systemic metabolism in the gastrointestinal wall. The luminal and brush border membrane protease activity of the colon is lower than that of the stomach and small intestine, which means that the colon is one of the most preferred gastrointestinal regions for peptide delivery [48].

Some of the most feasible colon-targeting approaches include the use of azo-bond or glycosidic prodrugs, time-controlled drug delivery systems, pressure-controlled systems, pH-controlled systems, and enzyme-controlled systems. Time-controlled systems cannot adapt to inter- and intra-individual variations in gastrointestinal transit time, while pH-dependent systems are often sensitive to food or disease induced changes in pH, and the efficacy of pressure-controlled systems has not been satisfactorily proven. The microflora in the colon produce reductive enzymes that are responsible for site-specific conversion of prodrugs to absorbable parent drug molecules, and degradation of susceptible polymers allows site-specific release of the drug. The enzyme-controlled approach, therefore, holds the highest potential for delivery of drugs to the colon [91, 92].

3.3.3.2 Targeting Receptors and Transporters

Different nutrient transporters and receptors are expressed on epithelial cell membranes and drug molecules can be chemically modified (e.g., by formation of prodrugs) in order to be recognized by these membrane transporters as substrates. These prodrugs are, therefore, used to target the transporters to be translocated across the cell membranes [93].

Two types of peptide transporters from the proton-coupled oligopeptide transporter family have been identified in mammals, namely PepT1 and PepT2, each differing in their specificity for substrates as well as affinity and transport capacity. PepT1 is capable of transporting di- and tri-peptides, as well as peptidomimetic analogs, in the small intestinal epithelium, while PepT2 is primarily located in the renal tubular epithelium [93, 94]. Linking of a drug molecule to an enzymatically stable dipeptide or single amino acid that is a substrate for PepT1 can, therefore, potentially be used to target this transporter. Proof of this concept has been demonstrated with different model drugs [95].

During receptor-mediated endocytosis in epithelial cells, a ligand binds to a surface receptor and the complex formed is invaginated into a coated pit. The endocytosed material may then be processed in any one of four ways. Transcytosis is one way of interest for protein delivery since the endocytosed material is shunted across the cell away from lysosomal degradation and is released from the cell at the basolateral side by means of exocytosis [96]. It was discovered that transcytosis is the natural mechanism of uptake of neonatal immunoglobulins, vitamin B_{12}, iron, certain viruses, plant lectins, and toxins. It was, therefore, hypothesized that chemical linking of a protein drug molecule to any of these molecules, in such a way that it does not interfere with their ability to bind to the intrinsic factor or receptor, would lead to co-uptake of the protein drug. It was, for example, found that the uptake mechanism of vitamin B_{12} showed potential to increase the oral absorption of α-interferon, erythropoietin, and granulosyte colony-stimulating factor by covalently linking them to the vitamin B_{12} molecule [96, 97].

3.3.4
Formulation Strategies

3.3.4.1 Particulate Carrier Systems

Microparticles (1–1000 μm) and nanoparticles (10–1000 nm) have been prepared from different polymeric materials to assist in the effective delivery of peptide and protein drugs through different mechanisms. These particulate carrier systems are capable of protecting the encapsulated peptide drug against degradation, prolonging the gastrointestinal residence time by means of mucoadhesion, promoting epithelial cell transport, expanding blood circulation time, and preventing self-aggregation of the peptide drug (e.g., insulin) [98, 99].

Particulate delivery systems that have been investigated as potential carriers include liposomes, polymer-lyposome conjugates, core–shell microparticles, nano-particles (which include nanocapsules that are vesicular systems and nanospheres that are matrix systems), polymersomes, and nanoreactors. Liposomes are vesicles composed of curved lipid bilayers formed by amphiphiles, which are orientated in such a way that their hydrophobic parts face the interior of the bilayer and hydro-philic parts face the exterior of the bilayer. Liposomes have experienced serious drawbacks, such as low encapsulation efficiency in general, disruption of the bilayer by interactions with high-density lipoproteins in the blood or surfactants in the lungs, and they are removed from the blood by the reticuloendothelial system that limits circulation time. One approach that is used to improve the drug delivery properties of liposomes is to coat them with polymers, such as polyethylene glycol, chitosan, or alginate, which proved to be successful *in vitro* to some extent. How-ever, more *in vivo* tests are needed to be conclusive in terms of their usefulness in effective protein delivery [100, 101].

Different methods have been applied to entrap peptide drug molecules inside micro- and nano-carriers, such as the single or double emulsion technique, solvent evaporation, a combination of emulsion and spray drying, extrusion/external gelation method, coacervation and the isoelectric precipitation method for encapsulation of bioactive substances. Several natural (e.g., albumin, alginate, chitosan, collagen, gelatine, rosin) and synthetic (e.g., poly(lactic acids), poly(lactic-co-glycolic acid) and poly (methacrylates)) polymers have been used in the formulation of particulate drug delivery systems. The drug release mechanism and profile from micro- and nano-particles depend on the physicochemical properties of the polymer used in the pre-paration of the dosage form [100, 101].

A relatively new technique that can be used to produce nanoparticles with precisely controlled sizes, shapes and compositions is called particle replication in non-wetting templates (PRINT). This PRINT technique is based on molds prepared from fluoropolymers that are liquids at room temperature, and that can be photochemically cross-linked on master templates made by advanced litho-graphic techniques. The nanoscale cavities in the molds can then be filled with an organic liquid precursor to form a solid particle by means of gentle chemical processes. The compatibility of PRINT with fragile biological molecules such as proteins, DNA, and anti-cancer drugs has already been demonstrated [102].

3.3.4.2 Enzyme Inhibition

This approach is based on the fact that peptidase and protease inhibitors included in drug delivery systems can prevent or reduce pre-systemic degradation of peptide drugs and, thereby, increase the fractional absorption of the drug. Although inhibition of enzymes in the gastrointestinal tract seems practically more feasible than in the liver, due to the systemic effect that may be elicited in the latter case, this strategy is faced by certain challenges when administered in the long term. These challenges include potential disturbances of the digestion of nutritive proteins as well as stimulation of enzyme secretion due to a feedback regulation [35, 103].

3.3.4.3 Mucoadhesive Systems

Formulations that prolong the residence time at the site of absorption and provide intimate contact with the absorptive cell surface can contribute to more successful mucosal absorption and enhanced bioavailability of peptide and protein drugs [104, 105]. This is accomplished by designing mucoadhesive drug delivery systems that form adhesive bonds with the mucus layer or with the epithelial cell surface, or a combination of the two [106]. Several polymers have been investigated for their mucoadhesion properties, such as chitosan and poly(acrylic acid), which were chemically modified by addition of thiol groups in an effort to improve their mucoadhesiveness by establishing an interaction with the cystein groups on the mucus glycoproteins [107]. However, in vivo studies revealed that these systems failed in their expectation to localize drugs for prolonged times at the site of absorption due to the relatively high mucus turnover rate and sloughing of epithelial cells [108]. This problem was thought to be overcome by using compounds that could bind specifically to carbohydrates on the cell surface, such as lectins. Unfortunately, cross-reactivity of the lectins with the mucus layer caused similar problems as experienced with the mucoadhesive polymers. Biomimetic mucoadhesive dosage forms have further advanced to employ fimbriae (i.e., filamentous protein projections on the surface of bacteria) as specific mucin-binding moieties [106, 109].

3.4
Conclusions

Although a variety of pharmacologically potent protein and peptide drugs have been discovered that can be produced on a large scale, their clinical use is negatively affected because they cannot be effectively delivered via the oral route of administration. Advances in pharmaceutical technology and innovations in drug delivery approaches have contributed to finding ways that have overcome many of the barriers that work against effective oral delivery of proteins and peptides. Strategies that have been investigated include co-administration of absorption enhancers, chemical modifications, targeting of specific absorption regions in the gastrointestinal tract, as well as receptors and transporters, particulate carrier systems, enzyme inhibitors, and mucoadhesive dosage forms. Although many of these strategies have been successful to varying extents in terms of improving the delivery of polypeptide drugs, especially as shown by means of *in vitro* transport studies, some issues still remain problematic and need further investigation, such as the potential toxicity of absorption enhancers and the effectiveness of most of the strategies investigated so far needs to be proven in the *in vivo* situation. However, measured by the progress made so far, it is realistic to accept that achievement of therapeutic levels of most orally administered peptide and protein drugs is a feasible possibility in the near future.

References

1 Antosova, Z., Mackova, M., Kral, V., and Macek, T. (2009) Therapeutic application of peptides and proteins: parenteral forever?. *Trends Biotechnol.*, **27** (11), 628–635.

2 Babu, V.R., Patel, P., Mundargi, R.C., Rangaswamy, V., and Aminabhavi, T.M. (2008) Developments in polymeric devices for oral insulin delivery. *Expert Opin. Drug Deliv.*, **5** (4), 403–415.

3 Aungst, B.J. (2000) Intestinal permeation enhancers. *J. Pharm. Sci.*, **89** (4), 429–442.

4 Shaji, J. and Patole, V. (2008) Protein and peptide delivery: oral approaches. *Ind. J. Pharm. Sci.*, **70** (3), 269–277.

5 Lu, Y., Yang, J., and Sega, E. (2006) Issues related to targeted delivery of proteins and peptides. *AAPS J*, **8** (3), E466–E478.

6 Singh, R., Shailesh, S., and Lillard, J.W. (2008) Past, present and future technologies for oral delivery of therapeutic proteins. *J. Pharm. Sci.*, **97** (7), 2497–2523.

7 Daugherty, A.L. and Mrsny, R.J. (1999) Transcellular uptake mechanisms of the intestinal epithelial barrier: part one. *Pharm. Sci. Technol. Today*, **2** (4), 144–151.

8 Fasano, A. (1998) Innovative strategies for the oral delivery of drugs and peptides. *Trends Biotechnol.*, **16** (4), 152–157.

9 Salama, N.N., Eddington, N.D., and Fasano, A. (2006) Tight junction modulation and its relationship to drug delivery. *Adv. Drug Deliv. Rev.*, **58** (1), 15–28.

10 Okano, T., Inui, K.-I., Maegawa, H., Takano, M., and Hori, R. (1986) H^+-coupled uphill transport of aminocephalosporins via the intestinal transport system in rabbit intestinal brush-border membranes. *J. Biol. Chem.*, **261** (30), 14130–14134.

11 Iseki, K., Sugawara, M., Sato, K., Naasani, I., Haykawa, T., Kobayashi, M., and Miyazaki, K. (1999) Multiplicity of the H^+-dependent transport mechanism of dipeptide and anionic β-lactam antibiotic ceftibuten in rat intestinal brush-border membrane. *J. Pharmacol. Exp. Ther.*, **289** (1), 66–71.

12 Rodewald, R. and Kraehenbuhl, J.-P. (1984) Receptor-mediated transport of IgG. *J. Cell Biol.*, **99** (1), 159s–164s.

13 Lee, V.H.L. and Yamamoto, A. (1989) Penetration and enzymatic barriers to peptide and protein absorption. *Adv. Drug Deliv. Rev.*, **4** (2), 171–207.

14 Pauletti, G.M., Gangwar, S., Knipp, G.T., Nerurkar, M.M., Okumu, F.W., Tamura, K., Siahaan, T.J., and Borchardt, R.T. (1996) Structural requirements for intestinal absorption of peptide drugs. *J. Control. Rel.*, **41** (1–2), 3–17.

15 Banga, A.K. and Chien, Y.W. (1988) Systemic delivery of therapeutic peptides and proteins. *Int. J. Pharm.*, **48** (1–3), 15–50.

16 Zhou, X.H. and Li Wan Po, A. (1991a) Peptide and protein drugs. I. Therapeutic applications, absorption and parenteral administration. *Int. J. Pharm.*, **75** (2–3), 97–115.

17 Lipka, E., Crison, J., and Amidon, G.L. (1996) Transmembrane transport of peptide type compounds: prospects for oral delivery. *J. Control. Rel.*, **39** (2–3), 121–129.

18 Aungst, B.J., Saitoh, H., Burcham, D.L., Huang, S.-M., Mousa, S.A., and Hussain, M.A. (1996) Enhancement of the intestinal absorption of peptides and non-peptides. *J. Control. Rel.*, **41** (1–2), 19–31.

19 Wang, W., Nema, S., and Teagarden, D. (2010) Protein aggregation – pathways and influencing factors. *Int. J. Pharm.*, **390** (2), 89–99.

20 Van Hoogdalem, E.J., De Boer, A.G., and Breimer, D.D. (1989) Intestinal drug absorption enhancement: an overview. *Pharmacol. Ther.*, **44** (3), 407–443.

21 Fagerholm, U. and Lennernäs, H. (1995) Experimental estimation of the effective unstirred water layer thickness in the human jejunum, and its importance in oral drug absorption. *Euro. J. Pharm. Sci.*, **3** (5), 247–253.

22 Verhoef, J.C., Boddé, H.E., De Boer, A.G., Bouwstra, J.A., Junginger, H.E., Merkus, F.W.H.M., and Breimer, D.D. (1990) Transport of peptide and protein drugs across biological membranes. *Eur. J. Drug Metab. Ph.*, **15** (2), 83–93.

23 Larhed, W.A., Artursson, P., Gråsjö, J., and Björk, E. (1997) Diffusion of drugs in native and purified gastrointestinal mucus. *J. Pharm. Sci.*, **86** (6), 660–665.

24 Norris, D.A., Puri, N., and Sinko, P.J. (1998) The effect of physical barriers and properties on the oral absorption of particulates. *Adv. Drug Deliv. Rev.*, **34** (2–3), 135–154.

25 Takatsuka, S., Kitazawa, T., Morita, T., Horikiri, Y., and Yoshino, H. (2006) Enhancement of the intestinal absorption of poorly absorbed hydrophilic compounds by simultaneous use of mucolytic agent and non-ionic surfactant. *Eur. J. Pharm. Biopharm.*, **62** (1), 52–58.

26 Schipper, N.G.M., Vårum, K.M., Stenberg, P., Ocklind, G., Lennernäs, H., and Artursson, P. (1999) Chitosans as absorption enhancers of poorly absorbable drugs 3: influence of mucus on absorption enhancement. *Eur. J. Pharm. Sci.*, **8** (4), 335–343.

27 Madara, J.L. and Trier, J.S. (1987) Functional morphology of the mucosa of the small intestine, in *Physiology of the Gastrointestinal Tract*, 2nd edn (ed. L.R. Johnson), Raven Press, New York, pp. 1209–1249.

28 Muranishi, M. and Yamamoto, Y. (1994) Mechanisms of absorption enhancement through gastrointestinal epithelium, in *Drug Absorption Enhancement: Concepts, Possibilities, Limitations and Trends* (ed. A.G. de Boer), Harwood Academic Press, pp. 66–100.

29 Washington, N., Washington, C., and Wilson, C.G. (eds) (2001) *Physiological Pharmaceutics: Barriers to Drug Absorption*, 2nd ed, Taylor and Francis, New York, pp. 312.

30 Sha'afi, R.I., Gary-Bobo, C.M., and Solomon, A.K. (1971) Permeability of red blood cell membranes to small hydrophilic and lipophilic solutes. *J. Gen. Physiol.*, **58**, 238–258.

31 Ward, P.D., Tippin, T.K., and Thakker, D.R. (2000) Enhancing paracellular permeability by modulating epithelial tight junctions. *Pharm. Sci. Technol. Today*, **3** (10), 346–358.

32 Salamat-Miller, N. and Johnston, T.P. (2005) Current strategies used to enhance the paracellular transport of therapeutic polypeptides across the intestinal epithelium. *Int. J. Pharm.*, **294** (1–2), 201–216.

33 Langguth, P., Bohner, V., Heizmann, J., Merkle, H.P., Wolffram, S., Amidon, G.L., and Yamashita, S. (1997) The challenge of proteolytic enzymes in intestinal peptide delivery. *J. Control. Rel.*, **46** (1–2), 39–57.

34 Carino, G.P. and Mathiowitz, E. (1999) Oral insulin delivery. *Adv. Drug Deliv. Rev.*, **35** (2–3), 249–257.

35 Aungst, B.J. (1993) Novel formulation strategies for improving oral bioavailability of drugs with poor membrane permeation or presystemic metabolism. *J. Pharm. Sci.*, **82** (10), 979–987.

36 Zhou, X.H. and Li Wan Po, A. (1991) Peptide and protein drugs. II. Non-parenteral routes of delivery. *Int. J. Pharm.*, **75** (2–3), 117–130.

37 Zhou, X.H. (1994) Overcoming enzymatic and absorption barriers to non-parenterally administered protein and peptide drugs. *J. Control. Rel.*, **29** (3), 239–252.

38 Alpers, D.H. (1987) Digestion and absorption of carbohydrates and proteins, in *Physiology of the Gastrointestinal Tract*, 2nd edn (ed. L.R. Johnson), Raven Press, New York, pp. 1469–1487.

39 Bernkop-Schnürch, A. (1998) The use of inhibitory agents to overcome the enzymatic barrier to perorally administered therapeutic peptides and proteins. *J. Control. Rel.*, **52** (1–2), 1–16.

40 Gardner, M.G. (1979) Superficial or membrane digestion of peptides in dinitrophenol-inhibited rat small intestine. *Clin. Sci.*, **57** (2), 217–220.

41 Burton, P.S., Goodwin, J.T., Conradi, R.A., Ho, N.F.H., and Hilgers, A.R. (1997) In vitro permeability of peptidomimetic drugs: the role of polarized efflux pathways as additional barriers to absorption. *Adv. Drug Deliv. Rev.*, **23** (1–3), 143–156.

42 Hunter, J. and Hirst, B.H. (1997) Intestinal secretion of drugs. The role of P-glycoprotein and related drug efflux systems in limiting oral drug absorption. *Adv. Drug Deliv. Rev.*, **25** (2–3), 129–157.

43 Chan, L.M.S., Lowes, S., and Hirst, B. H. (2004) The ABC's of drug transport in intestine and liver: efflux proteins limiting drug absorption and bioavailability. *Eur. J. Pharm. Sci.*, **21** (1), 25–51.

44 Benet, L.Z., Wu, C-Y., Hebert, M.F., and Wacher, V.J. (1996) Intestinal drug metabolism and antitransport processes: a potential paradigm shift in oral drug delivery. *J. Control. Rel.*, **39** (2–3), 139–143.

45 Zheng, Y., Qui, Y., Fu Lu, M., Hoffman, D., and Reiland, T.L. (1999) Permeability and absorption of leuprolide from various intestinal regions in rabbits and rats. *Int. J. Pharm.*, **185** (1), 83–92.

46 Morishita, I., Morishita, M., Takayama, K., Machida, Y., and Nagai, T. (1993) Enteral insulin delivery by microspheres in 3 different formulations using Eudragit L100 and S100. *Int. J. Pharm.*, **91** (1), 29–37.

47 Shantha Kumar, T.R., Soppimath, K., and Nachaegari, S.K. (2006) Novel delivery technologies for protein and peptide therapeutics. *Curr. Pharm. Biotechnol.*, **7**, 261–276.

48 Kagan, L. and Hoffman, A. (2008) Systems for region selective drug delivery in the gastrointestinal tract: biopharmaceutical considerations. *Exp. Opin. Drug Deliv.*, **5** (6), 681–692.

49 Ziv, E., Lior, O., and Kidron, M. (1987) Absorption of protein via the intestinal wall. A quantitative model. *Biochem. Pharmacol.*, **36** (7), 1035–1039.

50 Touitou, E. (1992) Enhancement of intestinal peptide absorption. *J. Control. Rel.*, **21**, 139–144.

51 Carino, G.P. and Mathiowitz, E. (1999) Oral insulin delivery. *Adv. Drug Deliv. Rev.*, **35**, 249–257.

52 Muranishi, S. (1990) Absorption enhancers. *Crit. Rev. Ther. Drug Carrier Syst.*, **7** (1), 1–33.

53 Whitehead, K. and Mitragotri, S. (2008) Mechanistic analysis of chemical permeation enhancers for oral drug delivery. *Pharm. Res.*, **25** (6), 1412–1419.

54 Fix, J.A. (1996) Strategies for delivery of peptides utilising absorption enhancing agents. *J. Pharm. Sci.*, **85** (12e), 1282–1285.

55 LeCluyse, E.L. and Sutton, S.C. (1997) In vitro models for selection of development candidates. Permeability studies to define mechanisms of absorption enhancement. *Adv. Drug Deliv. Rev.*, **23**, 163–183.

56 Catalioto, R.-M., Triolo, A., Giuliani, S., Altamura, M., Evangelista, S., and Maggi, C.A. (2008) Increased paracellular absorption by bile salts and P-glycoprotein stimulated efflux of otilonium bromide in Caco-2 cells monolayers as a model of intestinal barrier. *J. Pharm. Sci.*, **97** (9), 4087–4100.

57 Nerurkar, M.M., Ho, N.F.H., Burton, P.S., Vidmar, T.J., and Borchardt, R.T. (1997) Mechanistic roles of neutral surfactants on concurrent polarized and passive membrane transport of a model peptide in Caco-2 cells. *J. Pharm. Sci.*, **86** (7), 813–821.

58 Pauletti, G.M., Gangwar, S., Siahaan, T.J., Aubé, J., and Borchardt, R.T. (1997) Improvement of oral peptide bioavailability: peptidomimetics and prodrug strategies. *Adv. Drug Deliv. Rev.*, **27**, 235–256.

59 Xia, W.J. and Onyuksel, H. (2000) Mechanistic studies on surfactant induced membrane permeability enhancement. *Pharm. Res.*, **17** (5), 612–618.

60 Kotzé, A.F., De Leeuw, B.J., Lue en, H. L., De Boer, (A)Bert.G., Verhoef, J.C., and Junginger, H.E. (1997) Chitosans for enhanced delivery of therapeutic peptides across intestinal epithelia: *in vitro* evaluation in Caco-2 cell monolayers. *Int. J. Pharm.*, **159**, 243–253.

61 Kotzé, A.F., Luessen, H.L., De Boer, A. G., Verhoef, J.C., and Junginger, H.E. (1998) Chitosan for enhanced intestinal permeability: prospects for derivatives soluble in neutral and basic environments. *Eur. J. Pharm. Sci.*, **7**, 145–151.

62 Thanou, M., Verhoef, J.C., and Junginger, H.E. (2001) Oral drug absorption enhancement by chitosan and its derivatives. *Adv. Drug Deliv. Rev.*, **52**, 117–126.

63 Borchard, G., Luessen, H.L., De Boer, A.G., Verhoef, J.C., Lehr, C-M., and Junginger, J.E. (1996) The potential of mucoadhesive polymers in enhancing intestinal peptide drug absorption. III: effects of chitosan glutamate and carbomer on epithelial tight junctions in vitro. *J. Control. Rel.*, **39**, 131–138.

64 Di Colo, G., Zambito, Y., and Zaino, C. (2007) Polymeric enhancers of mucosal

epithelia permeability: synthesis, transepithelial penetration enhancing properties, mechanism of action, safety issues. *J. Pharm. Sci.*, **97**, 1–29.

65 Werle, M. (2008) Natural and synthetic polymers as inhibitors of drug efflux pumps. *Pharm. Res.*, **25** (3), 500–511.

66 Cano-Cebrián, M.J., Zornosa, T., Granero, L., and Polache, A. (2005) Intestinal absorption enhancement via the paracellular route by fatty acids, chitosans and others: a target for drug delivery. *Curr. Drug Deliv.*, **2**, 9–22.

67 Maher, S., Wang, X., Bzik, V., McClean, S., and Brayden, D.J. (2009) Evaluation of intestinal absorption and mucosal toxicity using two promoters. II. Rat instillation and perfusion studies. *Eur. J. Pharm. Sci.*, **38**, 301–311.

68 Johnson, P.H., Frank, D., and Costantino, H.R. (2008) Discovery of tight junction modulators: significance for drug development and delivery. *Drug Discov. Today*, **13** (5/6), 261–267.

69 Fasano, A. (1998) Novel approaches for oral delivery of macromolecules. *J. Pharm. Sci.*, **87** (11), 1351–1356.

70 Cox, D.S., Raje, S., Gao, H., Salama, N.N., and Edington, N.D. (2002) Enhanced permeability of molecular weight markers and poorly bioavailable compounds across Caco-2 cell monolayers using the absorption enhancer, zonula occludens toxin. *Pharm. Res.*, **19** (11), 1680–1688.

71 Salama, N.N., Eddington, N.D., and Fasano, A. (2006) Tight junction modulation and its relationship to drug delivery. *Adv. Drug Deliv. Rev.*, **58**, 15–28.

72 Matsuhisa, K., Kondoh, M., Takahashi, A., and Yagi, K. (2009) Tight junction modulator and drug delivery. *Exp. Opin. Drug Deliv.*, **6** (5), 509–515.

73 Maher, S., Devocelle, M., Ryan, S., McClean, S., and Brayden, D.J. (2010) Impact of amino acid replacements on in vitro permeation enhancement and cytotoxicity of the intestinal absorption promoter, melittin. *Int. J. Pharm.*, **387**, 154–160.

74 Fuller, E., Duckham, C., and Wood, E. (2007) Disruption of epithelial tight

junctions by yeast enhances the paracellular delivery of a model protein. *Pharm. Res.*, **24** (1), 37–47.

75 Chen, W., Lu, Z., Viljoen, A., and Hamman, J. (2009) Intestinal drug transport enhancement by Aloe vera. *Planta Medica*, **75**, 587–595.

76 Lu, Z., Chen, W., Viljoen, A., and Hamman, J.H. (2010) Effect of sinomenine on the in vitro intestinal epithelial transport of selected compounds. *Phytother. Res.*, **24**, 211–218.

77 Swenson, E.S., Milisen, W.B., and Curatolo, W. (1994) Intestinal permeability enhancement: efficacy, acute local toxicity and reversibility. *Pharm. Res.*, **11** (8), 1132–1142.

78 Fasano, A. (1998) Innovative strategies for the oral delivery of drugs and peptides. *Trends Biotechnol.*, **16**, 152–157.

79 Hamman, J.H., Schultz, C.M., and Kotzé, A.F. (2003) N-trimethyl chitosan chloride: optimum degree of quaternization for drug absorption enhancement across epithelial cells. *Drug Develop. Ind. Pharm.*, **29** (2), 161–172.

80 Oliyai, R. (1996) Prodrugs of peptides and peptidomimetics for improved formulation and delivery. *Adv. Drug Deliv. Rev.*, **19**, 275–286.

81 Borchardt, R.T. (1999) Optimizing oral absorption of peptides using prodrug strategies. *J. Control. Rel.*, **62**, 231–238.

82 Khandare, J. and Minko, T. (2006) Polymer drug conjugates: progress in polymeric prodrugs. *Prog. Polym. Sci.*, **31**, 359–397.

83 Ali, M. and Manolios, N. (2002) Peptide delivery systems. *Lett. Peptide Sci.*, **8**, 289–294.

84 Bailon, P. and Won, C.-Y. (2009) PEG-modified biopharmaceuticals. *Exp. Opin. Drug Deliv.*, **6** (1), 1–6.

85 Owens, D.R., Zinman, B., and Bolli, G. (2003) Alternative routes of insulin delivery. *Diabetic Med.*, **20**, 886–898.

86 Cefalu, W.T. (2004) Concept, strategies, and feasibility of noninvasive insulin delivery. *Diabetes Care*, **27**, 239–46.

87 Herce, H.D. and Garcia, A.E. (2007) Cell penetrating peptides: how do they do it?. *J. Biol. Phys.*, **33**, 345–356.

88 Snyder, E.L. and Dowdy, S.F. (2004) Cell penetrating peptides in drug delivery. *Pharm. Res.*, **21** (3), 389–393.

89 Patel, L.N., Zaro, J.L., and Shen, W.-C. (2007) Cell penetrating peptides: intracellular pathways and pharmaceutical perspectives. *Pharm. Res.*, **24** (11), 1977–1992.

90 Hassane, F.S., Saleh, A.F., Abes, R., Gait, M.J., and Lebleu, B. (2010) Cell penetrating peptides: overview and applications to the delivery of oligonucleotides. *Cell. Mol. Life Sci.*, **67**, 715–726.

91 Chourasia, M.K. and Jain, S.K. (2004) Polysaccharides for colon targeted drug delivery. *Drug Deliv.*, **11**, 129–148.

92 Roldo, M., Barbu, E., Brown, J.F., Laight, D.W., Smart, J.D., and Tsibouklis, J. (2007) Azo compounds in colon-specific drug delivery. *Exp. Opin. Drug Deliv.*, **4** (5), 547–560.

93 Mandava, N., Oberoi, R.K., Minocha, M., and Mitra, A.K. (2010) Transporter targeted drug delivery. *J. Drug Deliv. Sci. Technol.*, **20** (2), 89–99.

94 Majumdar, S., Duvvuri, S., and Mitra, A.K. (2004) Membrane transporter/receptor-targeted prodrug design: strategies for human and veterinary drug development. *Adv. Drug Deliv. Rev.*, **56**, 1437–1452.

95 Steffansen, B., Nielsen, C.U., Brodin, B., Eriksson, A.H., Andersen, R., and Frokjaer, S. (2004) Intestinal solute carriers: an overview of trends and strategies for improving oral drug absorption. *Eur. J. Pharm. Sci.*, **21**, 3–16.

96 Russell-Jones, G.J. (2001) The potential use of receptor-mediated endocytosis for oral drug delivery. *Adv. Drug Deliv. Rev.*, **46**, 59–73.

97 Russel-Jones, G.J., Arthur, L., and Walker, H. (1999) Vitamin B_{12}-mediated transport of nanoparticles across Caco-2 cells. *Int. J. Pharm.*, **179**, 247–255.

98 Yang, Y.-Y., Wang, Y., Powell, R., and Chan, P. (2006) Polymer core-shell nanoparticles for therapeutics. *Clin. Exp. Pharmacol. Physiol.*, **33**, 557–562.

99 Yamanaka, Y.J. and Leong, K.W. (2008) Engineering strategies to enhance nanoparticle-mediated oral delivery. *J. Biomater. Sci.– Polym. Ed.*, **19** (12), 1549–1570.

100 Des Rieux, A., Fievez, V., Garinot, M., Schneider, Y.-J., and Preat, V. (2006) Nanoparticles as potential oral delivery systems of proteins and vaccines: a mechanistic approach. *J. Control. Rel.*, **116**, 1–27.

101 Balasubramanian, V., Onaca, O., Enea, R., Hughes, D.W., and Palivan, C.G. (2010) Protein delivery: from conventional drug delivery carriers to polymeric nanoreactors. *Exp. Opin. Drug Deliv.*, **7** (1), 63–78.

102 Napier, M.E. and Desimone, J.M. (2007) Nanoparticle drug delivery platform. *Polym. Rev.*, **47**, 321–327.

103 Bernkop-Schnürch, A. (1998) The use of inhibitory agents to overcome the enzymatic barrier to perorally administered therapeutic peptides and proteins. *J. Control. Rel.*, **52**, 1–16.

104 Gabor, F., Bogner, E., Weissenboeck, A., and Wirth, M. (2004) The lectin-cell interaction and its implications to intestinal lectin-mediated drug delivery. *Adv. Drug Deliv. Rev.*, **56**, 459–80.

105 Peppas, N.A. and Huang, Y. (2004) Nanoscale technology of mucoadhesive interactions. *Adv. Drug Deliv. Rev.*, **56**, 1675–1687.

106 Vasir, J.K., Tambwekar, K., and Garg, S. (2003) Bioadhesive microspheres as a controlled drug delivery system. *Int. J. Pharm.*, **255**, 13–32.

107 Bernkop-Schnürch, A. (2005) Mucoadhesive systems in oral drug delivery. *Drug Discov. Today: Technol.*, **2** (1), 83–87.

108 Kompella, U.B. and Lee, V.H.L. (2001) Delivery systems for penetration enhancement of peptide and protein drugs: design considerations. *Adv. Drug Deliv. Rev.*, **46**, 211–245.

109 Peppas, N.A., Thomas, J.B., and McGinty, J. (2009) Molecular aspects of mucoadhesive carrier development for drug delivery and improved absorption. *J. Biomater. Sci.*, **20**, 1–20.

4

Rational Design of Amphipathic α-Helical and Cyclic β-Sheet Antimicrobial Peptides: Specificity and Therapeutic Potential

Wendy J. Hartsock and Robert S. Hodges

4.1
Introduction to Antimicrobial Peptides

The current lack of commercially available antibiotics that are effective at killing drug resistant microorganisms has rendered a therapeutic void and peptide-based antibiotics offer a unique opportunity to improve the antimicrobial pipeline.

Antimicrobial resistance to drug therapy is a major and growing concern that is further amplified by a lack in the development of new antimicrobial agents [1]. The so-called "ESKAPE" (*Enterococcus faecium, Staphylococcus aureus, Klebsiella pneumoniae, Acinetobacter baumannii, Pseudomonas aeruginosa,* and *Enterobacter species*) pathogens are responsible for the majority of drug-resistant nosocomial infections in the United States [1, 2]. These resistant pathogens lead to higher patient mortality and increased cost of patient care. Gram-negative infections caused by resistant microbes are a significant threat in intensive care units, especially in the light of the identification of pan-drug resistant (resistant to all commercially available antibiotics) *Pseudomonas* and *Acinetobacter* isolates [3, 4]. Despite the obvious need for drugs targeting these microbes, the current pipeline is limited and the development of new drugs targeting multi-resistant pathogens is critical.

Polymyxins, which are cyclic peptides typically included in topical ointments such as Neosporin, have enjoyed a re-emergence as last resort therapeutics to treat drug-resistant Gram-negative infections [5, 6]. The potential neurotoxic, dermatotoxic, and nephrotoxic liabilities, as well as the identification of *A. baumannii* isolates that exhibit resistance to these peptides, are potential limitations to the use of the polymyxins [4]. Thus, a serious and still unmet need to develop novel therapeutics targeting resistant pathogens, particularly Gram-negative microbes, subsists.

Antimicrobial peptides (AMPs) are a part of a large class of pore-forming peptides and proteins utilized by and targeted at multicellular and unicellular organisms alike [7]. AMPs, which are present in vertebrates, invertebrates,

Peptide Drug Discovery and Development: Translational Research in Academia and Industry, First Edition.
Edited by Miguel Castanho and Nuno C. Santos.
© 2011 WILEY-VCH Verlag GmbH & Co. KGaA, Weinheim.
Published 2011 by WILEY-VCH Verlag GmbH & Co. KGaA

bacteria, and plants are structurally diverse molecules and include α-helices, cyclic β-sheets, disulfide linked β-sheets, and disordered polypeptide chains. General features of AMPs include a net positive charge, high hydrophobic content, amphipathicity, and inducible secondary structure [8, 9].

Although, as their name suggests, the AMPs are antimicrobial in nature, they are also recognized as having important roles in other physiological processes [8, 10, 11]. The term "host defense peptide" is used interchangeably with AMP to identify peptides that act as a protective mechanism against invading species, either through direct interactions with the invading organism or by influencing other facets of the host immune response [8, 10]. The cathelicidins and defensins are key host defense peptides expressed by humans and are involved in several physiological processes in addition to acting as antimicrobial agents. These peptides have an effect on chemokine production and release, histamine release and subsequent neutrophil migration [7, 10, 11]. These AMPs also appear to play a role in skin diseases such as aptopic dermatitis and psoriasis, respiratory disorders such as cystic fibrosis and inflammatory bowel disease such as Chron's colitis. Their role in the management of infectious disease and in immunomodulation and inflammation has recently been reviewed by Guani-Guerra *et al.* 2010 [12].

Our laboratory and others have shown that amphipathic α-helical AMPs are a promising scaffold for the *de novo* design of therapeutics targeting drug resistant microbes including multi-drug resistant Gram-negative pathogens [13–19].

4.2
Antimicrobial and Hemolytic Activities of Amphipathic α-Helical Antimicrobial Peptides: Mechanisms and Selectivity

While the exact mechanism of action of amphipathic α-helical AMPs has yet to be elucidated, the target of these AMPs is generally considered to be the cellular membrane.

There are various models proposed for the interaction of AMPs with membranes including (i) barrel-stave [20] (ii) toroidal pore [21–24], and (iii) carpet [25] models, and others [7, 26]. In the barrel-stave model, a pore comprised of laterally interacting transmembrane peptides that are inserted perpendicular to the membrane yields a hydrophilic core through which cell leakage occurs. In the toroidal pore model, the hydrophilic portions of the peptide interact with the charged head groups of the membrane. The hydrophobic residues of the AMP interact with the lipid environment causing the inner and outer layers to connect, forming a bend in the membrane. The carpet model predicts aggregation of peptides parallel to the lipid bilayer, which solubilizes the membrane in a detergent-like fashion, and does not require the transmembrane insertion of the peptides [7, 11, 26]. Both the carpet and toroidal pore models do not require specific peptide–peptide interactions but rather lipid–peptide interactions to exert their mechanism of action.

Based on our results, to obtain AMPs with the desired properties (excellent antimicrobial activity and limited to no toxicity), we have proposed a "membrane discrimination" mechanism of action for antimicrobial peptides whose sole target is the biomembrane, based on a "barrel-stave" mechanism in eukaryotic cells and a "carpet" mechanism in prokaryotic cells [13–15]. We believe that specificity between the two types of membranes depends upon differences in lipid composition. In contrast to prokaryotic membranes, eukaryotic membranes are generally characterized by zwitterionic phospholipids, a relatively large amount of cholesterol and sphingomyelin, and the absence of the high negative transmembrane potential that is present in prokaryotic membranes [9, 15]. Prokaryotic membranes, in contrast, are largely comprised of negatively charged phospholipids and possess a negative transmembrane potential. Thus, if antimicrobial peptides form channels/pores in the hydrophobic core of the eukaryotic bilayer, they would cause hemolysis of human red blood cells; in contrast, for prokaryotic cells, the peptides would lyse cells in a detergent-like mechanism, as described by the carpet mechanism. Therefore, the ideal antimicrobial peptide therapeutic would not be able to penetrate the eukaryotic cell membrane (very low to no hemolytic activity) but would still be able to enter the prokaryotic membrane in the interface region of the bilayer parallel to the bilayer surface, with the non-polar face of the amphipathic helix interacting with the hydrophobicity of the lipids, and the polar and charged residues of the polar face interacting with the surface phospho-head groups of the lipids.

To be useful as antimicrobial agents for the treatment of infections in humans, AMPs must demonstrate selectivity between mammalian and microbial cellular membranes. Determining the hemolytic activity of AMPs from either the maximum concentration of peptide that results in no hemolysis (MHC) or the concentration of peptide required for 50% hemolysis (HC_{50}) of human erythrocytes is the standard assay used to determine toxicity to mammalian cells. The length of exposure of erythrocytes to AMPs has yet to be standardized and can range from minutes to hours, which limits one-to-one comparisons between values of hemolytic activity (MHC or HC_{50}) for various AMPs reported in the literature. In the Hodges laboratory, hemoglobin release from AMP exposed erythrocytes is determined over an 18-h time course experiment at $37\,^{\circ}C$ peptide concentrations ranging from 1 to 1000 µg ml^{-1}. This approach allows the assessment of acute (0–1 h) and chronic (1–18 h) toxicities as a result of AMP activity [9].

Selectivity for microorganisms over mammalian cells can be evaluated using the therapeutic index, which is determined from the ratio of hemolytic activity (HC_{50}) to antimicrobial activity (MIC) [9]. Using this definition of therapeutic index, a large number would signify high selectivity for the target microorganism, whereas a small number would imply low selectivity and, therefore, toxicity at mammalian cells. For example, a HC_{50} value of 500µM and a MIC value of 2 µM would yield a therapeutic index of 250.

AMPs targeted at microbes appear to exhibit selectivity for bacterial membranes over mammalian cells but the influence of experimental conditions on this conclusion has been called into question. Matsuzaki [27] reviewed the mechanisms of AMP selectivity for microorganisms over mammalian cells (mainly human erythrocytes) and suggested that the apparent selectivity of AMPs for microorganisms *in vitro* is an artifact of experimental conditions, namely that the typical cell content for bacterial assays is 5×10^5 colony-forming units/ml whereas hemolysis assays are typically performed using 6×10^8 cells/ml. In addition, since erythrocytes are typically 7 μm and bacterial cells are approximately 1 μm, a greater number of peptides may be required to produce toxic effects in erythrocytes compared to bacterial cells. However, as Matsuzaki points out, in the presence of invading microorganisms, AMPs have been shown to interact selectively with bacterial cell membranes over host cells [27]. Furthermore, the membranous environment of the cell varies, such that bacterial membranes are more negative compared to eukaryotic cell membranes. Since AMPs are, by and large, comprised of positively charged residues (in addition to having features such as hydrophobicity and amphipathicity), interaction with the bacterial cell membrane traps the peptides, thus sequestering them from host cells and adding a layer of selectivity to the interaction [27, 28]. Nevertheless, an AMP must demonstrate extremely low hemolytic activity, excellent antimicrobial activity, and a high therapeutic index to be useful as a clinical agent.

A number of strategies have been utilized to increase the selectivity of AMPs for microbes over host cells, including the manipulation of physiochemical properties of AMPs by modifying the number and position of hydrophobic residues, the overall hydrophobic moment (amphipathicity) and the net charge. Other modifications such as the incorporation of fluorinated amino acids and peptoids (N-substituted Gly) can also confer selectivity to the AMPs directed at microbial membranes in certain peptides by decreasing proteolytic degradation, enhancing antimicrobial activity, decreasing hemolysis, and/or combinations thereof [27, 29]. However, the most dramatic sequence modification to introduce selectivity was the concept of "specificity determinants", developed by Hodges and coworkers [13–19], whereby a single Lys substitution of a residue in the center of the non-polar face of amphipathic α-helical peptides dramatically reduced toxicity. Most recently, they demonstrated that the incorporation of two Lys residues into the center of the non-polar face could further reduce toxicity to mammalian cells. The requirement of one or two specificity determinants to reduce toxicity is dependent on the overall hydrophobicity of the non-polar face of the peptide.

4.3
Structure–Activity Relationship Studies of Amphipathic α-Helical and Cyclic β-Sheet Antimicrobial Peptides: Optimization of Pathogen Selectivity and Prevention of Host Toxicity

Our laboratory has demonstrated that there are distinct characteristics of amphipathic α-helical AMPs important for selective antimicrobial activity, and that these characteristics can be explicitly designed into our peptides. The features that can be manipulated to selectively target pathogens are (i) positive charge, (ii) hydrophobicity, (iii) amphipathicity, (iv) structural content in aqueous versus hydrophobic environments, (v) incorporation of specificity determinants, (vi) self-association,

(vii) chirality, and (viii) maintaining non-specific interactions with the membrane by avoiding stereochemical interactions with target molecules (enzymes, proteins, or lipids).

Cyclization can also modulate hemolytic and antimicrobial activity and has been applied to AMPs along with the incorporation of D-amino acids, resulting in peptides that demonstrated low hemolytic activity, high antimicrobial activity, and proteolytic stability.

Gramicidin S (GS, cyclo(Val-Orn-Leu-D-Phe-Pro)$_2$) is a naturally occurring cyclic 10-residue antimicrobial peptide (Figure 4.1) that demonstrates both antimicrobial and hemolytic activity. GS is an amphipathic antiparallel β-sheet with the hydrophobic side chains of Val and Leu protruding from the hydrophobic face and the basic side chain of the Orn residues projecting from the hydrophilic face. The impact of changing ring size on both antimicrobial and hemolytic activity of GS led to the discovery of a 14-residue analog, GS14 (cyclo-(VKLKVY$_d$PLKVKLY$_d$P), where Y$_d$ is Tyr in the D-conformation (Figure 4.1) that was essentially devoid of antimicrobial activity but demonstrated high hemolytic activity [30]. In contrast,

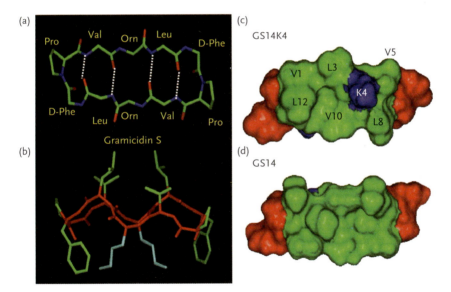

Figure 4.1 Structure of Gramicidin S (10-residue cyclic peptide) and analogs GS14 and GS14K4 (14-residue cyclic peptides). (a) Stick diagram of Gramicidin S and the corresponding intramolecular hydrogen bonds between the two strands of the beta-sheet in the cyclic peptide (dotted lines). (b) shows the amphipathic nature of Gramicidin S with 2 Val and 2 Leu residues (green) on the non-polar face and 2 Orn residues (blue) on the polar face. (c) Connolly surface representation of GS14K4 showing a D-Lys substituted for L-Lys at position 4 (the change in stereochemistry moves the Lys side-chain from the polar face to the center of the non-polar face) and GS14 (d). Green represents the hydrophobes in the non-polar face, red represents the residues in the beta-turns, D-Tyr and Pro in both turns of GS14 and GS14K4, and blue represents positively charged residues. The polar face of GS14 contains 4 Lys residues while the polar face of GS14K4 contains 3 Lys residues. Taken from Hodges *et al.* [9].

the 12 residue analog GS12 (cyclo-(VKLKY$_d$PKVKLY$_d$P) exhibited decreased hemolytic activity and a corresponding increase in Gram-negative selectivity compared to GS, but demonstrated a decrease in selectivity for Gram-positive bacteria. Both GS and GS14 maintained high β-sheet structure under aqueous conditions as opposed to GS12, which is disordered in the same aqueous medium. These results clearly demonstrated that hemolytic activity could be readily dissociated from antimicrobial activity by proper distribution of basic residues and control over the structural content of these peptides in aqueous versus hydrophobic media [31]. Further modification to the GS core by introducing a D-amino acid into each position of the sequence of GS14 resulted in diastereomers with disrupted β-sheet structures under aqueous conditions, as well as decreased amphipathicity (as determined by RP-HPLC). A 130-fold reduction in hemolytic activity and resulting 6500-fold increase in selectivity (therapeutic index) for Gram-negative bacteria (*P. aeruginosa* H188 and *E. coli* DC2) was observed for one analog GS14K4 (cyclo-(VKLK$_d$VY$_d$PLKVKLY$_d$P) compared to GS14. Analysis of GS14 and GS14K4 by nuclear magnetic resonance revealed that the single enantiomeric substitution of D-Lys for L-Lys at position 4 placed the basic side chain into the hydrophobic face of the β-sheet. This substitution decreased the hydrophobicity of the non-polar face, lowered the amphipathicity of the peptide, and disrupted the formation of the β-sheet secondary structure under aqueous conditions. The reduction in amphipathicity is correlated with reduced hemolytic activity, whereas lack of structure in an aqueous environment is proposed to enhance penetration of the peptides through the cell wall to reach the inner membrane (i.e., hydrophobic environment) of the bacterial cell where secondary structure is induced [31]. These studies were the first step that led to the concept of the specificity determinant, that is, placing a positively charged side-chain in the center of the non-polar face of amphipathic cyclic β-sheet and amphipathic α-helical AMPs to dramatically decrease toxicity [13, 31, 32].

The development of therapeutically relevant AMPs was further investigated in structure–activity relationship (SAR) studies of an α-helical AMP. V681 (also referred to as V13 in this chapter) is a 26-residue amphipathic α-helical peptide (Figure 4.2) that was prepared through random DNA mutagenesis of the antimicrobial peptide hybrid Cecropin A (1–8) Melittin B (1–18) [33, 34]. This amphipathic peptide has a hydrophilic face comprised of 14 residues and a non-polar face comprised of 12 residues. Peptide V13 has antimicrobial activity against both Gram-positive and Gram-negative bacteria but is also highly hemolytic.

To probe the dissociation of hemolytic and antimicrobial activity, Chen *et al.*, 2005 used *de novo* design to alter the biophysical properties of V13, including hydrophobicity, helicity, amphipathicity, and self-association [13].

Reversed-phase high performance liquid chromatography (RP-HPLC) and circular dichroism (CD) spectroscopy were used to measure the impact of selective modifications to specific biophysical properties of these peptides. RP-HPLC analysis is a useful technique to measure peptide hydrophobicity and self-association [13] as the retention time of a peptide reflects its ability to interact with the hydrophobic column matrix. RP-HPLC of peptides at 5, 35, and 80 °C (Figure 4.3)

(a)

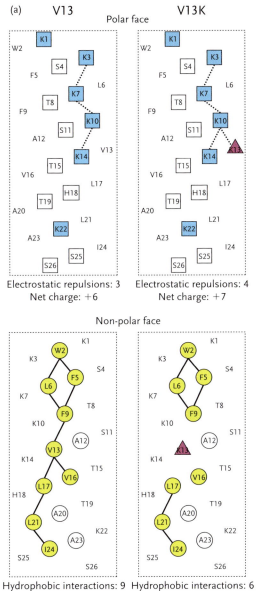

Electrostatic repulsions: 3   Electrostatic repulsions: 4
Net charge: +6   Net charge: +7

Hydrophobic interactions: 9   Hydrophobic interactions: 6
# of large hydrophobes 9   # of large hydrophobes 8

Figure 4.2 (Continued)

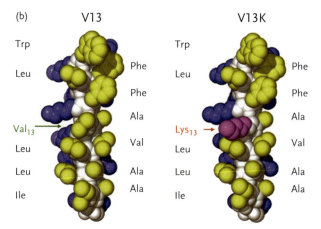

Figure 4.2 Helical net representations and space filling models of alpha-helical antimicrobial peptides V13 and V13K. In the helical nets (a) residues contributing to the polar face are boxed and displayed in the center of the net. Residues contributing to the non-polar face are circled and displayed in the center of the net. Large hydrophobes are colored yellow and positively charged residues are colored blue. The "specificity determinant " lysine residue at position 13 in the center of the non-polar face of V13K is denoted by a pink triangle. The i to i + 3 and i to i + 4 hydrophobic interactions between large hydrophobes along the helix are shown as black bars. The dotted bars denote potential electrostatic repulsions between i to i + 3 and i to i + 4 positively charged residues along the helix. In the space filling models (b) the positively charged residues are colored blue and the hydrophobic residues are colored yellow. The peptide backbone is colored white. The "specificity determinant" lysine residue at position 13 in the center of the non-polar face of peptide V13K is colored pink. The peptides shown here are in the all L-conformation. Adapted from Jiang *et al.* 2011 [19].

can be used to profile peptide self-association [35, 36] (dimerization/oligomerization at the hydrophobic face) based on the interaction of the available hydrophobic surface of peptide monomers versus dimers. Under RP-HPLC conditions peptides retain helicity, even at high temperatures, and, therefore, the ability to dimerize. At low temperatures the peptides favor dimerization via interactions between the non-polar face of each peptide during the partitioning between the mobile and stationary phases of RP-HPLC, which limits the hydrophobic surface available to interact with the reversed phase matrix and results in earlier elution times. At higher temperatures the peptides are predominantly in the monomeric α-helical state and interact more with the hydrophobic matrix, leading to later elution times. At temperatures above the association parameter, peptides are in equilibrium between α-helical and unstructured random coil states with the random coil structure dominating at the highest temperatures. Changes in elution times were used to characterize SAR of analogs of the amphipathic α-helical AMP V13 (Figure 4.4) [14].

Previous studies in the Hodges laboratory demonstrated that substitutions of centrally located residues in AMPs had the greatest impact on secondary structure [37, 38]. Therefore, the native Val at position 13 on the non-polar face and Ser at

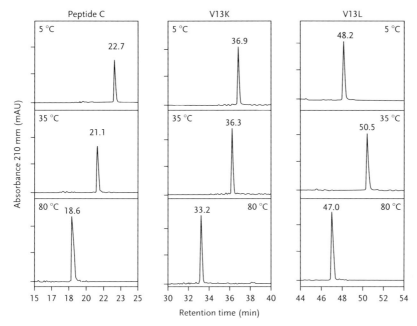

Figure 4.3 Effect of temperature on reversed-phase HPLC (RP-HPLC) elution profiles of control peptide C, peptide V13K and peptide V13L. Conditions are as follows: RP-HPLC, narrow-bore SB-C8 column (150 × 2.1 mm I.D.; 5 μm particle size, 300 Å pore size), linear AB gradient (1% acetonitrile/min.) at a flow rate of 0.25 ml min^{-1}, where eluent A is 0.05% aqueous trifluoroacetic acid (TFA) and eluent B is 0.05% TFA in acetonitrile. Only RP-HPLC profiles of peptide C, peptide V13K, and peptide V13L at 5, 35, and 80 °C were selected as examples to show the temperature effect. See Chen *et al.* 2005 for details [13].

position 11 on the polar face of V13 were substituted with Leu, Val, Ala, Gly, Ser, and Lys (given in order of decreasing hydrophobicity, Table 4.1). The relative hydrophobicity of amino acid side-chains is one of the most important factors in understanding peptide/protein structure, function, and biomolecular interactions. Thus, it is important to utilize the most accurate scale of the intrinsic hydrophilicity/hydrophobicity of amino acid side-chains [39, 40].

One of the most exciting analogs of peptide V13 resulted from the placement of Lys at position 13 (non-polar face) to give analog V13K (Figure 4.2). This substitution places the basic side-chain of Lys in the center of the hydrophobic face, thus interrupting the hydrophobic surface and yielding two distinct hydrophobic patches. While V13 is α-helical in benign media, V13K displays negligible structure under the same aqueous conditions (Figure 4.5). V13K also demonstrated an overall decrease in hydrophobicity, as determined by RP-HPLC, and decreased amphipathicity compared to the parent peptide V13. These characteristics led to a more than 32-fold decrease in hemolytic activity (undetectable in the assay) compared to V13 [13]. V13K demonstrated broad-spectrum antimicrobial activity and did not exhibit hemolytic activity after 8 h. Thus, incorporation of the basic

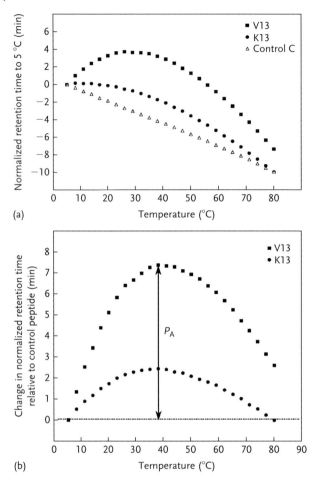

Figure 4.4 Measurement of peptide V13 and peptide K13 self-assembly using RP-HPLC temperature profiling. In (a) the retention time of each peptide at a given temperature is normalized to the retention time at 5 °C using the expression $(t_R{}^t - t_R{}^5)$, where $t_R{}^t$ is the retention time at a given temperature and $t_R{}^5$ is the retention time at 5 °C (26 elution profiles are obtained by running every 3 °C from 5 to 80 °C). In (b) the retention properties of each peptide were further normalized against a random-coil control peptide using the expression $(t_R{}^t - t_R{}^5$ for peptide X) $- (t_R{}^t - t_R{}^5$ for control peptide). The maximal change in retention time relative to the control peptide is defined as the association parameter (P_A). See Chen *et al.* 2006 for details [14].

side chain of Lys into the center of the hydrophobic face of the helix renders microbial specificity to the peptide and is, therefore, referred to as a "specificity determinant."

Further substitution of the non-polar face of V13 at position 13 with Leu increased the hydrophobicity and amphipathicity, while substitution with Ala decreased both of these parameters but maintained high helicity [13]. Substitution

Table 4.1 Antimicrobial activity and hemolytic activity of non-polar face and polar face substituted peptide analogs.

	1	11 13	26
V681 (V13)	Ac-K-W-K-S-F-L-K-T-F-K-S-A-V-K-T-V-L-H-T-A-L-K-A-I-S-S-amide		
S11X$_L$	Ac------------------------------------X$_L$--amide		
S11X$_D$	Ac------------------------------------X$_D$--amide		
V13X$_L$	Ac---X$_L$-------------------------------amide		
V13X$_D$	Ac---X$_D$-------------------------------amide		

	Gram-negative pathogens				Gram-positive pathogens		
Peptide	MIC$_{GM}$[a]	MHC[b]	Therapeutic index[c]	Peptide	MIC$_{GM}$[d]	MHC[b]	Therapeutic index[c]
V13	8.8	15.6	1.8	V13	6.3	15.6	2.5
V13L	12.7	7.8	0.6	V13L	10.9	7.8	0.7
V13A	3.8	31.2	8.1	V13A	4.5	31.2	6.9
V13G	4.1	125.0	30.2	V13G	7.4	125.0	16.9
V13S	4.2	125.0	30.1	V13S	7.4	125.0	16.9
V13K[e]	3.1	>250.0	163.0	**V13K**[e]	11.8	>250.0	42.3
V13V$_D$	3.3	62.5	19	V13V$_D$	2.8	62.5	22.7
V13L$_D$	5.5	7.8	1.4	V13L$_D$	3.3	7.8	2.4
V13A$_D$[e]	3.3	250.0	75.7	**V13A$_D$**[e]	4.3	250.0	57.8
V13S$_D$	6.3	>250.0	79.9	V13S$_D$	16.0	>250.0	31.3
V13K$_D$	7.7	>250.0	65.0	V13K$_D$	18.7	>250.0	26.8
V13	8.8	15.6	1.8	V13	6.3	15.6	2.5
S11L	16.6	4.0	0.2	S11L	14.8	4.0	0.3
S11V	9.7	7.8	0.8	S11V	6.9	7.8	1.1
S11A	8.3	15.6	1.9	S11A	6.6	15.6	2.4
S11G	5.2	7.8	1.5	S11G	4.5	7.8	1.7
S11K	13.7	4.0	0.3	S11K	10.5	4.0	0.4
S11V$_D$	6.1	125.0	20.5	S11V$_D$	6.6	125.0	19.0
S11L$_D$	5.0	31.2	6.2	S11L$_D$	4.7	31.2	6.7
S11A$_D$	4.3	15.6	3.6	S11A$_D$	3.8	15.6	4.1
S11S$_D$	2.9	15.6	5.3	S11S$_D$	2.3	15.6	6.7
S11K$_D$	2.6	31.2	11.8	S11K$_D$	2.8	31.2	11.0

[a]Antimicrobial activity (minimal inhibitory concentration) in µg ml^{-1} is given as the geometric mean (MIC$_{GM}$) of the minimal inhibitory concentration (MIC) values from triplicate experimental results against 6 strains of Gram-negative bacteria (*Escherichia coli* UB1005 wild type (wt), *E. coli* DC2 antibiotic sensitive (abs), *Salmonella typhimurium* C610 abs, *Pseudomonas aeruginosa* H187 wt, *P. aeruginosa* H188 abs).

[b]Hemolytic activity (minimal hemolytic concentration, MHC) in µg ml^{-1} was determined using human erythrocytes. A concentration of 500 µg ml^{-1} was used to determine the therapeutic index in cases where 250 µg ml^{-1} did not produce any detectable hemolysis.

[c]Therapeutic index was calculated by MHC (µg ml^{-1})/MIC$_{GM}$.

[d]Antimicrobial activity (minimal inhibitory concentration) in µg ml^{-1} is given as the geometric mean (MIC$_{GM}$) of the minimal inhibitory concentration (MIC) values from triplicate experimental results against against 6 strains of Gram-positive bacteria (*Staphylococcus aeureus* 25923 wt, *S. aereus* SAP0017 methicillin-resistant strain, *S. epidermidis* C621 wt, *Bacillus subtilis* C971 wt, *Enterococcus faecalis* C625 wt, *Corynebacterium xerosis* C875 wt).

[e]The compounds with the highest therapeutic indices for both Gram-negative and Gram-positive pathogens are highlighted in bold.

Data from Chen et al. 2005 [13]

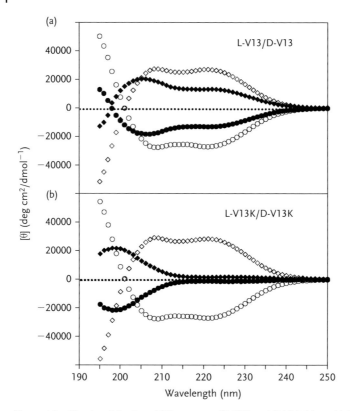

Figure 4.5 Circular dichroism (CD) spectra of L-V13 and D-V13 (a) and L-V13K and D-V13K peptides (b). Circles denote L-peptides (all residues in the L-conformation) and diamonds denote D-peptides (all residues in the D-conformation). Solid symbols show spectra obtained for peptides in 50 mM aqueous potassium phosphate buffer, pH 7, containing 100 mM KCl. Open symbols show spectra collected in the presence of aqueous buffer containing 50% trifluoroethanol (TFE is a non-polar helix-inducing solvent that mimics the hydrophobicity and helix-inducing properties of the membrane). See Chen *et al.* 2006 for details [14].

with either Ser or Lys resulted in decreased hydrophobicity of the non-polar face and, subsequently, decreased amphipathicity of the helix. Helicity of the peptide in benign media was significantly influenced by the hydrophobicity of the amino acid substituted on the non-polar face, such that helical content was higher when the amino acid was hydrophobic and decreased with decreasing hydrophobicity in the order V13L > V13V > V13A > V13S > V13K. Interestingly, while Ala has the highest helical propensity of the 20 naturally occurring amino acids [41], the helicity of V13A was lower than that of V13L, demonstrating the importance of the continuous hydrophobic surface of large hydrophobes on the non-polar face of the helix [13]. Non-polar environments, such as 50% trifluoroethanol (TFE), were capable of inducing helical structure in all of the peptides substituted at the non-polar face, regardless of the amino acid substitution.

Hemolytic activity was associated with the hydrophobicity of the amino acid substituted at position 13 of the non-polar face, such that hemolysis decreased in the order: L>V>A>S>K, which is in agreement with previous studies of Gramicidin S [30, 31]. The antimicrobial activity of the non-polar face substituted analogs against Gram-negative and Gram-positive pathogens was similar to V13 with V13K demonstrating the greatest improvement in activity against Gram-negative organisms. A slight decrease in activity against Gram-positive microbes was observed with the substitution of native Val with the more hydrophobic side chain of Leu [13]. Thus, the dramatic increase in the therapeutic index of V13K (90-fold improvement for Gram-negative pathogens) was a result of the significant decrease in hemolytic activity and a 2.8-fold improvement antimicrobial activity (Table 4.1).

On the polar face of V13 the native amino acid residue at position 11 is Ser and substitution with Leu, Val, and Ala increased the hydrophobicity of the polar face and, therefore, resulted in decreased amphipathicity. Lys substitution, on the other hand, increased the hydrophilicity of the polar face and led to a corresponding increase in amphipathicity [13]. The polar face substitutions led to a slight increase in hemolytic activity but maintained similar antimicrobial activity against Gram-negative and Gram-positive pathogens, with the exception of S11K which had decreased antimicrobial activity compared to the parent peptide V13.

The polar face substitutions of peptide V13 affected the helical content of the peptides differently than the non-polar face counterparts. As expected, the substitution of Leu on the polar face was more destabilizing to the helix compared to non-polar face substitution with Leu, which stabilized helical structure. Both Ala and Ser stabilized helical content when substituted on the polar face, as opposed to their destabilizing effects when incorporated at position 13 on the non-polar face [13].

The ability of peptides to self-associate in aqueous media was also linked with antimicrobial and hemolytic activity in that a lower ability to self-associate correlated with reduced hemolysis [15]. Self-association and helicity were positively correlated with peptide hydrophobicity (Figure 4.6 and Table 4.2).

In an effort to further disrupt the helical structure, single substitutions with D-amino acids were made at the center of the non-polar face of V13 at position 13 and position 11 on the polar face [13]. Kondejewski *et al.* 1999 [31] demonstrated that hemolytic activity could be dissociated from antimicrobial activity in Gramicidin S analogs by incorporation of a D-amino acid into the central portion of the β-sheet. In the case of alpha helical peptides, the substitution of a D-amino acid into a single position of an otherwise all L-peptide resulted in the disruption of the helical structure [13]. The amino acids substituted at positions 11 and 13 represented a spectrum of hydrophobicity in the order from most hydrophobic to least: Leu>Val>Ala>Gly>Ser>Lys [39, 40].

That helical content is also correlated with hemolysis was further confirmed by the observation that the single D-amino acid substitutions demonstrated decreased hemolysis compared to similar substitutions with L-amino acids [13].

The D-amino acid substitutions that led to decreased hydrophobic interactions on the non-polar face, disruption of helical structure and, therefore,

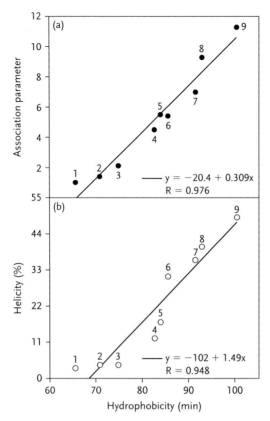

Figure 4.6 Relationship of self-association parameter and helicity versus overall peptide hydrophobicity. (a) The linear correlation of the association parameter and overall peptide hydrophobicity both measured by reversed-phase HPLC. (b) The linear correlation of peptide helicity determined by (CD) and overall hydrophobicity measured by RP-HPLC. Solid symbols, self-association parameter; open symbols, % helicity. The sequences of peptides 1–9, their % helix and hydrophobicity are shown in Table 4.2. See Chen *et al.* 2007 for details [15].

self-association, ultimately resulted in decreased hemolytic activity [13]. The substitution of Val at position 13 of peptide V13 with D-Ala (V13A$_D$) decreased hemolytic activity by sixteen-fold and either improved or maintained the MIC values of the parent peptide. This observation signifies the importance of structure on toxicity toward eukaryotic cells demonstrated by various amphipathic α-helical AMPs and extends the designation of the "specificity determinant" to include any amino acid substitution on the non-polar face of these peptides that results in a significant reduction in hemolytic activity.

Since the goal of these studies is to identify antimicrobial peptides that are capable of acting as therapeutic agents, these peptides (or their analogs) will ultimately be exposed to the proteolytic enzymes of both the host and the target microbe. To overcome degradation of the AMPs by natural proteases the

Table 4.2 Biophysical data of L-V13K$_L$ analogs.

No.	Denotation	Sequence	Hydrophobicity[a]		% Helicity[b]	$P_A{}^c$
			t_R (min)	Δt_R		
1	L6A/L21A	Ac-KWKSFAKTFKSAKKTVLHTAAKAISS-amide	65.6	−9.2	3	1.0
2	L6A	Ac-KWKSFAKTFKSAKKTVLHTAAKAISS-amide	70.8	−4.0	4	1.4
3	V13K$_L$	Ac-KWKSFLKTFKSAKKTVLHTAAKAISS-amide	74.8	0	4	2.1
4	A23L	Ac-KWKSFLKTFKSAKKTVLHTAAKLISS-amide	82.6	7.8	12	4.5
5	A12L	Ac-KWKSFLKTFKSLKKTVLHTAAKAISS-amide	83.9	9.1	17	5.5
6	A20L	Ac-KWKSFLKTFKSAKKTVLHTLAKAISS-amide	85.5	10.7	31	5.4
7	A12L/A23L	Ac-KWKSFLKTFKSLKKTVLHTAAKLISS-amide	91.4	16.6	36	7.0
8	A12L/A20L	Ac-KWKSFLKTFKSLKKTVLHTLAKAISS-amide	92.8	18.0	40	9.3
9	A12L/A20L/A23L	Ac-KWKSFLKTFKSLKKTVLHTLAKLISS-amide	100.4	25.6	49	11.3

^{a}The peptides are ordered by increasing hydrophobicity as determined by the retention time (t_R) of the peptides in RP-HPLC at room temperature and pH 2.$\Delta t_R{}^t$ is the difference in retention time between the peptide analog and the native peptide L-V13K (i.e., $t_{RX} - t_R$ $_{L-V13}$).

^{b}Helical content of the peptides reported as percent helicity in benign media.

^{c}Dimerization parameter (P_A) from RP-HPLC temperature profiling experiments calculated by the maximal retention time difference: ($t_R{}^t - t_R{}^5$ for peptide analogs) − ($t_R{}^t - t_R{}^5$ for a control peptide) where $t_R{}^t - t_R{}^5$ is the difference in retention time.

Adapted from Chen et al. 2007 [15].

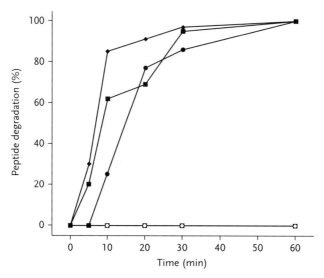

Figure 4.7 Peptide stability to proteolytic digestion by trypsin. Closed symbols denote L-peptides and open symbols D-peptides. The circles represent L-V13 and D-V13, the squares L-V13K and D-V13K and the diamonds L-V13A$_D$ and D-V13A$_L$. The prefix L- and D- represent all L and all D residues, respectively, except where noted. The two all D-peptides and D-V13A$_L$ (contains one L-amino acid at position 13) show no proteolysis. See Chen *et al.* 2006 for details [14].

enantiomers of V13 and V13K were prepared and subjected to proteolytic digestion, hemolysis assays, antimicrobial assays and biophysical characterization [14]. The L and D forms of the peptides yield mirror images in CD of the peptides in both benign and helix inducing environments (Figure 4.5). The L peptide (L-V13) and the D analog of V13 are helical in both media whereas the D and L enantiomers of V13K were unstructured random-coils under benign conditions (50 mM aqueous potassium phosphate buffer, pH 7, containing 100 mM KCl) and helical in 50% trifluoroethanol (TFE). The D enantiomer of V13K (denoted D-V13K or D1) exhibited complete proteolytic stability when incubated with trypsin for 8 h at 37 °C, while L-V13K was completely degraded within 60 min (Figure 4.7). Peptide D-V13K (D1) had either identical or greater antimicrobial activity over L-V13K, which further supports the assumption that the target of these peptides is the bacterial membrane, and so antimicrobial activity does not rely on specific chiral interactions with protein receptors, proteins, or lipid molecules. A slightly enhanced MIC for D1 over L-V13K was observed in assays with certain strains of *P. aeruginosa* and Gram-positive pathogens such as *S. aureus*, *S. epidermidis*, and *E. faecalis*, and is assumed to result from the proteolytic stability of D1, which is not possessed by L-V13K.

The rational design of peptides targeting Gram-negative bacteria was further examined by the incorporation of multiple specificity determinants in conjunction with the modulation of non-polar face hydrophobicity. Using D1 as a lead compound, various analogs were prepared and examined for MIC and hemolytic activity [16–19].

Helical net representations of the non-polar faces of the analogs of D1 are given in Figure 4.8. The hydrophobic residues that reside along the center of the non-polar face are colored green (Trp, Phe, Val, Ile) or yellow (Leu). The specificity determinant is defined by a pink triangle. The i to i + 3 and i to i + 4 hydrophobic interactions between large hydrophobes are denoted as solid black lines.

Analogs D1(K13) and D11 have identical non-polar faces comprised of eight large hydrophobic side-chains, six hydrophobic interactions and one specificity determinant located at position 13 [19]. However, these peptides differ in their polar face such that there is a cluster of four Lys residues incorporated into the center of the polar face of D11 (K11, K14, K15, and K18) and the positive charges extend linearly in both directions from the cluster to increase the net charge to +10 for D11 compared to +7 for D1. The result is an increase in antimicrobial activity (2.6-fold for *P. aeruginosa* and 1.8-fold for *A. baumannii*), a concomitant decrease in hemolytic activity (Table 4.3) by 1.8-fold and resulting increase in therapeutic index (3.3-fold for *A. baummanni* and 4.6-fold for *P. aeruginosa*). D11 demonstrated the weakest hemolytic activity of all the D analogs possessing one specificity determinant (D1(V13), D1(K13), D22, and D15). The overall hydrophobicity, amphipathicity, and association parameter was greater for D11 than for D1(K13) (Table 4.4).

An increase in the hydrophobic interactions of the non-polar face was achieved by substituting and re-arranging hydrophobic residues of D11 (Val16Ala and Ala20Leu) to give D22 which has eight hydrophobic interactions compared to six for D11 [19]. The polar face of these peptides is identical and both peptides possess a specificity determinant at position 13 on the non-polar face. The result is an increase in hydrophobicity, amphipathicity, and association parameter (Table 4.4), with a corresponding decrease in antimicrobial activity and increase in hemolytic activity and, therefore, a decreased therapeutic index. Thus, the increase in hydrophobicity led to a decrease in the therapeutic index of D22 compared to D11 (Table 4.3).

The incorporation of a second specificity determinant into position 16 of D22 (A16K) yielded analog D14, which has an identical polar face to D22 and two hydrophobic clusters on the non-polar face, the same as D22. The incorporation of the second specificity determinant (K16) into the peptide decreased the hydrophobicity by 8.9 min by RP-HPLC and the amphipathicity from 6.07 for D22 to 5.92 for D14. The resulting therapeutic index of D14 was similar to D11 (Table 4.3).

The substitution of residues W2, F5, F9, V16, and I24 in D11 with Leu to give peptide D15 resulted in an increase in hydrophobicity and a dramatic increase in self-association [19]. The change in hydrophobic side-chains of the hydrophobic cluster to all Leu had a minimal effect on MIC compared to D11 but increased hemolytic activity from 254.1 μM for D11 to 169.6 μM for D15 (Table 4.3).

Peptide D16, which is the Leu-substituted analog of D14, has a therapeutic index of 3355 for *A. baumannii* and 895 for *P. aeruginosa* as a result of a substantially

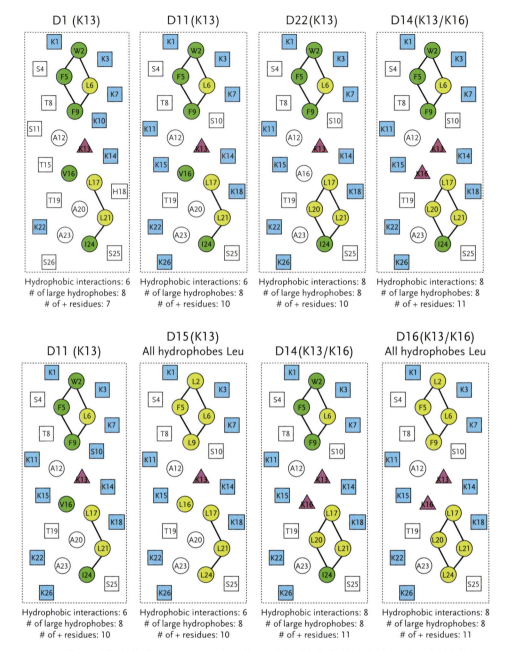

Figure 4.8 Helical net representations for peptides D1, D11, D22, D14, D15, and D16. The non-polar face of the alpha-helical antimicrobial peptide is displayed along the center of the helical net. The one letter code is used for amino acid residues. The D denotes that all residues in the peptides are in the D-conformation. The "specificity determinant(s)" lysine residue(s) at position 13 only or position 13 and 16 in the center of the non-polar face are denoted by pink triangle(s). The non-polar residues are displayed along the center of the helical nets and are circled. The large hydrophobes other than leucine residues (Trp, Phe, Val, and Ile) are colored green and the leucine residues are colored yellow. The i to i + 3 and i to i + 4 hydrophobic interactions between large hydrophobes along the helix are shown as black bars. The residues on the polar face are boxed and the positively charged residues are colored blue. Taken from Jiang et al. 2011 [19].

Table 4.3 Summary of biological activity of D1 analogs.

| | Hemolytic activity | | Antimicrobial activity | | | | | |
| | | | Acinetobacter baumannii | | | Pseudomonas aeruginosa | | |
Peptide name	HC$_{50}$^{a} (μM)	Fold^b	GM^c (μM)	T. I.^{d}	Fold^e	GM^c (μM)	T. I.^{d}	Fold^e
D1 (V13)	1.8	1.0	0.7	2.57	1.0	1.8	1.0	1.0
D1 (K13)	140.9	78.3	1.1	128.1	49.8	4.1	34.4	34.4
D11	254.1	141.2	0.6	423.5	164.8	1.6	158.8	158.8
D22	81.3	45.2	0.8	101.6	39.5	2.3	35.3	35.3
D14	351.5	195.3	0.8	439.4	171.0	2.5	140.6	140.6
D15	169.6	94.2	0.5	339.2	132.0	1.0	169.6	169.6
D16	1342.0^f	745.6	0.4	3355.0	1305.4	1.5	894.7	894.7

^{a}HC$_{50}$ is the concentration of peptide that results in 50% hemolysis after 18 h at 37 °C. The hemolytic activities that are lower than the original lead peptide D1 (K13) are in bold.
^{b}The fold improvement in HC$_{50}$ compared to that of D1 (V13).
^{c}MIC is the minimum inhibitory concentration of peptide that inhibits growth of bacteria after 24 h at 37 °C. GM is the geometric mean of the MIC values from 11 different isolates of A. baumannii or 6 different isolates of P. aeruginosa.
^{d}Therapeutic index (T.I.) is the ratio of the HC$_{50}$ value (μM) over the geometric mean MIC value (μM). Large values indicate greater antimicrobial specificity. The therapeutic indices with values ≥100 for A. baumannii and P. aeruginosa are bolded.
^{e}The fold improvement in therapeutic index compared to that of D1 (V13). Greater than 100-fold improvements are bolded.
^{f}The percent lysis for peptide D16 was only 10.7% after 18 h.
Data taken from Jiang et al. 2011 [19].

Table 4.4 Biophysical data of all D conformation analogs.

Peptide	Net charge	Hydrophobicity (t_R)^a	% Helicity^b	P$_A$^{c}	Amphipathicity^d
D1(V13)	+6	102.5	34	7.14	5.56
D1	+7	76.8	3	2.78	4.92
D11	+10	85.4	2	3.31	5.57
D22	+10	90.7	28	5.13	6.07
D14	+11	81.8	5	3.07	5.92
D15	+10	93.0	11	7.4	5.29
D16	+11	83.8	9	5.17	5.42

^{a}Retention time (t_R) of the peptides in RP-HPLC at room temperature and pH 2.
^{b}Helical content of the peptides reported as percent helicity in benign media.
^{c}Association parameter (P_A) from RP-HPLC temperature profiling experiments calculated by the maximal retention time difference: ($t_R{}^t - t_R{}^5$ for peptide analogs) − ($t_R{}^t - t_R{}^5$ for a control peptide) where $t_R{}^t - t_R{}^5$ is the difference in retention time.
^{d}Amphipathicity was determined by calculation of hydrophobic moment, see Jiang et al. 2011 [19] for details.

decreased hemolysis (HC$_{50}$ of 1342 µM for D16 compared to 351.5 for D14) even though the MIC is similar for both D14 and D16 (Table 4.3) [19].

Compared to our original starting peptide D1(V13), peptide D16 had a 746-fold improvement in the hemolytic activity, that is a decrease, maintained antimicrobial activity and improved therapeutic indices by 1305-fold and 895-fold against *A. baumannii* and *P. aeruginosa*, respectively (Table 4.3). D16 has now become an ideal candidate for the development of a commercial clinical therapeutic to treat Gram-negative bacterial infections.

These studies established three defining characteristics of the activity profile of these amphipathic α-helical peptides: (i) number, location, and pattern of positive charges on the polar face; (ii) number, location, and identity of the hydrophobic residues on the non-polar face; and (iii) number and location of specificity determinants. Figure 4.9 shows the difference between our original starting peptide D1 (V13) and our final lead peptide D16(K13/K16). On the polar face, peptide D1(V13) had a net charge of +6 whereas, D16(K13/K16) had a net charge of +11. In addition, the location and pattern of the positively charged residues was dramatically different between the two peptides. D1(V13) has an uninterrupted hydrophobic surface on its non-polar face of the helix (nine large hydrophobes and nine hydrophobic interactions between these hydrophobes), which stabilizes the α-helix and allows the helix to dimerize/oligomerize by this continuous hydrophobic surface (the ability to self-associate is high). In contrast, D16(K13/K16) has a dramatic change in the type of hydrophobes (8 Leu residues) compared to 1 Trp, 2 Phe, 2 Val, 1 Ile and 3 Leu residues for peptide D1(V13). The arrangement of the hydrophobes is also different with D16(V13/K16) where there are two hydrophobic patches separated by two specificity determinants (2 Lys residues) in the center of the non-polar face. In summary, these two peptides are dramatically different on both faces. These structural changes resulted in removing self-association and helical structure in aqueous solution, allowing inducible structure in hydrophobic media and giving the ideal activity profile for an antimicrobial peptide (limited or no hemolytic activity, excellent antimicrobial activity and exceptional therapeutic indices (Table 4.3)).

There is also an optimum hydrophobicity for antimicrobial activity (Figure 4.10) below and above which antimicrobial activity weakens [15]. For example, V13L is more hemolytic and has lower antimicrobial activity compared to V13K. Since V13L has a continuous hydrophobic face it is proposed to interact less with the water/lipid interface region of the lipid environment and have more transmembrane interactions with the lipid bilayer and, therefore, displays weaker antimicrobial activity compared to V13K, which is more restricted to the interface region. Hemolysis does not share a similar biphasic profile and hemolytic activity does not increase or decrease beyond a threshold of hydrophobicity but increases with increasing hydrophobicity.

Toxicity (i.e., hemolysis) associated with AMPs appears to be strongly dependent on the hydrophobicity, amphiphathicity, and helical content of the peptides. The ability to dissociate toxicity from antimicrobial activity in the α-helical peptide V13 through careful examination of biophysical characteristics appears to be the key to unlocking their therapeutic potential.

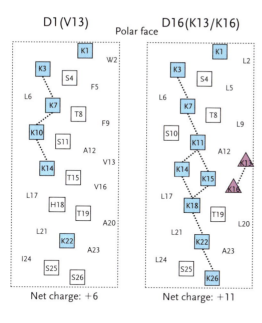

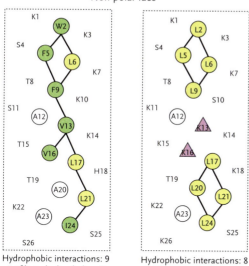

Figure 4.9 Helical net representations for peptides D1(V13) and D16(K13, K16). The upper panels display the polar face residues along the center of the helical net and the lower panels display the non-polar face residues along the center of the helical net. The polar face residues are boxed with the Lys residues colored blue. The non-polar face residues are circled and large hydrophobes Trp, Phe, Val, and Ile are colored green and Leu residues are colored yellow. The i to i + 3 and i to i + 4 hydrophobic interactions between large hydrophobes along the helix are shown as black bars. The specificity determinants, Lys residues, in the center of the non-polar face are denoted by pink triangles. The dotted bars denote potential electrostatic repulsions between i to i + 3 and i to i + 4 positively charged residues along the helix. Adapted from Jiang *et al.* 2011 [19].

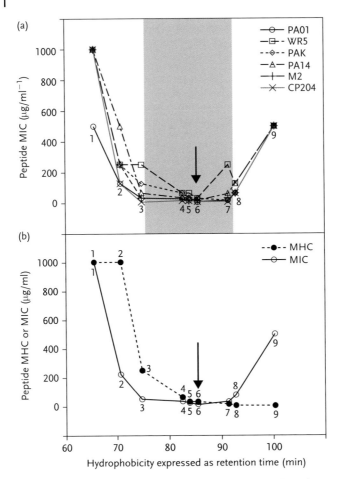

Figure 4.10 Relationship between peptide hydrophobicity, hemolytic activity (MHC), and antibacterial activity (MIC). (a) MIC values for 6 different strains of *Pseudomonas aeruginosa* versus overall peptide hydrophobicity (see Table 4.2). The shaded panel shows the optimal hydrophobicity zone for antimicrobial activity. (b) MIC values plotted as the geometric mean of the MICs for the six *P. aeruginosa* clinical isolates (solid line) and the MHC values (dotted line) versus peptide hydrophobicity. The numbers 1 to 9 denote the nine peptides varying systematically in hydrophobicity shown in Table 4.2. The arrow shows the optimal antimicrobial activity in both (a) and (b). MHC is the maximal peptide concentration that caused no hemolysis of human erythrocytes after 18 h. MIC is the lowest peptide concentration that inhibits growth after 24 h. Peptide 3 (V13K, Table 4.2) has the best therapeutic index of this hydrophobicity series of analogs. See Chen *et al.* 2007 for details [15].

4.4
Commercialization of Antimicrobial Peptides

Some of the concern regarding the development of AMPs as commercial antibiotics involves the potential for the development of resistance. Since the target of AMPs is presumably the cell membrane, and antimicrobial activity is dependent on general peptide–membrane interactions rather than specific peptide–receptor interactions, resistance is expected to be limited. When resistance has been shown to develop with other AMPs it has occurred by either constitutive or inducible mechanisms [11, 28]. Constitutive resistance mechanisms include changes to the electrostatic properties of the membrane that limit attraction to cationic AMPs, or changes to physical characteristics of the membrane that limit the penetration of AMPs. Inducible mechanisms typically involve protease activity or extracellular remodeling.

Other potential drawbacks to the commercialization of AMPs include toxicity, stability, cost of production, and formulation/delivery [42, 43]. Many of these issues are being addressed with the identification of minimal motifs, incorporation of D-amino acids, using branched peptides, employing retro-inverso design, immobilization of AMPs on medical implants, quantitative SAR, and sequence scrambling [8, 29].

4.5
Therapeutic Potential

We have demonstrated that toxicity can be engineered out of amphipathic α-helical peptides and amphipathic cyclic β-sheet peptides by the *de novo* design of peptides with an appropriate balance of specific characteristics. The factors we believe to be important for antimicrobial peptides to have the desired properties of a clinical therapeutic to treat bacterial infections include the following: (i) the presence of positively charged residues resulting in a net positive charge. Not only are the number of positively charged residues important but so is their location on the polar face; (ii) in the case of structured molecules, cyclic β-sheet peptides and α-helical peptides, have an amphipathic nature that segregates basic and polar residues to one face of the molecule (polar face) and hydrophobic residues to the other face (non-polar face). The degree of amphipathicity must also be regulated; (iii) an optimum overall hydrophobicity, including the number of hydrophobic i to $i+3$ / i to $i+4$ interactions between large hydrophobes along the helix; (iv) the importance of lack of structure in aqueous conditions but inducible structure in the presence of the hydrophobic environment of the membrane. The lack of a stable/rigid monomeric structure can prevent high affinity binding of the peptide to the negatively charged surface of lipopolysaccharide on the surface of gram-negative pathogens; (v) the presence of one or more "specificity determinant(s)," that is, a positively charged residue(s) in the center of the non-polar face of an amphipathic cyclic β-sheet and α-helical peptides which serve as a determinant(s) of specificity or selectivity between prokaryotic and eukaryotic cell membranes, that is, they reduce or eliminate toxicity as measured by hemolytic activity against human red blood cells. This can also be accomplished by changing the stereochemistry of the substituting residue in the center of the non-polar face of the molecule; (vi) these specificity determinants locate amphipathic peptides to the interface region of prokaryotic membranes and decrease or eliminate transmembrane penetration into eukaryotic membranes; (vii) the importance of eliminating or dramatically reducing peptide self-association in an aqueous environment to allow the monomeric unstructured peptide to pass more easily through the cell wall components to reach the cytopasmic bacterial membrane. Peptide self-association stabilizes structured dimers/oligomers which could hinder or prevent peptide translocation through the cell wall components to access the membrane in prokaryotic cells; (viii) the sole target for the antimicrobial peptide should be the bacterial membrane and the peptide should not be involved in any stereoselective interactions with chiral enzymes, lipids, or proteins; (ix) the use of the all D-enantiomer provides excellent peptide stability and resistance to proteolysis; and (x) if these AMPs are to be used as systemic therapeutics then the extent of serum binding to serum proteins must be modulated in the design process, since only the concentration of the unbound peptide is available to interact with the membrane as the therapeutic target.

There are a number of companies with AMP-based products in various stages of clinical development with activities ranging from the treatment of sepsis to non-small cell lung cancer [8, 42, 44–46]. These peptides are derived from a diverse array of sources including mammalian and plant host defense peptides.

AMPs offer numerous therapeutic prospects, especially for the treatment of diseases that lack effective medicines. The potential patent coverage of AMPs is vast and ranges from patenting AMPs themselves to AMP specific antibodies, peptide formulations and novel techniques for the identification of AMP susceptible microbes [45]. Peptide formulations covered under some recent patents include ointments, tablets, injections, depots, aerosols, and others, along with corresponding delivery options including oral, transdermal, injection, and rectal administration.

With so much potential for therapeutic development, AMPs are promising candidates for the next generation of antibiotics targeting multi-drug and pan-drug resistant pathogens.

References

1 Boucher, H.W.,Talbot, G.H., Bradley, J.S., Edwards, J.E., Gilbert, D., Rice, L. B., Scheld, M., Spellberg, B., and Bartlett, J. (2009) Bad bugs, no drugs: no ESKAPE! An update from the Infectious Diseases Society of America. *Clin. Infect. Dis.*, **48**, 1–12.

2 Rice, L.B. (2008) Federal funding for the study of antimicrobial resistance in nosocomial pathogens: no ESKAPE. *J. Infect. Dis.*, **197**, 1079–1081.

3 Maragakis, L.L. (2010) Recognition and prevention of multidrug-resistant Gram-negative bacteria in the intensive care unit. *Crit. Care Med.*, **38**, S345–S351.

4 Ho, J., Tambyah, P.A., and Paterson, D.L. (2010) Multiresistant Gram-negative infections: a global perspective. *Curr. Opin. Infect. Dis.*, **23**, 546–553.

5 Falagas, M.E. and Kasiakou, S.K. (2005) Colistin: the revival of polymyxins for the management of multidrug-resistant gram-negative bacterial infections. *Clin. Infect. Dis.*, **40**, 1333–1341.

6 Falagas, M.E. and Rafailidis, P.I. (2008) Re-emergence of colistin in today's world of multidrug-resistant organisms: personal perspectives. *Expert Opin. Investig. Drugs*, **17**, 973–981.

7 Anderluh, G. and Lakey, J. (Eds.) (2010) Proteins: membrane binding and pore formation. Austin, Texas, Landes Bioscience. *Advances in Experimental Medicine and Biology*, **677**, 1–167.

8 Kindrachuk, J. and Napper, S. (2010) Structure–activity relationships of multifunctional host defence peptides. *Mini Rev. Med. Chem.*, **10**, 596–614.

9 Hodges, R.S., Jiang, Z., Whitehurst, J., and Mant, C.T. Development of antimicrobial peptides as therapeutic agents, in *Development of Therapeutic Agents, Handbook in Pharmaceutical Sciences* (eds Gad, S. and Eventhal, M.), John Wiley and Sons, in press.

10 Shafer, W.M. (2006) SpringerLink (Online service). Antimicrobial peptides and human disease, in *Current Topics in Microbiology and Immunology*, Springer-Verlag, Berlin, Heidelberg.

11 Palffy, R., Gardlik, R., Behuliak, M., Kadasi, L., Turna, J., and Celec, P. (2009) On the physiology and pathophysiology of antimicrobial peptides. *Mol. Med.*, **15**, 51–59.

12 Guani-Guerra, E., Santos-Mendoza, T., Lugo-Reyes, S.O., and Teran, L.M. (2010) Antimicrobial peptides: general overview and clinical implications in human health and disease. *Clin. Immunol*, **135**, 1–11.

13 Chen, Y., Mant, C.T., Farmer, S.W., Hancock, R.E.W., Vasil, M.L., and Hodges R.S. (2005) Rational design of alpha-helical antimicrobial peptides with enhanced activities and specificity/therapeutic index. *J. Biol. Chem.*, **280**, 12316–12329.

14 Chen, Y., Vasil, A.I., Rehaume, L., Mant, C.T., Burns, J.L., Vasil, M.L., Hancock, R.E.W., and Hodges, R.S. (2006) Comparison of biophysical and biologic properties of alpha-helical enantiomeric antimicrobial peptides. *Chem. Biol. Drug Des.*, **67**, 162–173.

15 Chen, Y., Guarnieri, M.T., Vasil, A.I., Vasil, M.L., Mant, C.T., and Hodges, R. S. (2007) Role of peptide hydrophobicity in the mechanism of action of alpha-helical antimicrobial peptides. *Antimicrob. Agents Chemother.*, **51**, 1398–1406.

16 Jiang, Z., Kullberg, B.J., van der Lee, H., Vasil, A.I., Hale, J.D., Mant, C.T., Hancock, R.E.W., Vasil, M.L., Netea, M. G., and Hodges, R.S. (2008) Effects of hydrophobicity on the antifungal activity

of alpha-helical antimicrobial peptides. *Chem. Biol. Drug Des.*, **72**, 483–495.

17 Jiang, Z., Vasil, A.I., Hale, J.D., Hancock, R.E.W., Vasil, M.L., and Hodges, R.S. (2008) Effects of net charge and the number of positively charged residues on the biological activity of amphipathic alpha-helical cationic antimicrobial peptides. *Biopolymers*, **90**, 369–383.

18 Jiang, Z., Higgins, M.P., Whitehurst, J., Kisich, K.O., Voskuil, M.I., and Hodges, R.S. (2010) Anti-tuberculosis activity of -helical antimicrobial peptides: *de novo* designed L- and D-enantiomers versus L- and D-LL-. *Protein Pept. Lett.*, in press.

19 Jiang, Z., Vasil, A.I., Gera, L., Vasil, M. L., and Hodges, R.S. (2010) Rational design of -helical antimicrobial peptides to target Gram-negative pathogens, *Acinetobacter baumannii* and *Pseudomonas aeruginosa*: utilization of charge, "specificity determinants", total hydrophobicity, hydrophobe type and location as design parameters to improve therapeutic ratio. *Chem. Biol. Drug Des.*, Submitted.

20 Ehrenstein, G. and Lecar, H. (1977) Electrically gated ionic channels in lipid bilayers. *Q Rev. Biophys.*, **10**, 1–34.

21 Mor, A. and Nicolas, P. (1994) The NH2-terminal alpha-helical domain 1–18 of dermaseptin is responsible for antimicrobial activity. *J. Biol. Chem.*, **269**, 1934–1939.

22 Matsuzaki, K., Murase, O., Fujii, N., and Miyajima, K. (1995) Translocation of a channel-forming antimicrobial peptide, magainin 2, across lipid bilayers by forming a pore. *Biochemistry*, **34**, 6521–6526.

23 Matsuzaki, K., Murase, O., Fujii, N., and Miyajima, K. (1996) An antimicrobial peptide, magainin 2, induced rapid flip-flop of phospholipids coupled with pore formation and peptide translocation. *Biochemistry*, **35**, 11361–11368.

24 Ludtke, S.J., He, K., Heller, W.T., Harroun, T.A., Yang, L., and Huang, H. W. (1996) Membrane pores induced by magainin. *Biochemistry*, **35**, 13723–13728.

25 Pouny, Y., Rapaport, D., Mor, A., Nicolas, P., and Shai, Y. Interaction of

antimicrobial dermaseptin and its fluorescently labeled analogues with phospholipid membranes. *Biochemistry*, **31**, 12416–12423.

26 Shai, Y. (1999) Mechanism of the binding, insertion and destabilization of phospholipid bilayer membranes by alpha-helical antimicrobial and cell non-selective membrane-lytic peptides. *Biochim. Biophys. Acta*, **1462**, 55–70.

27 Matsuzaki, K. (2009) Control of cell selectivity of antimicrobial peptides. *Biochim. Biophys. Acta*, **1788**, 1687–1692.

28 Yeaman, M.R. and Yount, N.Y. (2003) Mechanisms of antimicrobial peptide action and resistance. *Pharmacol. Rev.*, **55**, 27–55.

29 Rotem, S. and Mor, A. (2009) Antimicrobial peptide mimics for improved therapeutic properties. *Biochim. Biophys. Acta*, **1788**, 1582–1592.

30 Kondejewski, L.H., Farmer, S.W., Wishart, D.S., Kay, C.M., Hancock, R.E.W., and Hodges, R.S. (1996) Modulation of structure and antibacterial and hemolytic activity by ring size in cyclic gramicidin S analogs. *J. Biol. Chem.*, **271**, 25261–25268.

31 Kondejewski, L.H., Jelokhani-Niaraki, M., Farmer, S.W., Lix, B., Kay, C.M., Sykes, B.D., Hancock, R.E.W., and Hodges, R.S. (1999) Dissociation of antimicrobial and hemolytic activities in cyclic peptide diastereomers by systematic alterations in amphipathicity. *J. Biol. Chem.*, **274**, 13181–13192.

32 Mc Innes, C., Kondejewski, L.H., Hodges, R.S., and Sykes, B.D. (2000) Development of the structural basis for antimicrobial and hemolytic activities of peptides based on gramicidin S and design of novel analogs using NMR spectroscopy. *J. Biol. Chem.*, **275**, 14287–14294.

33 Zhang, L., Falla, T., Wu, M., Fidai, S., Burian, J., Kay, W., and Hancock, R.E.W. (1998) Determinants of recombinant production of antimicrobial cationic peptides and creation of peptide variants in bacteria. *Biochem. Biophys. Res. Commun.*, **247**, 674–680.

34 Zhang, L., Benz, R., and Hancock, R.E.W. (1999) Influence of proline residues on the antibacterial and synergistic activities of alpha-helical peptides. *Biochemistry*, **38**, 8102–8111.

35 Mant, C.T., Chen, Y., and Hodges, R.S. (2003) Temperature profiling of polypeptides in reversed-phase liquid chromatography. I. Monitoring of dimerization and unfolding of amphipathic alpha-helical peptides. *J. Chromatogr. A*, **1009**, 29–43.

36 Lee, D.L., Mant, C.T., and Hodges, R.S. (2003) A novel method to measure self-association of small amphipathic molecules: temperature profiling in reversed-phase chromatography. *J. Biol. Chem.*, **278**, 22918–22927.

37 Chen, Y., Mant, C.T., and Hodges, R.S. (2002) Determination of stereochemistry stability coefficients of amino acid side-chains in an amphipathic alpha-helix. *J. Pept. Res.*, **59**, 18–33.

38 Monera, O.D., Sereda, T.J., Zhou, N.E., Kay, C.M., and Hodges, R.S. (1995) Relationship of sidechain hydrophobicity and alpha-helical propensity on the stability of the single-stranded amphipathic alpha-helix. *J. Pept. Sci.*, **1**, 319–329.

39 Kovacs, J.M., Mant, C.T., and Hodges, R.S. (2006) Determination of intrinsic hydrophilicity/hydrophobicity of amino acid side chains in peptides in the absence of nearest-neighbor or conformational effects. *Biopolymers (Peptide Science)*, **84**, 283–297.

40 Mant, C.T., Kovacs, J.M., Kim, H.M., Pollock, D.D., and Hodges, R.S. (2009) Intrinsic amino acid side-chain hydrophilicity/hydrophobicity coefficients determined by reversed-phase high-performance liquid chromatography of model peptides: comparison with other hydrophilicity/hydrophobicity scales. *Biopolymers (Peptide Science)*, **92**, 573–595.

41 Zhou, N.E., Monera, O.D., Kay, C.M., and Hodges, R.S. (1994) α-Helical propensities of amino acids in the hydrophobic face of an amphipathic α-helix. *Protein. Pept. Lett.*, **15**, 238–243.

42 Zhang, L. and Falla, T.J. (2006) Antimicrobial peptides: therapeutic

potential. *Expert. Opin. Pharmacother.*, **7**, 653–663.

43 Hancock, R.E.W. and Sahl, H.G. (2006) Antimicrobial and host-defense peptides as new anti-infective therapeutic strategies. *Nat. Biotechnol.*, **24**, 1551–1557.

44 Hirsch, T., Jacobsen, F., Steinau, H.U., and Steinstraesser, L. (2008) Host defense peptides and the new line of defence against multiresistant infections. *Protein. Pept. Lett.*, **15**, 238–243.

45 Pathan, F.K., Venkata, D.A., and Panguluri, S.K. (2010) Recent patents on antimicrobial peptides. *Recent. Pat. DNA Gene Seq.*, **4**, 10–16.

46 da Rocha Pitta, M.G. and Galdino, S.L. (2010) Development of novel therapeutic drugs in humans from plant antimicrobial peptides. *Curr. Protein Pept. Sci.*, **11**, 236–247.

5
Conotoxin-Based Leads in Drug Design

Muharrem Akcan and David J. Craik

5.1
Introduction

Peptides have recently been attracting much interest as leads for the development of new drugs because of their high potency for target receptors and low toxicity profiles. In this chapter, we focus on peptides derived from natural sources and, in particular, on peptides from the venoms of marine snails from the genus *Conus*. These snails use their venom either to capture prey or for defense purposes [1]. The venom contains a mixture of peptides, called conopeptides, with each conopeptide having selective pharmacological targeting properties [2–6]. Each cone snail venom typically contains more than 100 different conopeptides and it is estimated that there are about 1000 cone snail species worldwide [7, 8]. This natural resource provides a huge number of potent bioactive peptides that have potential to be developed into drug leads.

Conopeptides range in size from 10 to 40 amino acids and can be classified in two main classes: the disulfide-poor and the disulfide-rich peptides. In this chapter, we focus on disulfide-rich peptides, which are also referred to as conotoxins. They are the major class of conopeptides, and have the potential to provide drug leads for many neurological disorders, based on their potent activities on ion channels, membrane receptors, and transporters of many cell types [3].

5.1.1
Cone Snails

Cone snails are found mostly in tropical waters, especially in the Indo Pacific, East Atlantic, and Mediterranean regions [9]. Their beautifully patterned shells have long attracted the interest of collectors and have, in the past, been used to make jewellery [2]. Figure 5.1 shows some examples of cone shells and of the venom apparatus of the snails. These predatory marine mollusks feed on fish, worms, or other marine mollusks. Being slow-moving creatures, they use a special apparatus both to immobilize and to capture their prey. Specifically, they use a sharp harpoon, a radula-like structure, projected from a muscular tissue called the proboscis

Peptide Drug Discovery and Development: Translational Research in Academia and Industry, First Edition.
Edited by Miguel Castanho and Nuno C. Santos.
© 2011 WILEY-VCH Verlag GmbH & Co. KGaA, Weinheim.
Published 2011 by WILEY-VCH Verlag GmbH & Co. KGaA

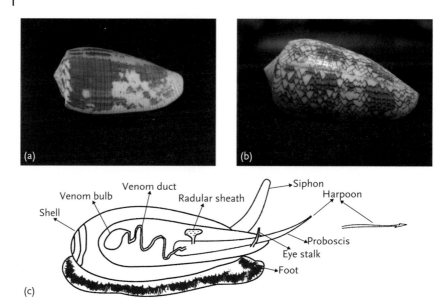

Figure 5.1 Cone snail shells and venom apparatus. (a) Cone shell of *Conus magus*; the source of MVIIA, marketed as Prialt, (b) Cone shell of *Conus textile*, (c) Schematic view of venom apparatus with a close-up of the harpoon on the right. (Cone shell photographs courtesy of Dr. David Wilson, The University of Queensland).

to inject their venom into prey [10]. As illustrated in Figure 5.1, the venom is produced in a long duct and arrives at the harpoon via pressure induced from the venom bulb.

5.1.2
Conotoxin Discovery and Characterization (MS, cDNA, Peptide Sequencing)

Cone snails began to attract the interest of neuroscientists after it was discovered that their venom, particularly that of *C. geographus*, is capable of causing human injury or death [11]. Scientists have since begun to characterize the venom components of the snails and analyze their effects on the human nervous system. In 1977 Spence *et al.* tested *C. geographus* venom at mammalian neuromuscular junctions and found that the peptidic constituents of the venom blocked muscle action potentials but this could be reversed [12]. These early studies have led to many efforts to discover and characterize new conopeptides from both structural and pharmacological perspectives.

Figure 5.2 gives an overview of the discovery and characterization process for conotoxins. It highlights that two approaches have been used: screening at the peptide level, and screening at the nucleic acid level. Edman sequencing and tandem mass spectrometry (MS/MS) have been the main technologies used to elucidate conotoxin sequences at the peptide level. As a precursor to these studies, the extracted venom is typically separated into its components by liquid

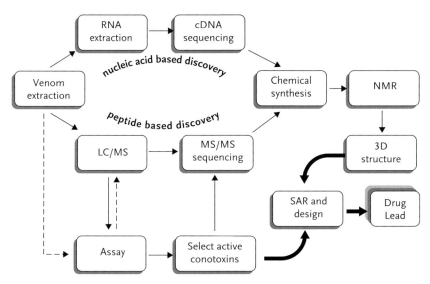

Figure 5.2 Flow chart of conotoxin characterization. Conotoxin-based drug leads can be discovered by two main routes, that is, as nucleic acid or peptide-based discoveries. In general, the determined peptide sequences are chemically synthesized for further structural analysis and bioassays.

chromatography-mass spectrometry (LC-MS) and biological assays are undertaken to select the active conotoxins for further study. The peptide sequences are then determined, mainly now by MS/MS but in early studies Edman sequencing was used. Typically, the determined sequence is then chemically synthesized for structural studies and/or biological assays.

cDNA sequence analysis of conotoxins is now also, or alternatively, used for sequencing efforts and has shown that conopeptides are the products of precursor proteins that have highly conserved signal sequences, and pro-peptide and mature peptide regions [13–15]. In addition to providing sequence information on the mature peptides, the cDNA approach provides information about precursor protein sequences and, potentially, about the processing events that lead to production of the mature peptides.

5.1.3
Conotoxin Classification and Targets

Conotoxins target voltage- and ligand-gated ion channels and membrane receptors and have been classified into pharmacological families (i.e., ω, μ, δ, κ, ι, α, ψ, χ, ε, γ, ρ, and σ), according to their targets and mechanism of action. As illustrated in Table 5.1, ω-conotoxins target voltage-gated calcium channels (VGCCs), whereas μ-, δ-, and ι-conotoxins target voltage-gated sodium channels (VGSCs), and κ-conotoxins target voltage-gated potassium channels (VGKCs). By contrast, α-conotoxins and ψ-conotoxins target nicotinic acetylcholine receptors (nAChRs),

Table 5.1 Conotoxin targets and pharmacological families.

Conotoxin target	Pharmacological family	Example	References
Voltage-gated calcium channel (VGCC)	ω	MVIIA	[19, 20]
Voltage-gated sodium channel (VGSC)	μ, μO, δ, ι	MrVIA	[21]
Voltage-gated potassium channel (VGKC)	κ, κJ, κM	PVIIA	[22]
Nicotinic acetylcholine receptors (nAChR)	α αA, αD, and ψ	Vc1.1	[61, 23]
Neuronal noradrenaline transporter	χ	MrIA	[24, 25]
Perisynaptic calcium channels or G protein coupled	ε	TxVA	[26]
Neuronal pacemaker cation currents	γ	PnVIIA	[27]
Alpha adrenoceptors (GPCR)	ρ	TIA	[28]
5-HT$_3$ receptor	σ	GVIIIA	[29]
Receptor?[a]	?	Gm9a	[30]

[a]Receptor has not been identified yet. Peptide causes spasmodic contractions in mouse brain.

which have been associated with many disorders, including Alzheimer's disease and Parkinson's disease. Their effects on ion channels and membrane receptors make conotoxins valuable as drug leads. For example, ω-conotoxin, MVIIA is already on the market for the treatment of chronic pain [16–18].

At a higher level of classification, conotoxins were initially classified into seven superfamilies (i.e., A, I, M, O, P, S, and T), according to their precursor peptide signal sequence and cystine motif [3]. To accommodate for discoveries in new conotoxin sequences, this superfamily number has expanded to include D, J, L, V, and Y superfamilies (Figure 5.3) [31]. In addition to these new superfamilies, the I and O superfamilies are now divided into three subgroups, that is the I1, I2, and I3 superfamilies and the O1, O2, and O3 superfamilies, respectively, according to differences in their cystine motifs.

Although the A and T superfamilies have the same cystine motif, their disulfide bond connectivities differ. Conversely, the M, O, and P superfamilies have the same disulfide connectivity but different cystine motifs. Conotoxins belonging to I, O, and P superfamilies have a cystine knot motif (i.e., an embedded ring formed by two disulfide bonds and connecting backbone segments threaded by a third disulfide bond), which is also present in spider, insect, fungi, and plant peptides and proteins [32–35]. The disulfide bond pattern of cystine knot peptides is Cys^I–Cys^{IV}, Cys^{II}–Cys^V, and Cys^{III}–Cys^{VI}.

5.1.4
Posttranslational Modifications (PTMs)

One feature that distinguishes conopeptides from many other classes of peptides is their extensive posttranslational modifications. Posttranslational modifications (PTMs) are chemical changes to the amino acid residues of a peptide that are not encoded in the corresponding gene. The two most common PTMs in conotoxins,

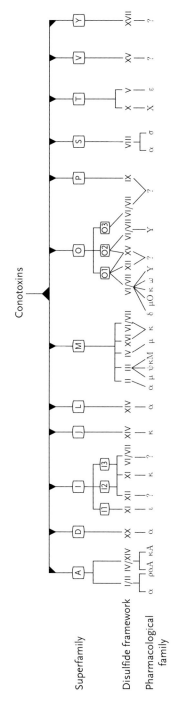

Figure 5.3 Conotoxin classification. Disulfide-rich conopeptides, referred to as conotoxins, are classified according to their gene superfamilies. The I superfamily is divided into three groups, as I1, I2, or I3, and the O superfamily as O1, O2, or O3. Conotoxins then further classified based on their disulfide frameworks and pharmacological families.

as in many other proteins, are disulfide bond formation and proteolytic cleavage. In addition to these classic PTMs, C-terminal amidation, hydroxylation of proline, and conversion of glutamate to γ-carboxy glutamic acid are the most common PTMs found in conotoxins. PTMs also include other changes, such as D–L residue substitutions. It is possible for one conotoxin to have multiple PTMs in its sequence while others have none [36]. A list of PTMs found in wild-type conotoxins is shown in Table 5.2. The roles of PTMs on conotoxin function are not fully understood, but it seems likely that they contribute to improving the activity and stability of these peptides.

5.1.5
Prospects for Drug Discovery

From the proceeding discussion it is clear that conotoxins are potent and exquisitely selective peptides and have exciting potential as drug leads. More broadly, peptides are generally regarded as great drug leads, but they have, typically, not yet translated this potential to the market widely, because they have some generic disadvantages, including poor stability, poor oral bioavailability and, potentially, high manufacturing costs. Conotoxins intrinsically overcome some of these generic disadvantages of peptides in that their disulfide-rich nature tends to make them more stable than corresponding linear peptides. Furthermore, conotoxins can be readily re-engineered to further enhance their stability using a variety of approaches, including cyclization [37, 38], the addition of non-peptidic moieties [39], or the addition of lipophilic moieties [40].

The ability to make these types of chemical changes arises from the fact that conotoxins are relatively small peptides, typically less than 40 amino acids, and, therefore, amenable to solid phase peptide synthesis (SPPS). The other factors that make conotoxins particularly suitable for drug design applications are their vast diversity of structures and wide range of pharmaceutical targets [4, 35]. With these general factors in mind we now discuss specific aspects of conotoxin chemical synthesis that underpin the applications of conotoxins as drug leads.

5.2
Conotoxin Synthesis, Folding, and Structure

5.2.1
Synthesis

To protect marine ecosystems and to avoid potential safety concerns in obtaining venom by milking, cone snail research has involved a significant focus on the chemical synthesis of conotoxins. Chemical synthesis allows the production of tens of milligrams amounts of conopeptides to conduct biological assays. The first chemically synthesized conotoxins were two α-conotoxins, GI and MI, achieved in the 1980s [41, 42]. In 1986, Nishiuchi *et al.* synthesized the first three disulfide-bonded ω-conotoxin GVIA [43]. These peptides were synthesized by SPPS, which

Table 5.2 Post-translational modifications in conotoxins.

PTM	Number of examples[a]	Example	Sequence[b,c]
C-terminal amidation	104	MVIIA	CKGKGAKCSRLMYDCCTGSCRSGKC[d]
4-hydroxy-proline	74	GIIIA	RDCC**TOO**KKCKDRQC**K**OQRCCA[d]
γ-carboxy glutamic acid	34	AsVIIA	TCKQKGEGCSLDVγCCSSSCKPGGPLFDFDC[d]
Pyroglutamic acid	12	PIB	**Z**SOGCCWNPACVKNRC[d]
Bromotryptophan	12	RVIIA	(**BTr**)FGHγγCTY(**BTr**)LGPCγVDDTCCSASCγSKFCGL(**BTr**)
Sulfotyrosine	6	AnIA	CCSHPACAANNQD(**sTy**)C[d]
D-Leucine	2	ArXIA	RTCSRRGHRCIRDSQCCGGMCCQGNRCFVAIRRCFHIPF
D-Phenylalanine	2	RXIA	GOSFCKADEKOCEYHADCCNCCLSGICAOSTNWILPGCSTSSF**f**KI
Glycosylated threonine	2	TxVA	γCCγDG(BTr)CC(**gTr**)AAO
5-Hydroxy-lysine	1	DeXIIIA	DCOTSCOTTCANG(**BTr**)ECC(**hLy**)GYOCVN(**hLy**)ACSGCTH[d]
Glycosylated serine	1	SIVA	ZKSLVP(**gSr**)VITTCCGYDOGTMCOOCRCTNSC

[a]As reported in 2010 by Kaas and Craik [31].
[b]Position of posttranslational modifications is indicated by bold print.
[c]Lower case letters are used to denote D-amino acids.
[d]C-terminal amidation, O: 4-hydroxyproline, BTr: bromotryptophan, hLy: 5-hydroxy-lysine, γ: gamma carboxylic glutamic acid, f: D-phenylalanine, l: D-leucine, O: 4-hydroxyproline, BTr: bromotryptophan, gTr: glycosylated serine, gSr: glycosylated serine, gTr: glycosylated threonine, Z: pyroglutamic acid, sTy: sulfotyrosine.

eliminates the solubility and purification problems that can occur during solution phase synthesis [44, 45].

The SPPS method involves the attachment of the first amino acid onto a solid polymer support and coupling of amino acids one-by-one to form the peptide sequence, as illustrated in Figure 5.4. To prevent unwanted couplings between individual amino acids, t-butoxycarbonyl (Boc) or fluoren-9-ylmethoxycarbonyl (Fmoc) protecting groups on the amine groups of each amino acid are used [46]. Boc and Fmoc groups have to be removed before the coupling of the next amino acid by trifluoroacetic acid (TFA) and piperidine/dimethylformamide (DMF) mixture, respectively.

After the assembly of the polypeptide chain, peptides synthesized with Boc chemistry are cleaved from the solid support using hydrofluoric acid (HF), whereas peptides synthesized with Fmoc chemistry are cleaved with TFA. Fmoc chemistry is often preferred to Boc chemistry because of the requirement to use hazardous HF during the cleavage step of Boc chemistry. However, deprotection and coupling yields of Fmoc chemistry are lower than in Boc chemistry [47].

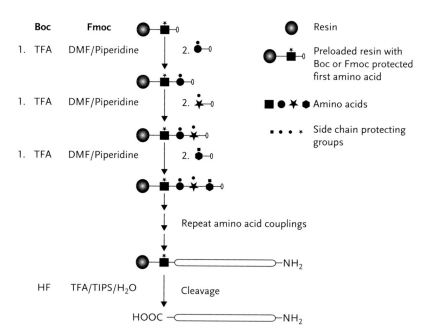

Figure 5.4 Conotoxin synthesis. Conotoxins are typically synthesized using SPSS, which includes repetitive deprotection and amino acid coupling steps. Deprotection of Fmoc and Boc groups can be achieved by treating the reaction mixture with DMF/piperidine and TFA respectively as shown on the left side of the reaction scheme. Deprotection steps are followed by amino acid couplings. After completion of the couplings, the peptide can be cleaved off from the resin by using TFA for Fmoc chemistry and HF for Boc chemistry.

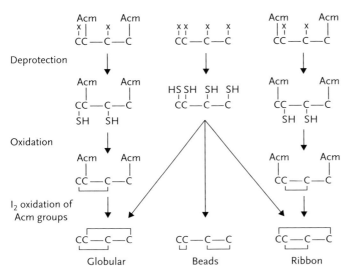

Figure 5.5 Schemes for the oxidative folding of α-conotoxins. The central scheme corresponds to one-step oxidative folding of α-conotoxins, which results globular, beads and ribbon isomers. The left and right schemes show regioselective oxidative folding in which two cysteine residues have acetamidomethyl (Acm) protecting groups. These side-chain protecting groups facilitate selective disulfide bond formation. Regioselective oxidative folding requires I_2 oxidation after the first oxidation to remove the Acm groups and produce either globular or ribbon isomers depending on the position of Acm groups.

5.2.2
Folding

Protein folding is the process whereby a linear amino acid sequence rearranges to form a characteristic three-dimensional structure, which is essential for the correct function of the protein [48]. For proteins containing cysteine residues the formation of the correct disulfide bonds is important for rigidity and conformational stability, but this oxidative folding process adds a degree of complexity to general protein folding. For example, folding of conotoxins having two disulfide bonds (i.e., α-conotoxins) can potentially produce three different isomers: globular (Cys^I–Cys^{III}, Cys^{II}–Cys^{IV}), ribbon (Cys^I–Cys^{IV}, Cys^{II}–Cys^{III}), and beads (Cys^I–Cys^{II}, Cys^{III}–Cys^{IV}), as illustrated in Figure 5.5. As the number of cysteine residues increases, the number of isomers also increases, so that there are 15 possible isomers for three-disulfide containing peptides. Despite this complexity, it has generally proved possible to correctly fold a wide range of two- or three-disulfide containing conotoxins.

5.2.3
Structure by NMR and X-Ray

Structural studies are important to understand the functions and therapeutic potential of conotoxins. Nuclear magnetic resonance (NMR) spectroscopy and X-Ray

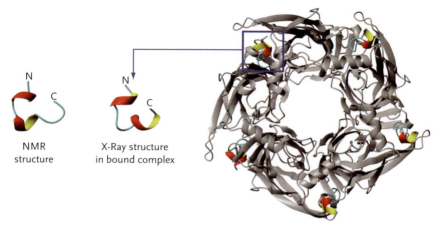

Figure 5.6 Structure of α-conotoxin ImI. The NMR structure of ImI in solution (PDB code 1im1) is compared with the crystal structure of ImI bound to the AChBP (PDB code 2c9t).

crystallography techniques enable high-resolution structure determinations by measuring the distances between atomic nuclei, or the electron density in a molecule, respectively. So far, 79 conotoxin structures have been determined by NMR, compared to only seven with X-Ray methods [49–53]. The relative dominance of NMR in the structure determination of conotoxins is primarily due to their comparatively small size, which minimizes peak overlap in NMR spectra, and the general difficulties of crystallizing small disulfide-rich peptides, which makes many inaccessible to X-ray methods.

Although the NMR technique is predominant in solution studies of conotoxins, X-ray crystallography studies have provided some very valuable structures of the complexes of conotoxins with model receptors. Figure 5.6 shows the crystal structure of α-conotoxin ImI bound to the acetylcholine binding protein, AChBP [53]. The overall fold of the peptide does not change between the free and bound states, highlighting the rigid nature of conotoxins, a characteristic that is an advantage in drug design studies.

5.3
Conotoxins as Drug Leads

5.3.1
Overview of Conotoxins in Drug Design

The exquisite potency and selectivity of conotoxins for a variety of pharmacologically important receptors is a key to their attractiveness as leads in the drug design process. Several conotoxins are in various stages of preclinical or clinical evaluation, and one is on the market. Conotoxins fill a size niche between that of small molecule drugs (typically less than 500 Da molecular weight) and biologics, which

Table 5.3 Conotoxins in clinical or preclinical development.

Conotoxin	Cone snail	Clinical stage	Company
ω-MVIIA (Prialt)	*C. magus*	Approved by FDA	Azur Pharma (www.prialt.com)
ω-CVID (AM336)	*C. catus*	Phase II	Zenyth Therapeutics [clinical development halted] CNSBio Pty Ltd (http://www.cnsbio.com)
κ-PVIIA (CGX-1051)	*C. purpurascens*	Preclinical	Cognetix Inc. (www.cognetix.com)
α-Vc1.1 (ACV1)	*C. victoriae*	Phase II	Metabolic Pharmaceuticals [clinical development halted] (http://www.metabolic.com.au)
χ-MrIA (Xen2174)	*C. marmoreus*	Phase II	Xenome (www.xenome.com)

are typically larger proteins (>5000 Da) such as growth factors, growth hormones, or hemopoietic agents. This unique size range has meant that conotoxin-based drug leads can target receptors that may be intractable with conventional small molecule drugs. In the following sections we describe specific examples of leads of conotoxins in drug design (Table 5.3).

5.3.2
ω-Conotoxins (MVIIA, CVID)

MVIIA is a 25-amino acid ω-conotoxin, originally isolated from the venom of *C. magus*. It blocks N-type VGCCs, which play a key role in neurotransmission release at synapses of the spinal cord [54]. A synthetic version of MVIIA, named Prialt or ziconotide, is the first conotoxin approved by the Food and Drug Administration (FDA) and the European Regulatory Agency for the treatment of severe chronic pain [16–18]. It has been used in hundreds of patients who are intolerant to other treatments such as morphine.

In addition to MVIIA, another ω-conotoxin, CVID, also targets VGCCs and was of early interest for its therapeutic potential. Adams *et al.* reported that CVID has a higher potency at N-type VGCCs but lower potency at P/Q-type VGCCs than other ω-conotoxins [55]. This favorable profile made it the most selective ω-conotoxin found at that time, but it has not advanced as far as MVIIA, which was the first-in-class compound. Figure 5.7 shows the three-dimensional structure of MVIIA and a comparison of the sequences of MVIIA and CVID.

5.3.3
α-Conotoxins (Vc1.1)

Neuronal nicotinic acetylcholine receptors (nAChRs) are ligand-gated ion channels which, as well as having profound physiological importance, have been

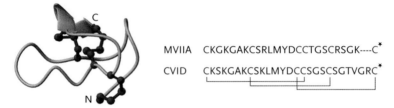

MVIIA   CKGKGAKCSRLMYDCCTGSCRSGK----C*

CVID   CKSKGAKCSKLMYDCCSGSCSGTVGRC*

Figure 5.7 3D structure of MVIIA and amino acid sequences of MVIIA and CVID. The β-strands are shown as arrows and the disulfide bonds are shown in ball-and-stick format. The asterisk at the end of each sequence indicates C-amidated termini.

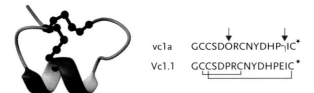

vc1a   GCCSDORCNYDHPᵧIC*

Vc1.1   GCCSDPRCNYDHPEIC*

Figure 5.8 3D structure of Vc1.1 and peptide sequences. The helical region is shown as a ribbon and the disulfide bonds are in ball and stick format. The post-translationaly modified amino acids are marked with arrows. The asterisk at the end of each sequence indicates C-amidated termini.

associated with many disorders, including Alzheimer's disease, depression, and schizophrenia. α-Conotoxins selectively inhibit nAChRs, which makes them valuable drug leads. One α-conotoxin of particular interest is the 16 amino acid peptide Vc1.1, which was first discovered from a cDNA sequence isolated from the venom duct of *C. victoriae*. The peptide has two disulfide bonds that brace a short helical structure, as shown in Figure 5.8. Recently, it was reported that Vc1.1 targets recombinant α9α10 nAChRs expressed in *Xenopus* oocytes [56, 57] and also activates GABA_B receptors, which cause the inhibition of N-type calcium channels in dorsal root ganglion (DRG) neurons [58, 59].

A synthetic version of Vc1.1, named ACV1, underwent preclinical trials for the treatment of neuropathic pain, and demonstrated that Vc1.1 has analgesic effects in several rat models [60, 61]. Development of the molecule was discontinued, however, as will be noted later in this chapter, a cyclized version of Vc1.1 has rekindled interest in this conotoxin.

5.3.4
χ-Conotoxins (MrIA)

The neuronal noradrenaline transporters (NETs) are important in learning and memory functions. Conotoxin MrIA from *C. marmoreus* belongs to the χ-pharmacological family and inhibits noradrenaline uptake, non-competitively,

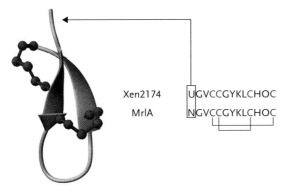

| Xen2174 | UGVCCGYKLCHOC |
| MrIA | NGVCCGYKLCHOC |

Figure 5.9 3D structure of MrIA. The β-strands are shown as arrows and disulfide bonds are in ball and stick format. The modified amino acid used to stabilize the clinical candidate Xen2174 is shown boxed.

through interacting with the NET. It comprises 13 amino acids and two disulfide bonds (Cys^I–Cys^{IV}, Cys^{II}–Cys^{III}), similar to the arrangement in the ribbon isomer of α-conotoxins (Figure 5.9).

A synthetic version of χ-conotoxin, MrIA (Xen2174), is being developed by Xenome Ltd. for patients suffering from cancer pain. It has completed Phase I/II clinical trials and has shown good stability and efficacy [62]. As illustrated in Figure 5.9, the only difference between MrIA and Xen2174 is the substitution of asparagine with a pyrogulutamate residue. This modification was made to replace a potentially unstable asparagine residue which degrades to aspartimide [63].

5.3.5
Re-engineered Conotoxins in Drug Design

The previous example (Xen2174) demonstrates the value of single residue modifications to improve the pharmaceutical properties of conotoxins. In this section we focus on more substantial re-engineering of conotoxins, and, in particular, on the use of head-to-tail cyclization to improve biopharmaceutical properties [37, 38]. These studies have been stimulated by recent discoveries of naturally occurring cyclic proteins that have exceptional stability [64]. It has long been known in the pharmaceutical industry that cyclic peptides are valuable drug leads because they are locked into a particular conformation, thereby minimizing entropic losses on binding; furthermore, the cyclic arrangement can enhance their stability. Until recently, cyclization technology had only been applied to small peptides, typically less than 12 amino acids, as guided by natural examples, such as cyclosporin. However, over the last few years there has been substantial effort in the re-engineering of larger peptides, to make them cyclic, including conotoxins. In designing cyclic derivatives of peptides, an examination of the 3D structure of the native acyclic peptide allows calculation of the number of residues required in an amino acid linker to join the N- and C-termini.

The first successful example reported was that of conotoxin MII, an inhibitor of α3β2 nAChRs [37]. Clark *et al.* (2005) showed that the use of six or seven amino acid linkers resulted in cyclic molecules having equivalent activity to the native (linear) peptide but improved stability in human plasma [37]. Interestingly, even though the initial predictions suggested that a linker of five amino acids would be sufficient to span the termini, the cyclized MII with five amino acid linker was inactive. This demonstrates the need for careful design of linkers to make sure that strain is not induced into the molecules by cyclization, which can cause loss of activity.

The work on α-conotoxin MII was followed by studies on the cyclization of the α-conotoxin Vc1.1, mentioned earlier [60]. Clark *et al.* (2010) reported recently that the cyclized version of Vc1.1 was more potent at the target receptor than the linear version [38], as indicated in Figure 5.10, and the cyclized molecule had

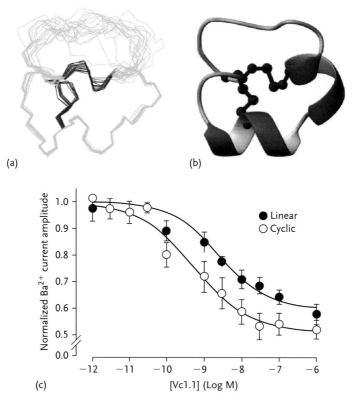

(a)   (b)

(c)   [Vc1.1] (Log M)

Figure 5.10 Cyclic Vc1.1. (a) The 20 low-energy structures of cVc1.1. (b) Ribbon representation of the average structure of cVc1.1. Disulfide bonds are shown in ball and stick format. (c) Concentration–response relationship for inhibition of high-voltage-activated Ca^{2+} channel currents in DRG neurons by linear and cyclic Vc1.1. The IC_{50} value for inhibition of Ca^{2+} channel currents by linear Vc1.1 is 1.7 and 0.3 nM for cyclic Vc1.1 [38].

substantially improved stability over the linear analog in simulated gastric fluid, simulated intestinal fluid, and human serum. This example, therefore, represents a case not only of improved stability, but also improvement in the potency of a cyclized molecule. In general, the termini of conotoxins are relatively close to one another, and, hence, there are many examples where similar technology could be applied for the stabilization of conotoxins.

5.4
Conclusions

We hope that this chapter has given an insight into the roles of conotoxins in drug design. In our opinion, conotoxins continue to be of interest as lead molecules in drug design, and although so far only one is on the market, the future looks promising for this class of peptides, given that a number of preclinical and clinical trials are currently underway. More broadly, the work described here shows the value of natural products as drug leads.

Acknowledgments

Work in our laboratory on conotoxins is supported by grants from the National Health & Medical Research Council (Australia) and the Australian Research Council. DJC is an NHMRC Professorial Fellow. We thank our colleagues listed in the references for their valuable contributions to conotoxin research.

References

1 Kohn, A.J., Saunders, P.R., and Wiener, S. (1960) Preliminary studies on the venom of the marine snail conus. *Ann. NY Acad. Sci.*, **90** (3), 706–725.

2 Olivera, B.M., Rivier, J., Clark, C., Ramilo, C.A., Corpuz, G.P., Abogadie, F.C., Mena, E.E., Woodward, S.R., Hillyard, D.R., and Cruz, L.J. (1990) Diversity of conus neuropeptides. *Science*, **249** (4966), 257–263.

3 Terlau, H. and Olivera, B.M. (2004) Conus venoms: a rich source of novel ion channel-targeted peptides. *Physiol. Rev.*, **84** (1), 41–68.

4 Adams, D.J., Alewood, P.F., Craik, D.J., Drinkwater, R.D., and Lewis, R.J. (1999) Conotoxins and their potential pharmaceutical applications. *Drug Devel. Res.*, **46** (3–4), 219–234.

5 Dutton, J.L. and Craik, D.J. (2001) Alpha-conotoxins: nicotinic acetylcholine receptor antagonists as pharmacological tools and potential drug leads. *Curr. Med. Chem.*, **8** (4), 327–344.

6 Halai, R. and Craik, D.J. (2009) Conotoxins: natural product drug leads. *Nat. Prod. Rep.*, **26** (4), 526–536.

7 Olivera, B.M., Gray, W.R., Zeikus, R., McIntosh, J.M., Varga, J., Rivier, J., Desantos, V., and Cruz, L.J. (1985) Peptide neurotoxins from fish-hunting cone snails. *Science*, **230** (4732), 1338–1343.

8 Mari, F. and Fields, G.B. (2003) Conopeptides: unique pharmacological agents that challenge current peptide methodologies. *Chimica Oggi-Chem. Today*, **21** (6), 43–48.

9 Kohn, A.J. (1959) The ecology of conus in Hawaii. *Ecol. Monog.*, **29** (1), 47–90.

10 Terlau, H., Shon, K.J., Grilley, M., Stocker, M., Stuhmer, W., and Olivera, B.M. (1996) Strategy for rapid immobilization of prey by a fish-hunting marine snail. *Nature*, **381** (6578), 148–151.

11 Endean, R., Parish, G., and Gyr, P. (1974) Pharmacology of venom of conus geographus. *Toxicon*, **12** (12), 131–138.

12 Spence, I., Gillessen, D., Gregson, R.P., and Quinn, R.J. (1977) Characterization of neurotoxic constituents of Conus-Geographus(L) venom, *Life Sci.*, **21**, 1759–1769.

13 Woodward, S.R., Cruz, L.J., Olivera, B. M., and Hillyard, D.R. (1990) Constant and hypervariable regions in conotoxin propeptides. *Embo J.*, **9** (4), 1015–1020.

14 Olivera, B.M., Walker, C., Cartier, G.E., Hooper, D., Santos, A.D., Schoenfeld, R., Shetty, R., Watkins, M., Bandyopadhyay, P., and Hillyard, D.R. (1999) Speciation of cone snails and interspecific hyperdivergence of their venom peptides potential – evolutionary significance of introns. *Ann. NY Acad. Sci.*, **870**, (Molecular Strategies in Biological Evolution), 223–237.

15 Yuan, D.D., Han, Y.H., Wang, C.G., and Chi, C.W. (2007) From the identification of gene organization of alpha conotoxins to the cloning of novel toxins. *Toxicon*, **49** (8), 1135–1149.

16 Miljanich, G.P. (2004) Ziconotide: neuronal calcium channel blocker for treating severe chronic pain. *Curr. Med. Chem.*, **11** (23), 3029–3040.

17 Rowbotham, M.C., Twilling, L., Davies, P.S., Reisner, L., Taylor, K., and Mohr, D. (2003) Oral opioid therapy for chronic peripheral and central neuropathic pain. *New Engl. J. Med.*, **348** (13), 1223–1232.

18 Canavero, S. and Bonicalzi, V. (2003) Chronic neuropathic pain. *New Engl. J. Med.*, **348** (26), 2688–2689.

19 Basus, V.J., Nadasdi, L., Ramachandran, J., and Miljanich, G.P. (1995) Solution structure of omega-conotoxin MVIIA using 2D NMR-spectroscopy. *FEBS Lett.*, **370** (3), 163–169.

20 Nielsen, K.J., Adams, D., Thomas, L., Bond, T., Alewood, P.F., Craik, D.J., and Lewis, R.J. (1999) Structure–activity relationships of omega-conotoxins MVIIA, MVIIC and 14 loop splice hybrids at N and P/Q-type calcium channels. *J. Mol. Biol.*, **289** (5), 1405–1421.

21 Zorn, S., Leipold, E., Hansel, A., Bulaj, G., Olivera, B.M., Terlau, H., and Heinermann, S.H. (2006) The mu O-conotoxin MrVIA inhibits voltage-gated sodium channels by associating with domain-3. *FEBS Lett.*, **580** (5), 1360–1364.

22 Jacobsen, R., Stocker, M., Terlau, H., Shon, K., Grilley, M., Gray, W.R., Stuhmer, W., and Olivera, B.M. (1996) Kappa-conotoxin PVIIA, a conus peptide targeted to potassium channels. *Soc. Neurosci. Abs.*, **22** (1–3), 351.

23 Clark, R.J., Fischer, H., Nevin, S.T., Adams, D.J., and Craik, D.J. (2006) The synthesis, structural characterization, and receptor specificity of the alpha-conotoxin Vc1.1 *J. Biol. Chem.*, **281** (32), 23254–23263.

24 Bryan-Lluka, L.J., Bonisch, H., and Lewis, R.J. (2003) Chi-conopeptide MrIA partially overlaps desipramine and cocaine binding sites on the human norepinephrine transporter. *J. Biol. Chem.*, **278** (41), 40324–40329.

25 Nilsson, K.P.R., Lovelace, E.S., Caesar, C.E., Tynngard, N., Alewood, P.F., Johansson, H.M., Sharpe, I.A., Lewis, R.J., Daly, N.L., and Craik, D.J. (2005) Solution structure of chi-conopeptide MrIA, a modulator of the human norepinephrine transporter. *Biopolymers*, **80** (6), 815–823.

26 Rigby, A.C., Lucas-Meunier, E., Kalume, D.E., Czerwiec, E., Hambe, B., Dahlqvist, I., Fossier, P., Baux, G., Roepstorff, P., Baleja, J.D., Furie, B.C., Furie, B., and Stenflo, J. (1999) A conotoxin from Conus textile with unusual posttranslational modifications reduces presynaptic Ca2+ influx. *Proc. Natl. Acad. Sci. USA*, **96** (10), 5758–5763.

27 Fainzilber, M., Nakamura, T., Lodder, J.C., Zlotkin, E., Kits, K.S., and

Burlingame, A.L. (1998) Gamma-conotoxin-PnVIIA, a gamma-carboxyglutamate-containing peptide agonist of neuronal pacemaker cation currents. *Biochemistry*, **37** (6), 1470–1477.

28 Lima, V., Mueller, A., Kamikihara, S.Y., Raymundi, V., Alewood, D., Lewis, R.J., Chen, Z.J., Minneman, K.P., and Pupo, A.S. (2005) Differential antagonism by conotoxin p-TIA of contractions mediated by distinct alpha(1)-adrenoceptor subtypes in rat vas deferens, spleen and aorta. *Eur. J. Pharmacol.*, **508** (1–3), 183–192.

29 England, L.J., Imperial, J., Jacobsen, R., Craig, A.G., Gulyas, J., Akhtar, M., Rivier, J., Julius, D., and Olivera, B.M. (1998) Inactivation of a serotonin-gated ion channel by a polypeptide toxin from marine snails. *Science*, **281** (5376), 575–578.

30 Miles, L.A., Dy, C.Y., Nielsen, J., Barnham, K.J., Hinds, M.G., Olivera, B.M., Bulaj, G., and Norton, R.S. (2002) Structure of a novel P-superfamily spasmodic conotoxin reveals an inhibitory cystine knot motif. *J. Biol. Chem.*, **277** (45), 43033–43040.

31 Kaas, Q., Westermann, J.C., and Craik, D.J. (2010) Conopeptide characterization and classifications: an analysis using ConoServer. *Toxicon*, **55** (8), 1491–1509.

32 McDonald, N.Q., Lapatto, R., Murrayrust, J., Gunning, J., Wlodawer, A., and Blundell, T.L. (1991) New protein fold revealed by a 2.3 Å resolution crystal structure of nerve growth factor. *Nature*, **354** (6352), 411–414.

33 Pallaghy, P.K., Nielsen, K.J., Craik, D.J., and Norton, R.S. (1994) A common structural motif incorporating a cystine knot and a triple stranded beta sheet in toxic and inhibitory polypeptides. *Protein Sci.*, **3** (10), 1833–1839.

34 Isaacs, N.W. (1995) Cystine knots. *Curr. Opin. Struct. Biol.*, **5** (3), 391–395.

35 Craik, D.J., Daly, N.L., and Waine, C. (2001) The cystine knot motif in toxins and implications for drug design. *Toxicon*, **39** (1), 43–60.

36 Craig, A.G., Bandyopadhyay, P., and Olivera, B.M. (1999) Post-translationally modified neuropeptides from conus venoms. *Eur. J. Biochem.*, **264** (2), 271–275.

37 Clark, R.J., Fischer, H., Dempster, L., Daly, N.L., Rosengren, K.J., Nevin, S.T., Meunier, F.A., Adams, D.J., and Craik, D.J. (2005) Engineering stable peptide toxins by means of backbone cyclization: stabilization of the alpha-conotoxin MII. *Proc. Natl. Acad. Sci. USA*, **102** (39), 13767–13772.

38 Clark, R.J., Jensen, J., Nevin, S.T., Callaghan, B.P., Adams, D.J., and Craik, D.J. (2010) The engineering of an orally active conotoxin for the treatment of neuropathic pain. *Angew. Chem. Int. Ed. Engl.*, **49** (37), 6545–6548.

39 Green, B.R., Catlin, P., Zhang, M.M., Fiedler, B., Bayudan, W., Morrison, A., Norton, R.S., Smith, B.J., Yoshikami, D., Olivera, B.M., and Bulaj, G. (2007) Conotoxins containing nonnatural backbone spacers: cladistic-based design, chemical synthesis, and improved analgesic activity. *Chem. Biol.*, **14** (4), 399–407.

40 Blanchfield, J., Dutton, J., Hogg, R., Craik, D., Adams, D., Lewis, R., Alewood, P., and Toth, I. (2001) The synthesis and structure of an N-terminal dodecanoic acid conjugate of alpha-conotoxin MII. *Lett. Pept. Sci.*, **8** (3–5), 235–239.

41 Nishiuchi, Y. and Sakakibara, S. (1982) Primary and secondary structure of conotoxin GI, a neurotoxic tridecapeptide from a marine snail. *FEBS Lett.*, **148** (2), 260–262.

42 Gray, W.R., Rivier, J.E., Galyean, R., Cruz, L.J., and Olivera, B.M. (1983) Conotoxin-MI – disulfide bonding and conformational states. *J. Biol. Chem.*, **258** (20), 2247–2251.

43 Nishiuchi, Y., Kumagaye, K., Noda, Y., Watanabe, T.X., and Sakakibara, S. (1986) Synthesis and secondary structure determination of omega-conotoxin GVIA – A 27-peptide with 3 intramolecular disulfide bonds. *Biopolymers*, **25**, S61–S68.

44 Merrifield, R.B. (1963) Solid phase peptide synthesis. 1. Synthesis of a tetrapeptide, *J. Am. Chem. Soc.*, **85**, 2149–2154.

45 Merrifield, R.B. (1964) Solid phase peptide synthesis. 2. Synthesis of bradykinin, *J. Am. Chem. Soc.*, **86**, 304–305.

46 Carpino, L.A. and Han, G.Y. (1972) 9-Fluorenylmethoxycarbonyl amino-protecting group, *J. Org. Chem.*, **37**, 3404–3409.

47 Schnölzer, M., Alewood, P., Jones, A., Alewood, D., and SBH, K. (2007) In situ neutralization in Boc-chemistry solid phase peptide synthesis: rapid, high yield assembly of difficult sequences. *Int. J. Peptide Res. Ther.*, **13** (1–2), 31–44.

48 Bulaj, G. and Olivera, B.M. (2008) Folding of conotoxins: formation of the native disulfide bridges during chemical synthesis and biosynthesis of conus peptides. *Antiox. Redox Signal.*, **10** (1), 141–155.

49 Marx, U.C., Daly, N.L., and Craik, D.J. (2006) NMR of conotoxins: structural features and an analysis of chemical shifts of post-translationally modified amino acids. *Magn. Reson. Chem.*, **44**, S41–S50.

50 Franco, A. and Mari, F. (1999) Three-dimensional structure of alpha-conotoxin EI determined by H-1 NMR spectroscopy. *Lett. Peptide Sci.*, **6** (4), 199–207.

51 Hu, S.H., Gehrmann, J., Guddat, L.W., Alewood, P.F., Craik, D.J., and Martin, J.L. (1996) The 1.1 angstrom crystal structure of the neuronal acetylcholine receptor antagonist, alpha-conotoxin PnIA from *Conus pennaceus*. *Structure*, **4** (4), 417–423.

52 Guddat, L.W., Martin, J.L., Shan, L., Edmundson, A.B., and Gray, W.R. (1996) Three-dimensional structure of the alpha-conotoxin GI at 1.2 angstrom resolution. *Biochemistry*, **35** (35), 11329–11335.

53 Ulens, C., Hogg, R.C., Celie, P.H., Bertrand, D., Tsetlin, V., Smit, A.B., and Sixma, T.K. (2006) Structural determinants of selective alpha-conotoxin binding to a nicotinic acetylcholine receptor homolog AChBP. *Proc. Natl. Acad. Sci. USA*, **103** (10), 3615–3620.

54 Olivera, B.M., Cruz, L.J., Desantos, V., Lecheminant, G.W., Griffin, D., Zeikus, R., McIntosh, J.M., Galyean, R., Varga, J., Gray, W.R., and Rivier, J.

(1987) Neuronal Ca channel antagonists. Discrimination between Ca channel subtypes using omega-conotoxin from *Conus magus* venom. *Biochemistry*, **26** (8), 2086–2090.

55 Adams, D.J., Smith, A.B., Schroeder, C.I., Yasuda, T., and Lewis, R.J. (2003) Omega-conotoxin CVID inhibits a pharmacologically distinct voltage sensitive calcium channel associated with transmitter release from preganglionic nerve terminals. *J. Biol. Chem.*, **278** (6), 4057–4062.

56 Vincler, M., Wittenauer, S., Parker, R., Ellison, M., Olivera, B.M., and McIntosh, J.M. (2006) Molecular mechanism for analgesia involving specific antagonism of alpha 9 alpha 10 nicotinic acetylcholine receptors. *Proc. Natl. Acad. Sci. USA*, **103** (47), 17880–17884.

57 Nevin, S.T., Clark, R.J., Klimis, H., Christie, M.J., Craik, D.J., and Adams, D.J. (2007) Are alpha 9 alpha 10 nicotinic acetylcholine receptors a pain target for alpha-conotoxins? *Mol. Pharmacol.*, **72** (6), 1406–1410.

58 Callaghan, B., Haythornthwaite, A., Berecki, G., Clark, R.J., Craik, D.J., and Adams, D.J. (2008) Analgesic alpha-conotoxins Vc1.1 and RgIA inhibit N-type calcium channels in rat sensory neurons via GABA(B) receptor activation. *J. Neurosci.*, **28** (43), 10943–10951.

59 Callaghan, B. and Adams, D.J. (2010) Analgesic alpha-conotoxins Vc1.1 and RgIA inhibit N-type calcium channels in sensory neurons of alpha 9 nicotinic receptor knockout mice. *Channels*, **4** (1), 51–54.

60 Sandall, D.W., Satkunanathan, N., Keays, D.A., Polidano, M.A., Liping, X., Pham, V., Down, J.G., Khalil, Z., Livett, B.G., and Gayler, K.R. (2003) A novel alpha-conotoxin identified by gene sequencing is active in suppressing the vascular response to selective stimulation of sensory nerves *in vivo*. *Biochemistry*, **42** (22), 6904–6911.

61 Satkunanathan, N., Livett, B., Gayler, K., Sandall, D., Down, J., and Khalil, Z. (2005) Alpha-conotoxin Vc1.1 alleviates neuropathic pain and accelerates functional recovery of injured neurones. *Brain Res.*, **1059** (2), 149–158.

62 Nielsen, C.K., Lewis, R.J., Alewood, D., Drinkwater, R., Palant, E., Patterson, M., Yaksh, T.L., McCumber, D., and Smith, M.T. (2005) Anti-allodynic efficacy of the chi-conopeptide, Xen2174, in rats with neuropathic pain. *Pain*, **118** (1–2), 112–124.

63 Brust, A., Palant, E., Croker, D.E., Colless, B., Drinkwater, R., Patterson, B., Schroeder, C.I., Wilson, D., Nielsen, C.K., Smith, M.T., Alewood, D., Alewood, P.F., and Lewis, R.J. (2009) Chi-conopeptide pharmacophore development: toward a novel class of norepinephrine transporter inhibitor (Xen2174) for pain. *J. Med. Chem.*, **52** (22), 6991–7002.

64 Craik, D.J. (2006) Chemistry – seamless proteins tie up their loose ends. *Science*, **311** (5767), 1563–1564.

6
Plant Antimicrobial Peptides: From Basic Structures to Applied Research

Suzana M. Ribeiro, Simoni C. Dias, and Octavio L. Franco

6.1
Introduction

Antimicrobial peptides (AMPs) are recognized as the first line of defense in several organisms against a wide array of pathogens [1]. These small molecules (<100 amino acid residue length) have been found in different forms of life including animals, microorganisms, and plants [2], being of particular interest due to their clinical and agricultural applicability.

Plants are able to synthesize an arsenal of antimicrobial, insecticidal [3], anti-tumor [4], and antiviral [5] peptides. With this in mind, many authors have tried to understand the physiological importance of some peptides to plant development and survival, asking questions like "why would a plant need to produce an anti-HIV agent?" [5]. Moreover, why do some plant AMPs also show deleterious activity in animal cells? The consensus is that these effects are fortuitous, and that AMPs are part of plant defense barriers, while they are also produced with other as yet unclear purposes. Apart from those questions, these "promiscuous molecules" present innovative prospects in the control of human and animal infections. Furthermore, they are promising tools in new biotechnological processes of crop protection. In this chapter we will summarize: the main classes, localization, structural folds, and biotechnological approaches to the use of antimicrobial peptides isolated from plants.

6.2
The Diversity of Plant Antimicrobial Peptides: Focusing on Tissue Localization and Plant Species Distribution

The natural production of AMPs in different plant organs has been notably associated with plant defense [6]. In the environment, plant pathogens and pre-dators, such as bacteria, fungi, nematodes, and insects, utilize plant compounds as

Peptide Drug Discovery and Development: Translational Research in Academia and Industry, First Edition.
Edited by Miguel Castanho and Nuno C. Santos.
© 2011 WILEY-VCH Verlag GmbH & Co. KGaA, Weinheim.
Published 2011 by WILEY-VCH Verlag GmbH & Co. KGaA

a source of nutrition [7]. Under these conditions, plants can provide a miscellany of chemical defenses, which include peptides. Some peptides are classified as pathogenesis-related (PR) proteins because they are detectable only after a pathogen attack, characterizing this strategy as an inducible defense [8]. The production of these molecules is not limited to the site of the infection by pathogens, but is instead commonly accumulated in healthy plant tissues, as reviewed in [18]. On the other hand, some peptides have been constitutively synthesized, as reviewed in [8]. Over 200 AMPs have been described in a vast number of plant families [11]. There are distinct groups of plant AMPs, such as cyclotides [5], defensins [9], impatiens [12], hevein-like peptides, knottins-like peptides, lipid-transfer proteins as reviewed in [18], myrosinase-binding proteins type 1 (MBP-1) [13], beta-barrelins [14], shepherins [15], snakins [10], and vicilin-like [16]. These molecules are categorized according to their function and relative structures [17], and especially according to the number and position of cysteine residues [18].

Moreover, this myriad of peptides can occur in different tissues, such as roots [19], leaves [20], flowers [21], tubers [10], and seeds [22]. Most AMPs have been reported in seeds, due to their large quantity of proteins. Furthermore, this tissue supports the embryo and, therefore, needs protection against potential pathogens present in the soil, explaining the presence of antimicrobial compounds [9].

Although AMPs are mainly found in seeds, they can also be expressed in vegetative tissues [23]. Evidence has shown that some cowpea defensins can be easily isolated from seeds, cotyledons, and leaves [24]. Defensins form a well known family, and they show potential applicability for plant and animal pathogen control [25]. It has recently been demonstrated that some defensins are non-toxic to mammalian cells [26], reinforcing the idea that AMPs from plants can contribute to drug development for the treatment of human infections caused by fungi.

Another interesting group of peptides found in different plant tissues consists of cyclotides, which present a wide range of applications and perspectives. Some peptides belonging to this group possess potent activity against human immunodeficiency virus (HIV) [27], Gram-negative bacteria [28], insects [3], molluscs [29], helmints [30], and cancer [31], making cyclotides suitable candidates for applications in drug design and agriculture [5].

Last but not least, flowers are still to be further investigated. They have received little attention, although they are also sources of peptides with inhibitory activities towards pathogens [21]. The flowers from ornamental tobacco (*Nicotiana alata*) and petunia (*Petunia hybrida*), show some defensins with the ability to control the development of phytopathogenic fungi *Fusarium oxysporum* and *Botrytis cinerea* [32].

6.3
Possible Structural Folds Found in Plant AMPs to Date

As previously described, AMPs are important components of the plant's natural defences toward invading pathogens. They are commonly related to properties such as amphipacity and cationicity. Although they have been commonly isolated from different species, only a few different structural scaffolds have been elucidated to date. Furthermore, several structures are in a single class, which mostly shows a typical structural fold such as that observed for cysteine-stabilized motifs (CSαβ) found in defensins [33] or cyclotides [34]. This fact decreases even more the number of known folds for plant AMPs. Since they are relatively small (< 10 kDa), the number of possible folds is also reduced. In this section we will examine these structural scaffolds, considering that the protein scaffold is a peptide framework that exhibits high tolerance of its residue modifications.

Initially, a classical fold is observed for CSαβ motifs, commonly found in plant defensins, also known as γ-thionins [33]. In the last few years several structures have been elucidated for this peptide class, including defensins from *Hordeum vulgareum, Triticum aestivum* [35], *Raphanus sativus* [36], *Aesculus hippocastanum* [37], *Pisum sativum* [38], and *Nicotiana alata* [32] In all cases, one α-helix and three anti-parallel β-sheets basically compose the three-dimensional structures of CSαβ peptides that have been investigated, creating a distinctive amphipatic two-layer αβ sandwich (Figure 6.1). However, the complete relationship between structure and function is still a mystery, because a single and typical structure has such a wide range of functions: it is able to cause mortality to pathogens such as bacteria and fungi or may inhibit digestive enzymes such as proteinases and α-amylases, as reviewed by Carvalho and Gomes [39]. Another important issue about defensins is that their cysteine-stabilized αβ (CSαβ) cores are extremely stable, especially due to the presence of large quantities of cysteines involved in disulfide bond formation, which confers several benefits on the use of this specific scaffold in the development of new drugs.

In summary, because of their low sequence identity, multiple biological functions, and high structural connection, plant proteins with the CSαβ motif are thought to be first-class candidates for peptide engineering. Some peptides containing this motif have been engineered to display novel functions by minimal residue replacement. For example, VrD1, a defensin from *Vigna radiata*, has been used as a model to understand the effects of residue substitution in defensin structure and function, and a methodical alanine substitution was performed to examine the amino acid tolerance of the CSαβ motif [40]. The alanine substitution of each location was ineffective in modifying the protein structure, although the biological activities of some mutants were altered or abolished. In short, amylase inhibitory function was significantly reduced when the amino acid residues located on the binding surface were changed, indicating that the scaffold was not directly related to function in the defensin family.

Another distinguished and well known biologically active plant peptide scaffold is found in the cyclotide class [34]. Cyclotides are a new and rising family of plant-derived backbone-cyclized polypeptides, approximately 30 amino acid residues long. These peptides show a highly conserved disulfide-stabilized core containing six cystines, commonly characterized by an atypical knotted structure (Figure 6.1). Cyclotides can be classified into two subfamilies: Möbius and bracelet. The first group is categorized by a twist formation in the peptide backbone and also by the

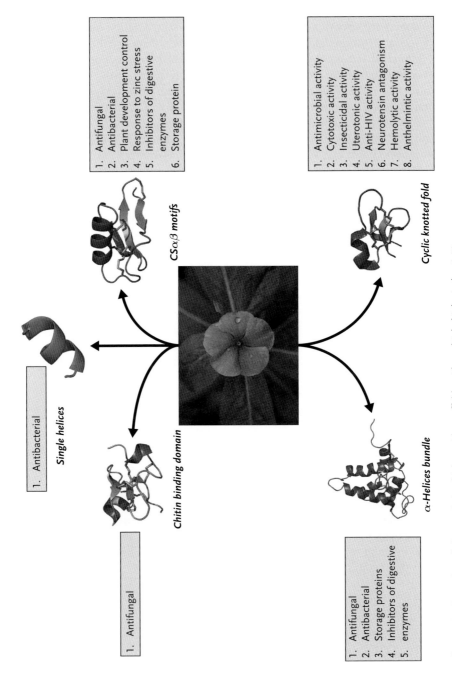

Figure 6.1 Examples of plant antimicrobial peptide scaffolds with multiple biological activities.

presence of a cis-Pro motif. The second group, known as the bracelet subfamily, is characterized by the absence of this twist feature, as reviewed in [41]. Besides bracelets and Möbius, there is a third group known for their activities as proteinase inhibitors. These peptides were first isolated from *M. cochincinensis*, and could not be classified into Möbius or bracelet subfamilies. Moreover, kalata B8 possess another type of cyclotide structure, which appears to be a hybrid between Möbius and bracelet subfamilies, suggesting that these families are closely related in evolutionary terms [34].

Cyclization seems to play an important role in peptide stability and activity. This observation has been reinforced by a study with kalata-B1, a Möbius member, where the cystine knot motif was shown to be important in the thermal stability, while the cyclic backbone was responsible for the complete enzymatic stability. However, an initial question is raised as to the advantages of these cyclic proteins compared to the usual acyclic ones. Indeed, one advantage is clear for cyclic peptides which, in general, are much more stable under the effects of temperature, chemicals, or enzymes than their linear counterparts; this suggests that cyclotides most probably evolved due to this stability. Moreover, as occurs with defensins, multiple biological activities including uterotonic activity, anti-HIV activity, neurotensin antagonism, hemolytic activity, antimicrobial activity, cytotoxic activity, insecticidal activity, and anthelmintic activity have been found in this unusual peptide class, establishing this group scaffold as peptide-base drugs [5].

Another important issue that supports the use of cyclotides as novel pharmaceuticals is that they can be readily synthesised *in vitro* using a variation of native chemical ligation technology [42]. In this procedure the backbone is initially cyclized and then the folding reaction occurs. Moreover, a library of cyclotides inside living bacterial cells has been constructed, raising the possibility of screening novel peptides into the cell with particular biological activities in a high-throughput fashion [43].

Another important structural scaffold found in plant antimicrobial peptides is related to a bundle of five α-helices, folded in a right-handed superhelix [44] (Figure 6.1). The folded protein is stabilized by two interchain disulfide bridges, since this is a heterodimeric group, and two extra bonds between cysteine residues in the large chain [45]. This specific fold has not been so thoroughly studied as cyclotides and defensins, but it can be directly related to 2S albumins and lipid-transfer proteins. Interestingly, *in vitro* investigations revealed that 2S albumins, a common protein storage family, can additionally play an important role in plant defense, acting as inhibitors of digestive enzymes and also as antimicrobial peptides [46]. The structural prototype of this family is named napin [44], but several other antimicrobial peptides have been assigned a similar scaffold.

If, on the one hand, folds that are able to complex to lipids are desirable for plant antimicrobial peptides, in order to cause a membrane disruption, on the other hand, carbohydrate binding-domains could also be valuable for the same function with a different strategy. With this in mind, some chitin-binding scaffolds have also been assigned to plant antimicrobial peptides, among them the peptide 2 purified from *Eucommia ulmoides* Oliv. This 41-residue long peptide exhibits chitin-binding activity and also inhibitory effects on both the development of cell wall chitin-containing fungi and chitin-free fungi [47]. The tertiary structure of EAFP2 represents a five-disulfide cross-linked structural fold, adopting a compact global structure formed by a 3_{10} helix (Cys3-Arg6), an α-helix and three-strand antiparallel β-sheets. Furthermore, the tertiary structure of this peptide shows a chitin-binding domain with a hydrophobic and a cationic surface, like most antimicrobial peptides previously described.

Finally, and no less important, we cite the plant AMPs that show simply helical structural folds. These peptides are less stable than other scaffolds previously cited, because of the absence or low quantity of disulfide bridges [48]. Nevertheless, they show higher flexibility due to an enhanced quantity of glycine residues. An important example is the dimeric peptide isolated from *P. guajava* seeds, named Pg-AMP1 [49]. The predicted structure was seen to be composed of two α-helices, one at N-termini and the other at C-termini, with a single flexible loop connecting them (Figure 6.1). Most glycine residues are found in this loop, conferring flexibility to peptide structure. Moreover, at the extremities of α-helices it is possible to find cationic arginine residues, providing the necessary positive charge to the active peptide. Hydrophobic residues are observed along the structure, being involved in dimer formation.

Another example of the same fold was observed in three antimicrobial peptides isolated from green coconut water [50]. These short peptides (1 kDa or less) are able to form a single amphiphilic helix that can probably penetrate and disrupt the bacterial membrane. In summary, all scaffolds presented here support simple properties on their surface, such as basic and hydrophobic residues, and these properties can probably be converted from one fold to another, helping to design new drugs over the mother protein chains. Moreover, these proteinaceous skeletons may also receive different sequences in the future, thus exposing different side chains and producing novel and intriguing pharmaceuticals.

6.4
New Biotechnological Products Produced from Plant Peptides

Finding curative powers in plants is a very old idea. People all over the world have long applied poultices and imbibed infusions of thousands of indigenous plants. It is impossible not to recall the traditional rhyme "An apple a day keeps the doctor away." In fact, the utilization of plants dates back to prehistory. There is evidence that Neanderthals used plants such as hollyhock *Alcea rosea* [51]. Currently, almost one-half of all pharmaceuticals dispensed in the Americas have higher-plant origins, but a very small number of them are intended for use as antibiotics, since we have so far relied on microorganism sources for these activities. Since the early use of antibiotics in the 1950s, the use of antimicrobial plant sources has been practically nonexistent. Nevertheless, plants show the ability to produce numerous compounds with antimicrobial properties, in addition to the plant AMPs previously described. In general, plants have an almost immeasurable capacity to produce aromatic compounds, such as phenols and other secondary metabolites, that show their ability to control infective pathogens. Additionally, plants are also able to synthesize quinones and tannins, which are responsible for plant pigmentation, and terpenoids, which are responsible for plant odors and flavors [52]. All of these compounds may be used by plants to avoid microorganism infections.

Considering all of these plant compounds, which obviously include the AMPs, an immediate question is raised. Why must plant compounds be chosen to the detriment of several other compounds from other sources? Clinical researchers and pharmaceutical companies have two main reasons for being interested in the issue of antimicrobial plant peptides. First, it is very likely that these phytochemicals will find their way into the arsenal of antimicrobial drugs prescribed by physicians. Secondly, the public is becoming progressively more conscious of problems with the over-prescription and misuse of commercial antibiotics. Moreover, many people would like to have more control over their medical care. This is partly why the use of plant peptides, as well as other forms of medical treatments, has enjoyed immense popularity since the late 1990s [51]. An additional reason to use plant antimicrobial peptides derives from their different mechanism of action than that of conventional antibiotics, as described in the first section of this chapter, which gives a clear alternative to the treatment of infections caused by resistant microorganisms in hospital environments [49].

Despite all this, until now no plant AMP has come onto the market, but the possibilities are enormous for biotechnology companies, since the use of peptides increases each day. Today, there are more than 50 marketed peptides worldwide, numerous peptides in the clinical trial phase, and thousands in late preclinical phases [53]. The potential of peptide therapeutics improves each year. This development has occurred thanks to manufacturing improvements, because now peptides can be produced through synthetic, recombinant, or transgenic methods (Figure 6.2).

The latter method can be utilized not only as a biofactory, but also to produce transgenic plants with enhanced resistance toward pathogens. With this in mind, a great variety of antibacterial peptides has been discovered in recent years. Protecting a host from various bacterial and fungal pathogens and from antimicrobial activity, these peptides have some other functions that attracted attention to new therapeutic opportunities. These include: (i) spectra-even tumoral cells; (ii) synergism with other AMPs and also with clinical therapeutics; (iii) ability to inactivate endotoxins and thus prevent septic shock; (iv) generally low toxicity to mammalian cells; (v) ability to modulate the innate immune response in mammals [54, 55].

However, isolation of plant peptides from natural sources is inefficient and time-consuming, while chemical synthesis is costly [56]. For pharmaceutical applications, an economical method to produce a large quantity of AMPs is needed, and preparation of peptide antibiotics on a large scale is a significant challenge in the development of commercial products [57]. Although the production of recombinant proteins is a very empirical system, modulating expression conditions can drastically alter protein yields. Different strategies have been developed

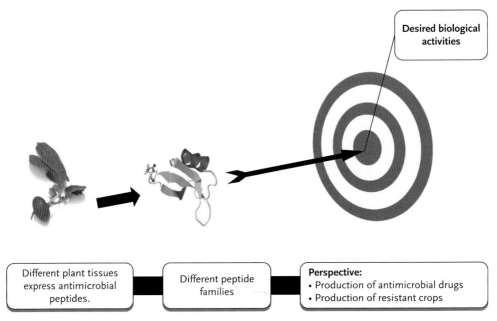

Desired biological
activities

Different plant tissues
express antimicrobial
peptides.

Different peptide
families

Perspective:
• Production of antimicrobial drugs
• Production of resistant crops

Figure 6.2 Flowchart of discovery and practical application of plant antimicrobial peptides.

to produce heterologous antimicrobial peptides sourced from plants in prokaryotic (*Escherichia coli*) and eukaryotic (yeasts, plants, and animal cells) systems [55] (Table 6.1).

In the prokaryotic system, the concentration of induction agents, different growth media conditions and multiple *Escherichia coli* strains employed for heterologous expression are factors that can contribute to expression levels and be systematically optimized. In general, *E. coli* is a safe strategy for heterologous recombinant protein studies due to the ease of genetic manipulation, relative inexpensiveness to culture, and very fast expression, typically producing protein in large quantities in a single day [66]. The importance of *E. coli* for heterologous protein production is perhaps best highlighted by the wide variety of commercial products available for the *E. coli* expression system [67]. Otherwise, some plant antimicrobial peptides have shown clear difficulties in being expressed in the prokaryotic system, since they have been proteolytically degraded, expressed at low levels and/or are sometimes insoluble and toxic to the host cell [56]. Plant defensin expression presents a challenge for *in vivo* synthesis because their structural features determine the unique biological properties of those proteins. Cysteine and arginine-high contents also affect expression levels, as well as recovery yield in some prokaryotic expression systems [65]. These residues seem to be essential for biological activity and their bridges are believed to be crucial for the maintenance of their three-dimensional structure, as well as for the thermodynamic and proteolytic stability of these peptides [10].

Table 6.1 Production of heterologous plant antimicrobial defensins.

Peptide name	Plant species/ tissue	Expression systems	Activity before heterologous expression	Activity after heterologous expression	References
TvD1	Tephrosia villosa/ leaf	Prokaryotic (Escherichia coli)	F;IR	F,IR:	[58]
VuD1	Vigna unguiculata/seeds	Prokaryotic (Escherichia coli)	A	IS, S	[48]
defensin-1 (pth1)	Solanum tuberosum/tuber	Prokaryotic (Escherichia coli)	BP;F	BP; F + +	[59]
Lm-def	Lepidium meyenii/ leaves	Prokaryotic (Escherichia coli)	ND	F	[60]
TDEF1	Trichosanthes kirilowii/leaves	Prokaryotic (Escherichia coli)	ND	F	[61]
PDC1	Zea mays/leaves	Prokaryotic (Escherichia coli) and Eukaryotic, yeast (Pichia pastoris)	ND	F	[62]
Tfgd1	Trigonella foenum-graecum /leaves	Prokaryotic (Escherichia coli)	ND	F	[63]
VaD1	Vigna angularis/ seeds	Prokaryotic (Escherichia coli)	F, IS, Ptn	F, BP;BN;Ptn; IS.	[64]
Psd1	Pisum sativum/ seeds	Eukaryotic, yeast (Pichia pastoris)	F	F – –	[65]

A: inhibitory activity against α-amylase (bacteria, fungi, insect or mammal); BN: inhibitory activity against Gram-negative bacteria; BP: inhibitory activity against Gram positive bacteria; F: inhibitory activity against fungi; IR: inhibitory activity against plant root growth; IS: inhibitory activity against insect; S: mammalian α-amylases from porcine pancreas and human saliva; – –: lower activity when compared to the authentic; + + with the synergistic and additive antimicrobial effects against phytopathogens previously reported; ND: not determined.

Furthermore, in the case of the prokaryotic system, *E. coli* is not capable of producing eukaryotic post-translational modifications, which can be critical for the production of folded active plant AMPs. Additionally, in the case of antibacterial peptides, it is not possible to achieve their expression directly in the *E. coli* system because they are toxic to host cells; there is also the problem of accumulation of the target proteins in insoluble aggregates known as inclusion bodies (IBs). IBs usually consist of almost pure, aggregated proteins which are typically misfolded and thus biologically inactive [67]. Different approaches can be utilized to solubilize inclusion bodies, including direct protein refolding from IBs using modified washing, solubilization, and different conditions such as protein expression under reduced temperatures, utilization of special strains of *E. coli* and derivatives of the BL21 parent. These special strains improve the stability of target plasmids with repetitive sequences, *lacy* mutants which have improved adjustable levels of protein expression. Therefore, the majority of these modifications do not fully guarantee increased solubility of recombinants [66]. To overcome these obstacles, several approaches in the biological expression systems have been developed by fusing the antibacterial peptide with a partner protein that has anionic properties [57]. The presence of an anionic segment was considered essential in the fusion partner for its ability to neutralize the positive charge of antibacterial peptides, thus resulting in efficient expression of the target protein. Such fusion partners include glutathione S-transferase (GST), maltose-binding protein (MBP), thioredoxin (Trx), ubiquitin [57], and chaperones [68]. The use of the partner protein could greatly improve the stability of the target proteins in host cells.

Despite the large numbers of plant AMPs isolated and characterized in the literature to date [39], few successes in recombinant protein expression in a prokaryotic system have been achieved (Table 6.1). One successful case is a defensin, TvD1, isolated from a weedy leguminous, *Tephrosia villosa* [58]. After being expressed in the *Escherichia coli* expression system, the recombinant peptide (rTvD1) was purified to exhibit potent antifungal activity on hyphae and spores/conidia of some species of phytopathogenic fungi, such as *P. personata* and several other soil-borne fungal pathogens, which cause economically significant diseases such as *Fusarium oxysporum* f. sp. vasinfectum (vascular wilt of tomato), *F. moniliforme* (root rot of rice), *Rhizoctonia solani* (sheath blight of rice), *Phytophthora parasitica* f. sp. nicotianae (leaf rot of tobacco), *Curvularia* spp (leaf spots), *Botrytis cinerea* (grape rot), and *Alternaria helianthi* (black or gray leaf spot of sunflower). The purified peptide also showed significant inhibition of root elongation in *Arabidopsis* seedlings, subsequently affecting the extension of growing root hairs; this indicates that it has the potential to disturb plant growth and development. Another example is the expression of an unusual defensin in the prokaryotic system, which was described in [48]. The defensin VuD1 was cloned from cowpea (*Vigna unguiculata*) seeds and further expressed in *E. coli* with potential application in the development of transgenic plants for insect pest control. Moreover, the coding regions of the potato snakin-1 (sn1) and defensin-1 (pth1) genes were amplified and cloned into the pCRII-TOPO_ Vector, and *E. coli* strain BL21 (DE3) was used as a host for expression of the target genes. However, the recombinant protein is accumulated in the form of insoluble aggregates (IBs) and was biologically inactive. After refolding, the proteins showed higher antimicrobial activities than peptides purified from plant tissues. Both peptides exhibited strong antibacterial activity against the phytopathogenic bacterium *Clavibacter michiganensis* subsp. *sepedonicus* (50%) and antifungal activity against the phytopathogenic fungi *Colletotrichum coccoides* and *Botrytis cinerea* [59].

Another option to solve the problems of insoluble aggregate formations and production of eukaryotic post-translational modifications involves the use of a eukaryotic expression system such as methylotrophic yeast, *Pichia pastoris*. The major advantages of fungal production include potential for high-level production (multiple grams per liter), secreted production facilitating downstream processing and purification, and a correctly matured and folded product with formation of the essential disulfide bridges [25]. In some cases, yeast expression requires several selection steps in various media. During the shake-flask cultivation, the recombinant protein was found to be sensitive to proteolytic degradation and the expression was very low [57]. The obvious disadvantage of fungal production is the inherent sensitivity of the host toward the peptides with antifungal activity [25].

Cabral et al. [65] obtained a large amount of functional recombinant Pisum sativum defensin1 (rPsd1), by expressing in Pichia pastoris. The antifungal potency of recombinant, by measuring the percentage of growth inhibition caused by serial dilutions of the protein sample, presented almost the same antifungal potency for N. crassa (IC50; 10 mg mL^{-1}) and A. versicolor (in the presence of 100 mg mL^{-1} of both Psd1 and rPsd1 the fungus growth was inhibited by about 30%). Nevertheless, the recombinant peptide presented a lower activity against A. niger and F. solani than the authentic Psd1. The expression systems can affect protein functionality. This was observed in [62] when the defensin PDC1 protein was expressed in E. coli and yeast and its antifungal activities were compared. The protein produced in P. pastoris was more effective in inhibiting growth of F. graminearum at all the protein levels that were tested. P. pastoris is believed to more effective in promoting disulfide bonding than E. coli, which would be expected to be important in the case of PDC1 protein. FTIR analysis of PDC1 protein expressed in the two expression systems showed that expression in P. pastoris gave a product with more β-sheets and less random unordered structure than when it was expressed in E. coli (Table 6.1).

The use of plants for expression and studies of AMPs has become a reality and is established as a valuable biotechnological approach. AMPs could also be used in model plants and in transgenic plants of different crop species. This approach could offer a solution for creating crops resistant to a wide range of bacterial and fungal pathogens [69]. Recent studies show that the use of plants for production of recombinant proteins offers considerable advantages over the prokaryote and other conventional systems, such as mammalian cell culture and microbial fermentation. In addition, the recombinant protein produced in plants can perform most of the post-translational modifications required for protein stability, bioactivity, and favorable pharmacokinetics [70]. The major limitation of this system is its low level of protein expression. This aspect is important and involves parameters which affect the economics of protein production and purification [71, 72]. Some plant peptides have been expressed in tobacco [15, 40], Arabidopsis [69], rice [73], potato [72], barley [74], tomato [75], and potato [72]. Most transgenic plants are driven by constitutive promoters such as UBQ or CaMV35S [76]. Using a light-regulated leaf specific promoter, Oard et al. [69] produced transgenic plants carrying the extracellular targeting of antimicrobial peptides and achieved effective inhibition of initial pathogen attack.

In the case of fungus-resistant plants, it has been demonstrated that agronomically useful levels of control can be achieved by the rough expression of a single transgene in agricultural crops [77]. This was shown when the alfalfa antifungal peptide (alfAFP) defensin, isolated from seeds of Medicago sativa, was expressed in transgenic potato, displaying strong activity against the agronomically important fungal pathogen Verticillium dahliae. Transgenic potato plants provide robust resistance in the greenhouse, and this resistance is maintained under field conditions. Here, the transgenic crop showed the same level of resistance as it would after fumigation, and it was significantly different from the unfumigated control. All the information above reinforces the fact that plant defensins may be used as an efficient tool to inhibit yeasts or filamentous fungi and bacterial pathology by serving as a source of new antibacterial products, working as well as the construction of bacterial/fungi resistant transgenic plants. Moreover, these plants could be utilized as bio-factories, producing large quantities of antibiotics with activity toward bacteria with enhanced resistance to classic antibiotics [78].

Additionally, an important study using a previously developed plant expression system, MAR, based on a plant transformation vector and expressed in post-transcriptional gene silencing (PTGS), was developed by Sels *et al.* [79]. It was capable of cloned expression and purifying one PR peptide that was homogeneous with *A. thaliana* ecotype Columbia-0. After the correct folding was confirmed, the recombinant peptide demonstrated inhibitory activity against several yeasts being considered as strong candidates for pharmaceutical antimycotics. It is expected that novel studies will use PTGS-MAR and other expression systems in order to obtain large amounts of bioactive, correctly processed plant defensins from transgenic bio-factories [8].

Some studies have shown that plant peptides may also be used to genetically improve animals. With this goal, a defensin from *Capsicum chinense* that showed fungicidal and cytotoxic activity was expressed in bovine endothelial cells, con-ferring impenetrability to *Candida albicans* in transfected cells BVE-E6E7 [80]. The medium for cultivation was clones of transfected cells which, when developed, exhibited inhibitory properties against germ tube formation, viability, and inter-nalization of *Candida albicans*, and cytotoxic effects against the human tumor cell line, HeLa. Results from this work point to the enormous potential of the use of defensins from plants in the treatment of animal mycoses, in the *in vitro* study of host–pathogen interaction, and in the development of novel drugs.

References

1 Zasloff, M. (2002) Antimicrobial peptides of multicellular organisms. *Nature*, **415**, 389–395.

2 Yount, N.Y. and Yeaman, M.R. (2004) Multidimensional signatures in antimicrobial peptides. *Proc. Natl. Acad. Sci. USA*, **101**, 7363–7368.

3 Jennings, C.V., Rosengren, K.J., Daly, N.L., Plan, M., Stevens, J., Scanlon, M.J., Waine, C., Norman, D.G., Anderson, M.A., and Craik, D.J. (2005) Isolation, solution structure, and insecticidal activity of kalata B2, a circular protein with a twist: do Mobius strips exist in nature?. *Biochemistry*, **44**, 851–860.

4 Wong, J.H. and Ng, T.B. (2005) Sesquin, a potent defensin-like antimicrobial peptide from ground beans with inhibitory activities toward tumor cells and HIV-1 reverse transcriptase. *Peptides*, **26**, 1120–1126.

5 Craik, D.J., Mylne, J.S., and Daly, N.L. (2010) Cyclotides: macrocyclic peptides with applications in drug design and agriculture. *Cell Mol. Life Sci.*, **67**, 9–16.

6 Benko-Iseppon, A.M., Galdino, S.L., Calsa, T. Jr, Kido, E.A., Tossi, A., Belarmino, L.C., and Crovella, S. Overview on plant antimicrobial

peptides. *Curr. Protein Pept. Sci.*, **11**, 181–188.

7 Dangl, J.L. and Jones, J.D. (2001) Plant pathogens and integrated defence responses to infection. *Nature*, **411**, 826–833.

8 Sels, J., Mathys, J., De Coninck, B.M., Cammue, B.P., and De Bolle, M.F. (2008) Plant pathogenesis-related (PR) proteins: a focus on PR peptides. *Plant Physiol. Biochem.*, **46**, 941–950.

9 Terras, F.R., Schoofs, H.M., De Bolle, M.F., Van Leuven, F., Rees, S.B., Vanderleyden, J., Cammue, B.P., and Broekaert, W.F. (1992) Analysis of two novel classes of plant antifungal proteins from radish (*Raphanus sativus* L.) seeds. *J. Biol. Chem.*, **267**, 15301–15309.

10 Berrocal-Lobo, M., Segura, A., Moreno, M., Lopez, G., Garcia-Olmedo, F., and Molina, A. (2002) Snakin-2, an antimicrobial peptide from potato whose gene is locally induced by wounding and responds to pathogen infection. *Plant Physiol.*, **128**, 951–961.

11 Hammami, R., Ben Hamida, J., Vergoten, G., and Fliss, I. (2009) PhytAMP: a database dedicated to antimicrobial plant peptides. *Nucleic Acids Res.*, **37**, D963–D968.

12 Tailor, R.H., Acland, D.P., Attenborough, S., Cammue, B.P., Evans, I.J., Osborn, R.W., Ray, J.A., Rees, S.B., and Broekaert, W.F. (1997) A novel family of small cysteine-rich antimicrobial peptides from seed of *Impatiens balsamina* is derived from a single precursor protein. *J. Biol. Chem.*, **272**, 24480–24487.

13 Duvick, J.P., Rood, T., Rao, A.G., and Marshak, D.R. (1992) Purification and characterization of a novel antimicrobial peptide from maize (*Zea mays* L.) kernels. *J. Biol. Chem.*, **267**, 18814–18820.

14 McManus, A.M., Nielsen, K.J., Marcus, J.P., Harrison, S.J., Green, J.L., Manners, J.M., and Craik, D.J. (1999) MiAMP1, a novel protein from *Macadamia integrifolia* adopts a Greek key beta-barrel fold unique amongst plant antimicrobial proteins. *J. Mol. Biol.*, **293**, 629–638.

15 Koo, J.C., Chun, H.J., Park, H.C., Kim, M.C., Koo, Y.D., Koo, S.C., Ok, H.M., Park, S.J., Lee, S.H., Yun, D.J., Lim, C.O., Bahk, J.D., Lee, S.Y.. and Cho, M. J. (2002) Over-expression of a seed specific hevein-like antimicrobial peptide from *Pharbitis* nil enhances resistance to a fungal pathogen in transgenic tobacco plants. *Plant Mol. Biol.*, **50**, 441–452.

16 Marcus, J.P., Green, J.L., Goulter, K.C. and Manners, J.M. (1999) A family of antimicrobial peptides is produced by processing of a 7S globulin protein in *Macadamia integrifolia* kernels. *Plant J.*, **19**, 699–710.

17 Garcia-Olmedo, F., Molina, A., Alamillo, J.M., and Rodriguez-Palenzuela, P. (1998) Plant defense peptides. *Biopolymers*, **47**, 479–491.

18 Lay, F.T. and Anderson, M.A. (2005) Defensins – components of the innate immune system in plants. *Curr. Protein Pept. Sci.*, **6**, 85–101.

19 Asiegbu, F.O., Choi, W., Li, G., Nahalkova, J., and Dean, R.A. (2003) Isolation of a novel antimicrobial peptide gene (Sp-AMP) homologue from *Pinus sylvestris* (Scots pine) following infection with the root rot fungus *Heterobasidion annosum*. *FEMS Microbiol. Lett.*, **228**, 27–31.

20 Teixeira, F.R., Lima, M.C.O.P., Almeida, H.O., Romeiro, R.S., Silva, D.J.H., Pereira, P.R.G., Fontes, E.P.B., and Baracat-Pereira, M.C. (2006) Bioprospection of cationic and anionic antimicrobial peptides from bell pepper leaves for inhibition of *Ralstonia solanacearum* and *Clavibacter michiganensis* ssp. michiganensis growth. *J. Phytopathol.*, **154**, 418–421.

21 Tavares, L.S., Santos Mde, O., Viccini, L.F., Moreira, J.S., Miller, R.N., and Franco, O.L. (2008) Biotechnological potential of antimicrobial peptides from flowers. *Peptides*, **29**, 1842–1851.

22 Pelegrini, P., Farias, L., Saude, A., Costa, F., Bloch, C., Silva, L., Oliveira, A., Gomes, C., Sales, M., and Franco, O. (2009) A novel antimicrobial peptide from *Crotalaria pallida* seeds with activity against human and

phytopathogens. *Curr. Microbiol.*, **59**, 400–404.

23 Terras, F.R., Eggermont, K., Kovaleva, V., Raikhel, N.V., Osborn, R.W., Kester, A., Rees, S.B., Torrekens, S., Van Leuven, F., Vanderleyden, J. *et al.* (1995) Small cysteine-rich antifungal proteins from radish: their role in host defense. *Plant Cell*, **7**, 573–588.

24 Franco, O.L., Murad, A.M., Leite, J.R., Mendes, P.A., Prates, M.V., and Bloch, C. Jr (2006) Identification of a cowpea gamma-thionin with bactericidal activity. *FEBS J.*, **273**, 3489–3497.

25 Thevissen, K., Kristensen, H.H., Thomma, B.P., Cammue, B.P., and Francois, I.E. (2007) Therapeutic potential of antifungal plant and insect defensins. *Drug Discov. Today*, **12**, 966–971.

26 Tavares, P.M., Thevissen, K., Cammue, B.P.A., Francois, I.E.J.A., Barreto-Bergter, E., Taborda, C.P., Marques, A. F., Rodrigues, M.L., and Nimrichter, L. (2008) In vitro activity of the antifungal plant defensin RsAFP2 against *Candida* isolates and its *in vivo* efficacy in prophylactic murine models of candidiasis. *Antimicrob. Agents Chemother.*, AAC.00448–AAC.00408.

27 Gustafson, K.R., Sowder, R.C., Henderson, L.E., Parsons, I.C., Kashman, Y., Cardellina, J.H., McMahon, J.B., Buckheit, R.W., Pannell, L.K., and Boyd, M.R. (1994) Circulins A and B. Novel human immunodeficiency virus (HIV)-inhibitory macrocyclic peptides from the tropical tree *Chassalia parvifolia*. *J. Am. Chem. Soc.*, **116**, 9337–9338.

28 Pranting, M., Loov, C., Burman, R., Goransson, U., and Andersson, D.I. The cyclotide cycloviolacin O2 from *Viola odorata* has potent bactericidal activity against Gram-negative bacteria. *J. Antimicrob. Chemother.*, **65**, 1964–1971.

29 Plan, M.R., Saska, I., Cagauan, A.G., and Craik, D.J. (2008) Backbone cyclised peptides from plants show molluscicidal activity against the rice pest *Pomacea canaliculata* (golden apple snail). *J. Agric. Food Chem.*, **56**, 5237–5241.

30 Colgrave, M.L., Kotze, AC, Kopp, S., McCarthy, J.S., Coleman, G.T., and

Craik, D.J. (2009) Anthelmintic activity of cyclotides: *in vitro* studies with canine and human hookworms. *Acta Trop.*, **109**, 163–166.

31 Lindholm, P., Goransson, U., Johansson, S., Claeson, P., Gullbo, J., Larsson, R., Bohlin, L., and Backlund, A. (2002) Cyclotides: a novel type of cytotoxic agents. *Mol. Cancer Ther.*, **1**, 365–369.

32 Lay, F.T., Schirra, H.J., Scanlon, M.J., Anderson, M.A., and Craik, D.J. (2003) The three-dimensional solution structure of NaD1, a new floral defensin from *Nicotiana alata* and its application to a homology model of the crop defense protein alfAFP. *J. Mol. Biol.*, **325**, 175–188.

33 Pelegrini, P.B. and Franco, O.L. (2005) Plant gamma-thionins: novel insights on the mechanism of action of a multi-functional class of defense proteins. *Int. J. Biochem. Cell Biol.*, **37**, 2239–2253.

34 Daly, N.L., Rosengren, K.J., and Craik, D.J. (2009) Discovery, structure and biological activities of cyclotides. *Adv. Drug Deliv. Rev.*, **61**, 918–930.

35 Bruix, M., Jimenez, M.A., Santoro, J., Gonzalez, C., Colilla, F.J., Mendez, E., and Rico, M. (1993) Solution structure of gamma 1-H and gamma 1-P thionins from barley and wheat endosperm determined by 1H-NMR: a structural motif common to toxic arthropod proteins. *Biochemistry*, **32**, 715–724.

36 Fant, F., Vranken, W., Broekaert, W., and Borremans, F. (1998) Determination of the three-dimensional solution structure of *Raphanus sativus* antifungal protein 1 by 1H NMR. *J. Mol. Biol.*, **279**, 257–270.

37 Fant, F., Vranken, W.F., and Borremans, F.A. (1999) The three-dimensional solution structure of *Aesculus hippocastanum* antimicrobial protein 1 determined by 1H nuclear magnetic resonance. *Proteins*, **37**, 388–403.

38 Almeida, M.S., Cabral, K.M., Kurtenbach, E., Almeida, F.C., and Valente, A.P. (2002) Solution structure of *Pisum sativum* defensin 1 by high resolution NMR: plant defensins, identical backbone with different

mechanisms of action. *J. Mol. Biol.*, **315**, 749–757.

39 Carvalho A.O. and Gomes, V.M. (2009) Plant defensins – prospects for the biological functions and biotechnological properties. *Peptides*, **30**, 1007–1020.

40 Yang, X., Xiao, Y., Wang, X., and Pei, Y. (2007) Expression of a novel small antimicrobial protein from the seeds of motherwort (*Leonurus japonicus*) confers disease resistance in tobacco. *Appl. Environ. Microbiol.*, **73**, 939–946.

41 Pelegrini, P.B., Quirino, B.F., and Franco, O.L. (2007) Plant cyclotides: an unusual class of defense compounds. *Peptides*, **28**, 1475–1481.

42 Kent, S.B. (2009) Total chemical synthesis of proteins. *Chem. Soc. Rev.*, **38**, 338–351.

43 Jagadish, K. and Camarero, J.A. (2010) Cyclotides, a promising molecular scaffold for peptide-based therapeutics. *Biopolymers*, **94**(5): 611–616.

44 Pantoja-Uceda, D., Bruix, M., Santoro, J., Rico, M., Monsalve, R., and Villalba, M. (2002) Solution structure of allergenic 2 S albumins. *Biochem. Soc. Trans.*, **30**, 919–924.

45 Rico, M., Bruix, M., Gonzalez, C., Monsalve, R.I., and Rodriguez, R. (1996) 1H NMR assignment and global fold of napin BnIb, a representative 2S albumin seed protein. *Biochemistry*, **35**, 15672–15682.

46 Pelegrini, P.B., Noronha, E.F., Muniz, M.A., Vasconcelos, I.M., Chiarello, M.D., Oliveira, J.T., and Franco, O.L. (2006) An antifungal peptide from passion fruit (*Passiflora edulis*) seeds with similarities to 2S albumin proteins. *Biochim. Biophys. Acta*, **1764**, 1141–1146.

47 Huang, R.H., Xiang, Y., Tu, G.Z., Zhang, Y., and Wang, D.C. (2004) Solution structure of *Eucommia* antifungal peptide: a novel structural model distinct with a five-disulfide motif. *Biochemistry*, **43**, 6005–6012.

48 Pelegrini, P.B., Lay, F.T., Murad, A.M., Anderson, M.A., and Franco, O.L. (2008) Novel insights on the mechanism of action of alpha-amylase inhibitors from the plant defensin family. *Proteins*, **73**, 719–729.

49 Pelegrini, P.B., Murad, A.M., Silva, L.P., Dos Santos, R.C., Costa, F.T., Tagliari, P.D., Bloch, C. Jr, Noronha, E.F., Miller, R.N., and Franco, O.L. (2008) Identification of a novel storage glycine-rich peptide from guava (*Psidium guajava*) seeds with activity against Gram-negative bacteria. *Peptides*, **29**, 1271–1279.

50 Mandal, S.M., Dey, S., Mandal, M., Sarkar, S., Maria-Neto, S., and Franco, O.L. (2009) Identification and structural insights of three novel antimicrobial peptides isolated from green coconut water. *Peptides*, **30**, 633–637.

51 Cowan, M.M. (1999) Plant products as antimicrobial agents. *Clin. Microbiol. Rev.*, **12**, 564–582.

52 Mahomoodally, M.F., Gurib-Fakim, A., and Subratty, A.H. (2010) Screening for alternative antibiotics: an investigation into the antimicrobial activities of medicinal food plants of Mauritius. *J. Food Sci.*, **75**, M173–M177.

53 Saladin, P.M., Zhang, B.D., and Reichert, J.M. (2009) Current trends in the clinical development of peptide therapeutics I. *Drugs*, **12**, 779–784.

54 Giuliani, A., Pirri, G., and Nicoletto, S. (2007) Antimicrobial peptides: an overview of a promising class of therapeutics. *Cent. Eur. J. Biol.*, **2**, 1–33.

55 Stotz, H.U., Thomson, J.G., and Wang, Y. (2009) Plant defensins: defense, development and application. *Plant Signal Behav.*, **4**, 1010–1012.

56 Pazgier, M. and Lubkowski, J. (2006) Expression and purification of recombinant human alpha-defensins in *Escherichia coli*. *Protein Expr. Purif.*, **49**, 1–8.

57 Xu, X., Jin, F., Yu, X., Ren, S., Hu, J., and Zhang, W. (2007) High-level expression of the recombinant hybrid peptide cecropin A(1–8)-magainin2(1–12) with an ubiquitin fusion partner in *Escherichia coli*. *Protein Expr. Purif.*, **55**, 175–182.

58 Vijayan, S., Guruprasad, L., and Kirti, P.B. (2008) Prokaryotic expression of a constitutively expressed *Tephrosia villosa* defensin and its potent antifungal activity. *Appl. Microbiol. Biotechnol.*, **80**, 1023–1032.

59 Kovalskaya, N. and Hammond, R.W. (2009) Expression and functional characterization of the plant antimicrobial snakin-1 and defensin recombinant proteins. *Protein Expr. Purif.*, **63**, 12–17.

60 Solis, J., Medrano, G., and Ghislain, M. (2007) Inhibitory effect of a defensin gene from the Andean crop maca (*Lepidium meyenii*) against *Phytophthora infestans*. *J. Plant Physiol.*, **164**, 1071–1082.

61 Da-Hui, L., Gui-Liang, J., Ying-Tao, Z., and Tie-Min, A. (2007) Bacterial expression of a *Trichosanthes kirilowii* defensin (TDEF1) and its antifungal activity on *Fusarium oxysporum*. *Appl. Microbiol. Biotechnol.*, **74**, 146–151.

62 Kant, P., Liu, W.-Z., and Pauls, K.P. (2009) PDC1, a corn defensin peptide expressed in *Escherichia coli* and *Pichia pastoris* inhibits growth of *Fusarium graminearum*. *Peptides*, **30**, 1593–1599.

63 Olli, S. and Kirti, P.B. (2006) Cloning, characterization and antifungal activity of defensin Tfgd1 from *Trigonella foenum-graecum* L.J. *Biochem. Mol. Biol.*, **39**, 278–283.

64 Chen, G.H., Hsu, M.P., Tan, C.H., Sung, H.Y., Kuo, C.G., Fan, M.J., Chen, H.M., Chen, S., and Chen, C.S. (2005) Cloning and characterization of a plant defensin VaD1 from azuki bean. *J. Agric. Food Chem.*, **53**, 982–988.

65 Cabral, K.M., Almeida, M.S., Valente, A. P., Almeida, F.C., and Kurtenbach, E. (2003) Production of the active antifungal *Pisum sativum* defensin 1 (Psd1) in *Pichia pastoris*: overcoming the inefficiency of the STE13 protease. *Protein Expr. Purif.*, **31**, 115–122.

66 Peti, W. and Page, R. (2007) Strategies to maximize heterologous protein expression in *Escherichia coli* with minimal cost. *Protein Expr. Purif.*, **51**, 1–10.

67 Cunningham, F. and Deber, C.M. (2007) Optimizing synthesis and expression of transmembrane peptides and proteins. *Methods*, **41**, 370–380.

68 Sorensen, H.P. and Mortensen, K.K. (2005) Advanced genetic strategies for recombinant protein expression in

Escherichia coli. *J. Biotechnol.*, **115**, 113–128.

69 Oard, S. and Enright, F. (2006) Expression of the antimicrobial peptides in plants to control phytopathogenic bacteria and fungi. *Plant Cell Reports*, **25**, 561–572.

70 Twyman, R.M., Schillberg, S., and Fischer, R. (2005) Transgenic plants in the biopharmaceutical market. *Expert Opin. Emerg. Drugs*, **10**, 185–218.

71 Desai, P.N., Shrivastava, N., and Padh, H. (2010) Production of heterologous proteins in plants: strategies for optimal expression. *Biotechnol. Adv.*, **28**, 427–435.

72 Almasia, N.I., Bazzini, A.A., Hopp, H. E., and Vazquez-Rovere, C. (2008) Overexpression of snakin-1 gene enhances resistance to *Rhizoctonia solani* and *Erwinia carotovora* in transgenic potato plants. *Mol. Plant Pathol.*, **9**, 329–338.

73 Iwai, T., Kaku, H., Honkura, R., Nakamura, S., Ochiai, H., Sasaki, T., and Ohashi, Y. (2002) Enhanced resistance to seed-transmitted bacterial diseases in transgenic rice plants overproducing an oat cell-wall-bound thionin. *Mol. Plant Microbe Interact.*, **15**, 515–521.

74 Molina, A. and Garcia-Olmedo, F. (1997) Enhanced tolerance to bacterial pathogens caused by the transgenic expression of barley lipid transfer protein LTP2. *Plant J.*, **12**, 669–675.

75 Kostov, K., Christova, P., Slavov, S., and Batchvarova, R. (2009) Constitutive expression of a radish defensin gene Rs-Afp2 in tomato increases the resistance to fungal pathogens. *Biotechnol. Biotec. Eq.*, 1121–1125.

76 Zhu, Y.J., Agbayani, R., and Moore, P.H. (2007) Ectopic expression of *Dahlia merckii* defensin DmAMP1 improves papaya resistance to *Phytophthora palmivora* by reducing pathogen vigor. *Planta*, **226**, 87–97.

77 Gao, A.-G., Hakimi, S.M., Mittanck, C.A., Wu, Y., Woerner, B.M., Stark, D.M., Shah, D.M., Liang, J., and Rommens, C.M.T. (2000) Fungal pathogen protection in potato by expression of a plant defensin peptide. *Nat. Biotechnol.*, **18**, 1307–1310.

78 Murad, M., Pelegrini, P., Neto, S., and Franco, O. (2007) Novel findings of defensins and their utilization in construction of transgenic plants. *Trans. Plant J.*, **1**, 39–48.

79 Sels, J., Delaure, S.L., Aerts, A.M., Proost, P., Cammue, B.P., and De Bolle, M.F. (2007) Use of a PTGS-MAR expression system for efficient in planta production of bioactive *Arabidopsis thaliana* plant defensins. *Transgenic Res.*, **16**, 531–538.

80 Anaya-Lopez, J.L., Lopez-Meza, J.E., Baizabal-Aguirre, V.M., Cano-Camacho, H., and Ochoa-Zarzosa, A. (2006) Fungicidal and cytotoxic activity of a *Capsicum chinense* defensin expressed by endothelial cells. *Biotechnol. Lett.*, **28**, 1101–1108.

Part II

Peptide Drugs' Translational Tales – Peptide Drugs Before, Through and After Industry Pipelines

Peptide Drug Discovery and Development: Translational Research in Academia and Industry, First Edition.
Edited by Miguel Castanho and Nuno C. Santos.
© 2011 WILEY-VCH Verlag GmbH & Co. KGaA, Weinheim.
Published 2011 by WILEY-VCH Verlag GmbH & Co. KGaA

7
Omiganan Pentahydrochloride: A Novel, Broad-Spectrum Antimicrobial Peptide for Topical Use

Evelina Rubinchik and Dominique Dugourd

7.1
Omiganan: A Novel Anti-Infective Agent for Topical Indications

As the arsenal of effective antimicrobials wanes in the face of increasing drug resistance, antimicrobial peptides have emerged as a novel class of therapies for the prevention and treatment of infections. Antimicrobial peptides are evolutionarily ancient weapons – widely produced by microbes themselves, invertebrate, plant, and animal species – that exhibit features desirable for potential antimicrobial therapeutics. Namely, antimicrobial peptides act by mechanisms different than those of classical antibiotics, kill rapidly, exhibit broad spectrum activity, show synergy with classical antibiotics, and are significantly less likely to develop resistance [1]. Additional favorable characteristics have elevated some antimicrobial peptides, such as omiganan, to the top of the developmental pipeline [2]. These peptides are small in size, easy to manufacture, possess favorable properties of solubility and stability, and exhibit broad-spectrum killing activity. Although highly active *in vitro*, the action of antimicrobial cationic peptides typically requires high concentrations in order to aggregate and induce membrane perturbations and this requirement limits the development of these agents for the treatment of systemic infections. Therefore, most efforts have been devoted to developing antimicrobial peptides as topical agents, where local concentrations ideal for optimal killing activity can be successfully achieved [1]. Topical application also ensures that peptides are not exposed to proteolytic enzymes which can rapidly degrade peptides if these are administered systemically.

Omiganan pentahydrochloride (omiganan, previously referred to as MBI 226 and MX-594AN) is a novel synthetic cationic peptide analog derived from the naturally occurring antimicrobial peptide indolicidin. Omiganan is relatively small in size, highly soluble and stable in aqueous solutions, and exhibits a wide spectrum of activity and potent killing effect [3–7]. Omiganan demonstrates rapid microbicidal activity against a wide variety of microorganisms, including gram-positive, gram-negative, and fungal pathogens [4–7]. Omiganan is an amphipathic

Peptide Drug Discovery and Development: Translational Research in Academia and Industry, First Edition.
Edited by Miguel Castanho and Nuno C. Santos.
© 2011 WILEY-VCH Verlag GmbH & Co. KGaA, Weinheim.
Published 2011 by WILEY-VCH Verlag GmbH & Co. KGaA

molecule that carries a net positive charge, which drives omiganan's affinity for negatively charged targets associated with microbial membranes, and perturbs membrane integrity, leading to rapid cell death [4, 8]. The unique characteristics and killing activity of omiganan have made it an attractive candidate for the treatment and prevention of topical infections. Specifically, a 1% aqueous gel formulation of omiganan (Omigard^{TM}) is currently in clinical development for the prevention of catheter-related infections. Omiganan 1–5% hydroalcoholic solutions have been evaluated for the treatment of acne vulgaris while omiganan 1% and 2.5% gel formulations are undergoing testing as a topical treatment for rosacea.

7.2
Structure and Mechanism of Action

Omiganan is a 12-amino-acid synthetic peptide analog of indolicidin, a naturally occurring antimicrobial peptide isolated from bovine neutrophil granules. The primary structure of omiganan is shown in Figure 7.1. The secondary structure of omiganan is thought to be also related to that of indolicidin since it retains many of its core elements [2, 8]. Indolicidin exhibits an unordered structure in aqueous environments but adopts a unique and flexible poly-L-proline-type II helix conformation, together with β-turn behavior when it interacts with lipid analogs [9, 10]. The mechanistic studies performed with indolicidin suggest that it forms, in a dose-dependent manner, discrete channels in lipid planar bilayers, resulting in membrane depolarization [10]. In gram-positive organisms, indolocidin depolarizes the membrane and forms mesosomal, intracellular membrane-like structures [11]. In gram-negative organisms, indolicidin must first permeabilize the gram-negative lipopolysaccharide-enriched outer membrane to gain access to the cytoplasmic membrane. Interestingly, in both gram-positive and gram-negative organisms, indolicidin induces cell death without complete or notable cellular lysis, suggesting that other cytoplasmic targets, possibly related to indolicidin's ability to bind DNA [12] and inhibit DNA synthesis [13], may contribute to cellular death.

The proposed mechanism of action of omiganan is in agreement with that suggested in the literature for indolicidin and similar cationic peptides. The primary mechanism of action is believed to be related to its ability to affect the cytoplasmic membranes of gram-negative and gram-positive bacteria and yeasts, resulting in membrane depolarization and cell death [14]. The membrane effect on

Omiganan	I	L	R			W	P	W	W	P	W	R	R	K	-CONH$_2$
Indolicidin	I	L	P	W	K	W	P	W	W	P	W	R	R		-CONH$_2$

Figure 7.1 Primary sequence of omiganan. Sequence alignment of the synthetic omiganan antimicrobial peptide compared to its parental and naturally occurring antimicrobial peptide, indolicidin (I = isoleucine, L = leucine, K = lysine, P = proline, R = arginine, and W = tryptophan).

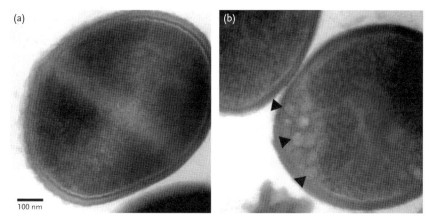

Figure 7.2 Effect of omiganan treatment on *S. aureus*. Transmission electron micrographs of *S. aureus* cells treated with either (a) vehicle control (isotonic saline) or (b) 64 µg mL^{-1} omiganan for 30 min. Cells treated with omiganan were less likely to show signs of cell division and contained more debris; cell walls of omiganan-treated cells appeared morphologically altered but intact. Omiganan treatment resulted in more granulated intracellular material and the formation of micelle-like structures (denoted with arrowheads in (b)).

the microorganisms is clearly observed by electron microscopy (Figure 7.2), which shows that exposure of bacteria to omiganan results in the formation of micelles and mesosomes [15]. Additional research confirms that the specific structure of omiganan – the presence of both positively charged and hydrophobic amino acids – creates a foundation for its ability to interact with bacterial membranes. This research was focused on the mechanism of action of omiganan at the molecular level and revealed that omiganan preferentially partitions in membranes simulating those of microorganisms over cholesterol-containing membranes simulating those of mammalian cells [8]. Furthermore, this research indicated that omiganan may have a membrane saturation–triggered mechanism of antimicrobial action. A proposed model for the action of omiganan is shown in Figure 7.3. Further research suggested that, in addition to membrane effects, the antibacterial activity of omiganan may be associated with its ability to inhibit, in a dose-dependent manner, macromolecular synthesis of DNA, RNA, and proteins [8, 16].

Because the primary target of omiganan is the broadly conserved microbial membrane, specific receptors are not thought to be involved in its mechanism of action. Additional supportive evidence for the non-receptor-mediated mechanism comes from the exceptionally rapid killing action of omiganan [4]. These features clearly distinguish the physical membrane-disrupting mechanism of action of antimicrobial peptides from the specific target-based mechanism of many conventional antibiotics (e.g., peptidoglycan enzyme inhibition). The latter mechanism requires the bacteria to be metabolically active in order for the antibiotics to exert their effect, resulting in greater time lapses prior to the development of bactericidal activity as compared to omiganan.

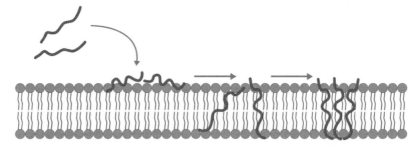

Figure 7.3 Model for omiganan-induced killing. The electrostatic characteristics of omiganan help drive its interaction with the microbial cytoplasmic membrane. Once bound, the peptide likely undergoes a conformational change, stabilizing its interaction with the polar lipid heads, and possibly initiating its insertion into the bilayer. Peptide aggregation destabilizes the membrane integrity, leading to membrane depolarization and cell death.

This non-receptor-mediated mechanism of action makes the acquisition of resistance to omiganan less likely to occur because significant hurdles will need to be overcome. Developing resistance will likely require multiple mutations and/or acquisitions of new genes to help make the necessary changes at the membrane level while still retaining the organism's inherent virulence and robustness [4]. It is important to mention that in some microbes resistance, linked to a decreased susceptibility to antimicrobial peptides, has evolved against naturally occurring antimicrobial peptides. This resistance usually occurs because the electrostatic charge of external structures (teichoic acids, phospholipids, or lipid A) is modified, and this reduces the affinity of antimicrobial peptides for these structures [17, 18]. However, these adaptations do not confer wide-spectrum resistance to all antimicrobial peptides, and are typically achieved at great cost to other essential biological processes. At present, all data generated in pre-clinical and clinical studies confirm that the acquisition of resistance to omiganan is unlikely to occur. For example, studies have shown that bacteria remain sensitive to omiganan even after multiple serial passaging in its presence [19]. For all gram-positive and gram-negative isolates tested, there was no, or minimal, increase in minimal inhibitory concentrations (MIC) after repeated exposure to omiganan at sub- to supra-MIC concentrations; a fourfold increase was seen in only one methicillin-resistant *Staphylococcus aureus* isolate [19], however, it was rapidly lost after passaging in media without omiganan. In comparison, MICs for ciprofloxacin or fusidic acid increased up to 128-fold. These results are supported by data obtained from clinical studies: analysis of *Propionibacterium acnes* isolates collected from human subjects with significant *P. acnes* skin colonization indicated that the organism did not develop decreased susceptibility to omiganan after 6 weeks of daily treatments with 1% omiganan solution [20]. Pre- and post-exposure omiganan $MIC_{50}s$ (MIC at which 50% of the isolates of a species are inhibited) remained the same (2 $\mu g\,mL^{-1}$) and the pre- and post-exposure omiganan $MIC_{90}s$ (MIC at which 90% of the isolates of a species are inhibited) were within one dilution of each other (2 and 4 $\mu g\,mL^{-1}$, respectively). No subject carried isolates with more than a twofold increase from baseline in omiganan MICs. Similar results were observed in patients exposed to a placebo solution [20].

7.3
Spectrum of Activity

Since omiganan is undergoing clinical development for the prevention of catheter-related infections, its antifungal and antibacterial activity against all major pathogens associated with catheter-related infections has been well characterized. In a recent study of omiganan against more than 1600 microbial isolates, a potent dose-dependent killing activity was displayed against gram-positives, gram-negatives, and fungal species [3, 4]. MIC_{90} ranged from 4 to $256 \, \mu g \, mL^{-1}$ for gram-positives, $8-256 \, \mu g \, mL^{-1}$ for gram-negatives, and $32-512 \, \mu g \, mL^{-1}$ for *Candida* species. Minimal bactericidal concentrations (MBCs) were the same or two- to fourfold greater than the MICs and rapid killing was observed within 2 to 6 h for all organisms tested [4]. A more recent study addressed the efficacy of omiganan against a collection of contemporary bacterial and fungal isolates commonly responsible for catheter-associated infections [5, 6]. All gram-positive ($n = 390$), gram-negative ($n = 167$), and fungal ($n = 126$) isolates tested were inhibited by ≤ 128, ≤ 1024, and $\leq 1024 \, \mu g \, mL^{-1}$ of omiganan, respectively. The agent was most active against coagulase-negative staphylococci ($MIC_{50-90} = 4 \, \mu g \, mL^{-1}$) and inhibited all *S. aureus* at $MIC_{50-90} = 16 \, \mu g \, mL^{-1}$. There were small or no increases in MICs observed against drug-resistant bacterial and fungal isolates. Even against methicillin- and vancomycin-resistant *S. aureus* isolates (MRSA and VRSA), the MIC_{90} of omiganan was virtually identical to their wild-type counterparts [7]. The omiganan 1% (10 000 $\mu g \, mL^{-1}$) topical gel formulation, at 10–2500 times the MIC for all microbial isolates tested, should be expected to inhibit all major microorganisms colonizing human skin, including those with drug-resistant phenotypes.

Given that omiganan is undergoing clinical development for the treatment of acne vulgaris and rosacea, its activity against *P. acnes* has also been comprehensively characterized [20]. The results of these studies indicated that omiganan exhibited potent antimicrobial activity against isolates of *P. acnes* ($MIC_{50} = 2 \, \mu g \, mL^{-1}$, $MIC_{90} = 4 \, \mu g \, mL^{-1}$, $n = 28$) as well as against *Propionibacterium* spp. ($MIC_{50} = 2 \, \mu g \, mL^{-1}$, $MIC_{90} = 4 \, \mu g \, mL^{-1}$, $n = 512$).

7.4
Preclinical Efficacy Studies

To determine the efficacy and potency of omiganan under conditions more relevant to the clinical situation, a study was performed to assess the dose-dependent activity of omiganan (0.1%, 0.25%, 0.5%, 1%, and 2% gels) in an *ex vivo* (pig skin) model of skin colonization by gram-positive, gram-negative, and fungal isolates [21]. Omiganan was tested against organisms associated with catheter-related infections including *S. aureus* (methicillin-resistant and -sensitive strains), *S. epidermidis*, *Escherichia coli*, *Enterobacter cloacae*, *Enterococcus faecium*, and *Candida albicans*. The drug exhibited a dose-dependent killing activity with maximal eradication (up to 2.9–3.9 $\log_{10}$ colony forming unit (CFU) per site reduction) occurring at the 1–2% dose [21]. Kill curve studies with *S. epidermidis*, the major organism colonizing human skin, demonstrated that 1% omiganan exerts a rapid bactericidal effect with a 2.7 $\log_{10}$ CFU/site reduction of bacterial counts at 1 h post-application and a 5.2 $\log_{10}$ CFU/site reduction at 24 h. No significant difference was noted in activity toward methicillin-resistant and -sensitive *S. aureus* and the drug activity was not affected by the inoculum size, suggesting that the 1% dose will be equally effective against skin infections of various severities. Omiganan efficacy was also tested in an *in vivo* guinea pig colonization model with the animal skin challenged with either *S. aureus*, *S. epidermidis*, or *C. albicans*. Topically applied omiganan showed potent antimicrobial and antifungal activity at levels comparable to the *ex vivo* pig colonization model [21].

The pig skin colonization model was also used to characterize the activity of omiganan against *P. acnes* organisms [20]. These studies revealed that 0.1–5.0% omiganan solution and gel formulations exhibited potent, dose-dependent activity against *P. acnes*. The effect was characterized by 2.1–4.1 $\log_{10}$ CFU/site reduction in bacterial counts at 24 h post-treatment whereas the placebo formulations demonstrated either no effect or minor inhibitory activity (due to the presence of alcohol in the solution formulation). The effects of the 0.75–5.0% omiganan formulations were equal or superior to 1.0% clindamycin (Dalacin T$^{\circledR}$ Topical Solution). The kill kinetic study conducted in the pig skin model demonstrated that the antibacterial effect of 2.5% omiganan solution was very rapid with more than 99% killing observed at 1 h post treatment.

Recent studies showed that, in addition to antimicrobial action, some antimicrobial peptides may exhibit anti-inflammatory activity [22]. These properties make cationic peptides attractive drug candidates for the treatment of acne vulgaris, a disease with both bacterial and inflammatory components. Since there are no reliable models of acne-induced dermal inflammation, the activity of omiganan in the irritant model of dermatitis (ear inflammation induced by 12-*O*-tetradecanoylphorbol acetate) that reproduces some elements of *P. acnes*-induced inflammation was determined. When tested in this model, 0.5% and 5% omiganan solutions reduced the ear inflammation by 31% and 40%, respectively, versus placebo, suggesting that the drug may have some anti-inflammatory activity [20].

7.5
Preclinical Toxicology Studies

The safety of omiganan formulations has been evaluated in various *in vitro* and *in vivo* studies conducted under good laboratory practice (GLP) conditions. Topical application of omiganan 1% gel resulted in no adverse local or systemic effects in repeated-dose (14-day and 28-day, rat and rabbit) animal toxicity studies [23]. No skin irritation was observed when omiganan gel was applied repeatedly to either intact or abraded animal skin, nor were there any indications of delayed hypersensitivity responses. Omiganan also offered a benign genotoxocity profile, demonstrating no clastogenic effects or genetic mutations when evaluated in *in vitro* and *in vivo* genotoxicity tests.

7.6
Clinical Studies

Omiganan is currently undergoing clinical development for the prevention of catheter-related infections and for the treatment of acne vulgaris and rosacea.

Catheter-related infections have become a serious public health threat and are one of the leading causes of nosocomial infection [24, 25]. Eliminating catheter-related infections has emerged as a frontline public health initiative since these infections are frequently life-threatening, even when treated, with high-risk patients suffering a >30% mortality rate [26]. The Center for Disease Control and Prevention has estimated that 250 000 catheter-related bloodstream infections occur each year in the United States [27], resulting in healthcare interventions that may cost as much as $2.3 billion annually [26].

Catheter-related infections include: local catheter site infections, which are infections at the catheter insertion site; catheter colonization, which is the growth of microorganisms on the portion of the catheter below the skin surface; and catheter-related bloodstream infections, which are infections in the bloodstream caused by microorganisms associated with the catheter. The vast majority of catheter-related infections are initiated by the patient's own endogenous microflora [28]. They occur when bacteria and/or fungi that colonize the patient's skin around the catheter insertion site migrate down to colonize the catheter and then break away seeding into the blood and causing subsequent bloodstream infections. Successful interventions which prevent catheter colonization and reduce incidence of catheter-related infections could provide a substantial benefit to patients and significantly reduce the high costs associated with such infections. Currently available topical antimicrobials suffer from limited duration of effect and increasingly widespread antimicrobial resistance, which have contributed to inconsistent efficacy in preventing catheter-related infections [27–30].

Omiganan 1% gel is designed to prevent catheter-related infections by killing organisms on the skin surface surrounding the catheter entry site. When evaluated in the phase I study in healthy volunteers, omiganan 1% gel effectively reduced skin colonization, with a 3-log reduction in bacterial counts observed 24 h after dermal application. The antibacterial activity of omiganan was retained for 48 and 72 h, demonstrating a robust 6- and 3.5-log decrease in bacterial counts, respectively [31, 32]. When omiganan 1% gel was applied around the insertion site of the peripheral catheter for five consecutive days, no catheter colonization was found in the catheter-tip cultures from any of the six subjects who received omiganan. In contrast, 83.3% (5/6) of the catheter-tip cultures of subjects who received the placebo showed colonization, illustrating a benefit of omiganan in preventing catheter colonization [31, 32].

Two phase III, randomized, evaluation-committee blinded studies were conducted to further evaluate the efficacy and safety of omiganan 1% gel in comparison to the standard of care, 10% povidone-iodine. Omiganan 1% gel demonstrated significant antimicrobial efficacy compared to povidone-iodine, as evidenced by a statistically significant reduction in the secondary end points of catheter colonization and microbiologically-confirmed local catheter site infections. In one phase III study, omiganan 1% gel was also superior to povidone-iodine in preventing clinically-diagnosed local catheter site infections. In addition, there was a positive trend in favor of omiganan for reducing the incidence of catheter-related bloodstream infections compared to povidone-iodine in both phase III studies. In all clinical studies, omiganan 1% gel was well tolerated, did not induce clinically significant irritation or contact sensitization, and was not systemically absorbed [2, 23, 32].

In addition to prevention of catheter-related infections, omiganan has also been evaluated for the treatment of acne vulgaris and rosacea. Rosacea is a medically unsatisfied chronic inflammatory condition that primarily affects the facial skin of an estimated 14 million Americans. Currently, the cause of rosacea is unknown and there is no cure for the disease [33]. The clinical signs and symptoms of rosacea include: facial flushing and erythema, inflammatory papules and pustules, hypertrophy of the sebaceous glands of the nose, and ocular changes. None of the therapies available currently treat all of these signs and symptoms, and the length of their treatment can be limited due to undesirable side effects. To determine an optimal dose and treatment regimen of omiganan gel formulations, a phase II study was conducted in subjects with papulopustular rosacea. Once daily omiganan 2.5% gel has demonstrated superior lesion count reductions and Treatment Success (as defined by Investigator Global Assessment scores) compared to 1% gel and placebo at nine weeks of treatment. Omiganan gel was well-tolerated at all doses tested.

Acne vulgaris is a chronic inflammatory disorder of the pilosebaceous unit that widely affects adolescents and young adults. The pathogenesis of acne vulgaris is multifactorial with the following key factors responsible for the development of acne lesions: follicular epidermal hyperproliferation, excessive sebum formation and subsequent plugging of the follicle, presence and activity of *P. acnes*, and development of dermal inflammation [34, 35]. Currently available options for the treatment of acne vulgaris include therapies with retinoids, benzoyl peroxide, and antibiotics. However, the use of topical and systemic antibiotics is complicated by the development of resistant strains of *P. acnes* [36], and isotretinoin is a known teratogen [37]. Therefore, there is a need to develop new acne vulgaris therapies and recent research suggests that cationic peptides may be attractive novel drug candidates for this indication [22]. When omiganan 2.5% and 5% hydroalcoholic solutions were evaluated for 6 weeks in a phase II study in patients with substantial facial acne lesions, omiganan demonstrated clinical benefit by reducing counts of inflammatory and non-inflammatory lesions and improving physician's Global Severity Assessment scores [2, 38]. In the second phase II study in subjects with mild to moderate acne vulgaris, omiganan 2.5% solution demonstrated statistical superiority over the vehicle control in reducing inflammatory, non-inflammatory, and total lesion counts and improving physician's Global Severity Assessment scores at 6 weeks of treatment [2]. In all clinical studies conducted with 1–5% omiganan solutions, the drug was well tolerated and non-irritating, there were no serious adverse events related to the study drug and no systemic absorption after topical application.

7.7
Conclusions

The *in vivo* and *in vitro* preclinical studies demonstrated that the antimicrobial peptide omiganan exhibits broad spectrum activity, is rapidly bactericidal and fungicidal, has a mechanism of action that is different from that of the currently approved antibiotics, and is significantly less likely to develop resistance as compared to the conventional antibiotics. The drug was well tolerated in preclinical toxicology studies and in clinic. Omiganan demonstrated promising activity in several clinical trials, however, additional studies are needed to further evaluate its potential as a novel antimicrobial drug.

References

1 Giuliani, A., Pirri, G., and Nicoletto, S.F. (2007) Antimicrobial peptides: an overview of a promising class of therapeutics. *Cent. Eur. J. Biol.*, **2**, 1–33.

2 Melo, M.N., Dugourd, D., and Castanho, M.A. (2006) Omiganan pentahydrochloride in the front line of clinical applications of antimicrobial peptides. *Recent Patents Anti-Infect. Drug Disc.*, **1**, 201–207.

3 Anderegg, T.R., Fritsche, T.R., and Jones, R.N. (2004) Quality control guidelines for MIC susceptibility testing of omiganan pentahydrochloride (MBI 226), a novel antimicrobial peptide. *J. Clin. Microbiol.*, **42**, 1386–1387.

4 Sader, H.S., Fedler, K.A., Rennie, R.P., Stevens, S., and Jones, R.N. (2004) Omiganan pentahydrochloride (MBI 226), a topical 12-amino-acid cationic peptide: spectrum of antimicrobial activity and measurements of

bactericidal activity. *Antimicrob. Chemother.*, **48**, 3112–3118.

5 Fritsche, T.R., Rhomberg, P.R., Sader, H.S., and Jones, R.N. (2008) Antimicrobial activity of omiganan pentahydrochloride against contemporary fungal pathogens responsible for catheter-associated infections. *Antimicrob. Chemother.*, **52**, 1187–1189.

6 Fritsche, T.R., Rhomberg, P.R., Sader, H.S., and Jones, R.N. (2008) Antimicrobial activity of omiganan pentahydrochloride tested against contemporary bacterial pathogens commonly responsible for catheter-associated infections. *Antimicrob. Chemother.*, **61**, 1092–1098.

7 Fritsche, T.R., Rhomberg, P.R., Sader, H.S., and Jones, R.N. (2008) *In vitro* activity of omiganan pentahydrochloride tested against

vancomycin-tolerant, -intermediate, and -resistant *Staphylococcus aureus. Diagn. Microbiol. Infect. Dis.*, **60**, 399–403.

8 Melo, M.N. and Castanho, M.A. (2007) Omiganan interaction with bacterial membranes and cell wall models. Assigning a biological role to saturation. *Biochim. Biophys. Acta*, **1768**, 1277–1290.

9 Rozek, A., Friedrich, C.L., and Hancock, R.E. (2000) Structure of the bovine antimicrobial peptide indolicidin bound to dodecylphosphocholine and sodium dodecyl sulfate micelles. *Biochemistry*, **39**, 15765–15774.

10 Falla, T.J., Karunaratne, D.N., and Hancock, R.E. (1996) Mode of action of the antimicrobial peptide indolicidin. *J. Biol. Chem.*, **271**, 19298–12303.

11 Friedrich, C.L., Rozek, A., Patrzykat, A., and Hancock, R.E. (2001) Structure and mechanism of action of an indolicidin peptide derivative with improved activity against gram-positive bacteria. *J. Biol. Chem.*, **276**, 24015–24022.

12 Hsu, C.H., Chen, C., Jou, M.L., Lee, A. Y., Lin, Y.C., Yu, Y.P., Huang, W.T., and Wu, S.H. (2005) Structural and DNA-binding studies on the bovine antimicrobial peptide, indolicidin: evidence for multiple conformations involved in binding to membranes and DNA. *Nucleic Acids Res.*, **33**, 4053–4064.

13 Subbalakshmi, C., Krishnakumari, V., Sitaram, N., and Nagarj, R. (1998) Interaction of indolicidin, a 13-residue peptide rich in tryptophan and proline and its analogues with model membranes. *J. Biosci.*, **23**, 9–13.

14 Dugourd, D., Pasetka, C., Erfle, D., Rubinchik, E., Lee, L., Friedland, H.D., and McNicol, P. (2002) MBI 226 antimicrobial peptide interacts with Gram-positive and Gram-negative cell membranes. Abstr. 102nd General meeting of American Society for Microbiology, May 18–23, 2002, Salt Lake City, USA. Abstr.A-46.

15 Dugourd, D., Brinkman, J., Pasetka, C., Guarna, M., Friedland, H.D., and Clement, J. (2003) Omiganan pentahydrochloride (MBI 226) affects *Staphylococcus aureus* cell membrane.

Abstr. 43rd annual Interscience Conference on Antimicrobial Agents and Chemotherapy, September 14–17, 2003, Chicago , USA. Abstr. C1–1811.

16 Dugourd, D., Pasetka, C., Erfle, D., Rubinchik, E., Guarna, M., McNicol, P., and Friedland, H.D. (2002) MBI 226 antimicrobial peptide inhibits Staphylococcus aureus macromolecular synthesis. Abstr. 102nd General meeting of American Society for Microbiology, May 18–23, 2002, Salt Lake City, USA. Abstr. A-47.

17 Peschel, A. (2002) How do bacteria resist human antimicrobial peptides?. *Trends Microbiol.*, **10**, 179–186.

18 Shi, Y., Cromie, M.J., Hsu, F.F., Turk, J., and Groisman, E.A. (2004) PhoP-regulated *Salmonella* resistance to the antimicrobial peptides magainin 2 and polymyxin B. *Mol. Microbiol.*, **53**, 229–241.

19 Hoban, D., Witwicki, E., Zhanel, G., Workman, L., Clement, J., Friedland, H. D., and Dugourd, D. (2003) In-vitro resistance development of clinically relevant bacteria to omiganan pentahydrochloride. 43rd Annual Interscience Conference on Antimicrobial Agents and Chemotherapy, September 14–17, 2003, Chicago, USA. Abstr. E-1706.

20 Rubinchik, E., Friedland, H.D., and Dugourd, D. (2010) The novel cationic peptide omiganan: evaluation of antimicrobial (*Propionibacterium acnes*) and anti-inflammatory effects, in (ed. D. Roth), *Dermatology Research: Focus on Acne, Melanoma and Psoriasis*, Novapublishers, pp. 229–244.

21 Rubinchik, E., Dugourd, D., Algara, T., Pasetka, C., and Friedland, H.D. (2009) Antimicrobial and antifungal activity of a novel cationic antimicrobial peptide, omiganan, when tested in experimental skin colonization models. *Int. J. Antimicrob. Agents*, **34**, 457–461.

22 Guarna, M.M., Coulson, R., and Rubinchik, E. (2006) Anti-inflammatory activity of cationic peptides: application to the treatment of acne vulgarus. *FEMS Lett.*, **257** (1), 1–6.

23 Friedland, H.D, Sharp, D.D., Erfle, D.J., and Rubinchik, E. (2003) Omiganan (MBI 226) 1% gel: a novel topical antimicrobial agent with a favorable safety profile. Abstr. 43rd Annual Interscience Conference on Antimicrobial Agents and Chemotherapy, Sept 14–17, 2003, Chicago, USA.

24 Mermel, L.A. (2000) Prevention of intravascular catheter-related infections. *Ann. Intern. Med.*, **132**, 391–402.

25 Pittet, D., Tarara, D., and Wenzel, R.P. (1994) Nosocomial bloodstream infection in critically ill patients. Excess length of stay, extra costs, and attributable mortality. *JAMA*, **271**, 1598–1601.

26 Pronovost, P., Needham, D., Berenholtz, S., Sinopoli, D., Chu, H., Cosgrove, S., Sexton, B., Hyzy, R., Welsh, R., Roth, G., Bander, J., Kepros, J., and Goeschel, C. (2006) An intervention to decrease catheter-related bloodstream infections in the ICU. *N. Engl. J. Med.*, **355**, 2725–2732.

27 O'Grady, N.P., Alexander, M., Dellinger, E.P., Gerberding, J.L., Heard, S.O., Maki, D.G., Masur, H., McCormick R. D., Mermel, L.A., Pearson, M.L., Raad, I.I., Randolph, A., and Weinstein, R.A. (2002) Guidelines for the prevention of intravascular catheter-related infections. *Clin. Infect. Dis.*, **35**, 1281–1307.

28 Hibbard, J.S., Mulberry, G.K., and Brady, A.R. (2002) A clinical study comparing the skin antisepsis and safety of chloraPrep, 70% isopropyl alcohol, and 2% aqueous chlorhexidine. *J. Infus. Nurs.*, **25**, 244–249.

29 Hibbard, J.S. (2005) Analyses comparing the antimicrobial activity and safety of current antiseptic agents: a review. *J. Infus. Nurs.*, **28**, 194–207.

30 Ho, K.M. and Litton, E. (2006) Use of chlorhexidine-impregnated dressing to prevent vascular and epidural catheter colonization and infection: a meta-analysis. *J. Antimicrob. Chemother.*, **58**, 281–287.

31 McNicol, P., Friedland, H., Fraser, J., and Krieger, T. (1999) MBI 226 antimicrobial peptide prevents colonization of intravenous catheters. Abstr. 39th Annual Interscience Conference on Antimicrobial Agents and Chemotherapy, September 26–29, 1999, San Francisco, USA. Abstr. 1674.

32 Isaacson, R.E. (2003) MBI-226 Micrologix/Fujisawa. *Curr. Opin. Investig. Drugs*, **4**, 999–1003.

33 Korting, H.C. and Schollmann, C. (2009) Current topical and systemic approaches to treatment of rosacea. *J. Eur. Acad. Dermatol. Venereol.*, **8**, 876–882.

34 Burkhart, C.G., Burkhart, C.N., and Lehmann, P.F. (1999) Acne: a review of immunologic and microbiologic factors. *Postgrad. Med.*, **75**, 328–331.

35 Koreck, A., Pivarcsi, A., Dobozy, A., and Kemeny, L. (2003) The role of innate immunity in the pathogenesis of acne. *Dermatology*, **206**, 96–105.

36 Eady, E.A., Cove, J.H., Holland, K.T., and Cumliffe, W.J. (1989) Erythromycin resistant propionibacteria in antibiotic treated acne patients: association with therapeutic failure. *Br. J. Dermatol.*, **121**, 51–57.

37 Ellis, C.N. and Krach, K.J. (2001) Uses and complications of isotretinoin therapy. *J. Am. Acad. Dermatol.*, **45**, S150–S157.

38 Friedland, H.D., Sharp, D.D., and Robinson, J.R. (2003) Double-blind, randomized, vehicle-controlled study to assess the safety and efficacy of MBI 594An in the treatment of acne vulgaris. 61st Annual Meeting of American Academy of Dermatology, March 21–26, 2003, San Francisco, USA. Abstr. P51.

8
Turning Endogenous Peptides into New Analgesics: The Example of Kyotorphin Derivatives

Marta M.B. Ribeiro, Isa D. Serrano, and Sónia Sá Santos

8.1
Introduction

According to the World Health Organization statistics in 2004, "one in five people worldwide suffer from moderate to severe chronic pain, and one in three of those are unable to maintain an independent lifestyle due to their pain" [1].

In the light of the huge global burden of chronic pain, that has a trend to increase as the average lifespan increases, the "holy grail" of biomedical research has long been the development of effective treatment options for pain relief. However, few novel analgesics have entered clinical use in the past decades. Can analgesic peptides help solve this crisis?

8.2
Peptides as Future Drug Candidates

Increasing attention has been dedicated recently to peptides as future drug candidates [2]. The unraveling of the human genome, in particular, proteomic, are the precursors of this renewed interest. Peptidic molecules have some key advantages as drug candidates: (i) low toxicity: they are made of amino acid residues which control numerous body processes, therefore their metabolic cleavage products are non-toxic and (ii) facilitated synthesis: peptides are heteropolymers of up to 40 amino acid residues in a defined sequence. Due to their small size they can be artificially synthesized more straightforwardly than other compounds, and unnatural residues can be introduced in order to optimize their performance [3]. Alternatively, they can be manufactured through transgenic and recombinant methods.

Peptide drugs represent an annual market of $300–500 millions and a growth rate of up to 25% per year [4]. At present, there are more than 70 therapeutic peptides on the market [3]. Among the approved peptide drugs are natural peptides such as insulin, vancomycin, oxytocin, and cyclosporine, synthetic peptides such as

Peptide Drug Discovery and Development: Translational Research in Academia and Industry, First Edition.
Edited by Miguel Castanho and Nuno C. Santos.
© 2011 WILEY-VCH Verlag GmbH & Co. KGaA, Weinheim.
Published 2011 by WILEY-VCH Verlag GmbH & Co. KGaA.

Fuzeon (enfuvirtide) and Integrilin (eptifibatide), and the recombinant peptidic hormone Humalog (rDNA origin insulin) [2]. There are approximately 400 peptides in the drug discovery pipelines [3], 150 of which are in clinical trials [3]. Among these, the ones which are in phase I trial were designed for Central Nervous System Applications (32%), cancer therapy (30%), metabolic diseases (20%), inflammation (13%), and virology (5%) [2]. Considering peptides designed for central nervous system applications, 20% are applied in therapy and diagnostic tools, while 12% are applied in other fields [2] such as analgesia, representing up to 18 out of the 150 in clinical trials. Regarding scientific publications, based on a PubMed search (February 2011), there were 31 819 articles published in the last 10 years displaying "peptide" in the title, 25 of which combined "peptide" and "analgesic." Why are these numbers so modest? The discovery of novel therapeutic analgesic peptides is hindered by challenges in their synthesis, poor bioavailability (some cell body barriers are impermeable to peptidic compounds), inefficient oral formulations, and reduced stability, mainly due to the susceptibility to peptidases of the serum and cells [4–6].

Significant improvements in the synthetic strategies are being achieved and should turn the industrial large-scale production of peptides into a less expensive process in the near future [3]. A novel and highly efficient method for large-scale manufacture, yielding highly pure peptides, is called DioRaSSP® (Diosynth Rapid Solution Synthesis of Peptides, WO 00/71569, [7]). It combines the advantages of the homogenous character of classical solution-phase synthesis with the generic character and the amenability to automation inherent to the solid-phase approach and is being widely used in industry [4].

Improvements are also being made to increase bioavailability peptides, including the development of cell-penetrating peptides [8, 9], and of novel formulations comprising different delivery systems, such as intra-nasal or transdermal. Novel modifications, pegylated peptides (with a polyethylene glycol derivative) and lipidated peptides for instance, will increase peptide stability and selectivity yielding the desired final product: a highly potent therapeutic peptide with minimal drug–drug interactions and low toxicity [3, 10].

Furthermore, promising results have been reported, both *in vitro* and *in vivo*, concerning the application of peptides as a trafficking moiety to deliver drugs selectively to a specific tissue and/or cell type. For instance, paclitaxel–peptide conjugates are currently undergoing phase I clinical trials for effective delivery to treat brain tumors [11].

8.3
Central Nervous System Analgesic Peptides

With regard to analgesic drugs, peptides are very promising candidates, mainly for CNS analgesia. Interest in the role of peptides in the brain began as early as the 1930s and, thereafter, extensive research has been carried out [12–15]. Most of the peptide-derived analgesics display opioid-like properties, either due to their structure and/or specific mechanism of action and/or analgesic efficacy.

8.4
Endogenous Opioid System

Opium and its derivative alkaloids (e.g., morphine) have been used for thousands of years as powerful central agents in the treatment of chronic pain. Besides their analgesic effect, opioids can induce several unwanted side effects such as respiratory depression, reduced gastrointestinal motility, clouding of consciousness, nausea, tolerance liability, and addiction, which often hamper their widespread use in clinical practice [16].

Over the last three decades, the pharmacology of the endogenous opioid system has been extensively explored. Such endogenous system is mainly composed of naturally occurring opioid peptides (i.e., enkephalins, endomorphins, dynorphins, and endorphins) and their corresponding receptors. Besides the well-known functions relative to nociceptive transmission, the endogenous opioid system also regulates many other physiological responses such as gastrointestinal motility, respiration, endocrine and immune functions [17]. It is also involved in the regulation of stress response, of several behavioral and emotional effects, such as memory, learning, mental illness, and mood [15]. Opioid receptors belong to the G protein-coupled receptor family, and from the three main classes of opioid receptors already identified (μ, δ, and κ-opioid receptors), the most potent analgesic effects have been shown to be mediated by the μ-receptor (MOR) [18]. In fact, the lack of morphine antinociception in MOR-knockout mice demonstrates the importance of this receptor in morphine-induced analgesia [19]. However, the endogenous ligands to the μ-receptor were only discovered in 1997, when two tetrapeptides, named as endomorphins (endomorphin-1, EM-1, and endomorphin-2, EM-2), were identified and isolated in bovine brain [20], and subsequently in human cortex [21]. Endomorphins are structurally quite different from the so-called "typical opioids" (enkephalins, dynorphins, and endorphins, which all share the Tyr-Gly-Gly-Phe sequence at the N-terminus), since they have a Pro residue in position 2 which joins the two pharmacophoric residues Tyr^1 and Trp/Phe (i.e., EM-1: Tyr-Pro-Trp-Phe-NH_2 and EM-2: Tyr-Pro-Phe-Phe-NH_2). Both EM-1 and EM-2 showed remarkable affinity and selectivity towards the μ-receptor, having also a potent and specific antinociceptive effect in mice [20]. In fact, they act as strongly as morphine in acute pain and are more effective than the majority of the opioid peptides against neuropathic pain, even at low doses [15]. Therefore, the finding that endomorphins could serve as substitutes for opioids, without their undesired side effects, opened new avenues to discover new potentially applicable drugs for the treatment of moderate to severe chronic pain. Recently, the advances achieved in endomorphin research over the past decade have been reviewed [18, 22].

In spite of the *in vivo* efficacy of opioid drugs like morphine for pain control, prolonged treatment with such drugs is not practical since antinociceptive tolerance develops such that, to achieve the same pharmacological effect, the opioid dose escalation also increases the incidence and severity of the adverse effects. In fact, there is still a great need to discover and/or develop drugs that result in effective analgesia with lesser or, ideally, without the detrimental effects of morphine.

8.5
Strategies to Deliver Analgesic Peptides to the Brain

As mentioned above, strategies to improve metabolic stability and decrease the clearance of peptide drugs are of major importance in pharmaceutical research. In the specific case of CNS-targeted molecules, crossing of the blood–brain barrier (BBB) adds an extra – and, most of the time, the most complex – problem. The BBB is formed by a continuous layer of the brain endothelium lining brain capillaries which is highly restrictive to the crossing of molecules [23]. Since BBB limits the passage of up to 95% of the drugs to the brain [24], few treatments are available for most CNS pathologies. A limited capacity to cross the BBB is frequently related to insufficient drug lipophilicity [25].

Multiple approaches have been described to enhance drug delivery to the brain, such as [26]: (i) invasive procedures, which include direct injection or infusion, biodegradable implants, and transient osmotic opening of the BBB; (ii) chemical delivery systems, such as lipid-mediated transport (lipidization of small molecules), prodrug approach, and the lock-in system; (iii) biological delivery systems, in which pharmaceuticals are re-engineered to cross the BBB via specific endogenous transporters localized in the brain capillary endothelium; (iv) employing "Trojan horse" technology to allow, for instance, the transport of large molecules across the BBB; and (v) encapsulation via the use of particular carrier systems, such as nanoparticles and liposomes.

One must not forget that endogenous peptidases are present not only in the serum but also on the capillary endothelial cells of the BBB which, therefore, reduces the ability of enzymatically labile peptides to enter the brain. However, enzyme inhibition to increase BBB-crossing efficiency is not a realistic approach because of the large number (and concentration) of enzymes involved in the degradation of each peptide-based drug [5] and all the possible consequences of inhibiting enzymes essential for metabolism. The solution instead is to redesign each peptide in order to improve resistance to degradation and/or use prodrugs, which are the most successful techniques employed nowadays.

A strategy to improve the CNS delivery, in particular of poorly permeable, highly polar, compounds, is via the lipidization of molecules [27, 28]. A successful example of this approach is heroin, a diacyl derivative of morphine, that crosses the BBB about 100-fold better than its parent drug just by being more lipophilic [27]. The increase in lipophilicity can be achieved by addition of lipophilic groups and/or reduction of hydrogen bonding potential (e.g., via methylation) [29]. However, structural modification to enhance the lipid solubility of a peptide may affect its therapeutic efficiency. That is the case for the synthetic opioid peptide [D-

Pen^2,D-Pen^5]-enkephalin (DPDPE; Tyr-D-Pen-Gly-Phe-D-Pen-OH): the incorporation of two methyl groups on the Tyr of DPDPE significantly enhances both lipophilicity and analgesia, whereas trimethylation on the Phe of DPDPE improved delivery but not its analgesic effect (for references see [28]). Another possible strategy to enhance peptide lipophilicity involves removal of amino acid side-chains by polar groups; however, care should also be taken because, for opioid peptides, the deletion of the hydroxy group of Tyr, for instance, leads to a total loss of bioactivity [13]. This is probably due to the importance of Tyr residues for adoption of the correct peptide conformation and docking constraints towards receptor binding.

Peptide drug modification via glycosylation has also been used to improve biodistribution to the brain. The attachment of carbohydrate moieties to opioid peptides has been shown to improve their transport across the BBB [29]. Evidence also suggests that glycosylation reduces clearance [30] and increases metabolic stability [31] which, in combination with the improved BBB transport, contributes to the improved analgesia exhibited by glycosylated opioids [5]. Glycosylation-based strategies may also prove highly useful in conditions requiring prolonged administration of drugs, such as chronic pain or depression [29].

8.6
Development of New Opioid-Derived Peptides

Opioid ligands can be classified into two types: agonists and antagonists, both of which would bind the opioid receptor with good affinities. Therefore, the major difference between them is that agonists stabilize the receptor conformation in an active form, and trigger a specific response by the cell, whereas antagonists stabilize the receptor conformation in an inactive form and, therefore, act against the effects of agonists [14]. Naloxone, a universal opioid antagonist, has a binding affinity for the receptor that is similar to that of the agonist morphine [32].

Two different approaches have been explored to design and synthesize new or improved opioid ligands: (i) modification of known morphine analogs (for details see [14]) and (ii) the modification of naturally occurring ligands, such as enkephalin, dermorphin, and endomorphin.

Enkephalins are linear peptides displaying a slight selectivity for δ- over μ-opioid receptors [15]. The cyclization of [Met^5]-enkephalin (Tyr-Gly-Gly-Phe-Met-OH) plus the inclusion of two D-penicillamine residues resulted in the derivative DPDPE, which was found to be highly potent and selective for δ-receptors [33] and also to be resistant to proteolytic breakdown. Moreover, a significant increase in BBB permeability was detected after addition of chlorine to the Phe residue(s) of DPDPE and biphalin, another enkephalin analog [28].

Biphalin is a dimeric peptide [(Tyr-D-Ala-Gly-Phe-NH)$_2$] with two enkephalin sequences that are connected "tail-to-tail" (C-terminal to C-terminal) by a hydrazine bridge [34]. The affinity of biphalin for δ-opioid receptors is significantly higher than that for μ-opioid receptors. When administered intra-cerebroventricularly it is more potent than morphine at eliciting antinociception [35], probably as a result of a synergic interaction between both opioid receptors [36]. On the other hand, when given intra-venously, it produced inferior analgesia than that with morphine, suggesting that biphalin may suffer some enzymatic breakdown in the periphery before crossing the BBB [37]. However, it should be highlighted that due to the insertion of D-Ala residues in the 2 and 2′ positions (instead of the Gly residue) and also to the presence of the amino-linker, biphalin is more stable against enzymatic degradation when compared to endogeneous opioid peptides. Alteration of the structure of biphalin to include a CH_2–CH_2–CH_2 chain between the –NH–NH– linker, produces a compound that displays lower biological activity, indicating that the spacer plays a vital role in activity [38].

The dermorphin-derived tetrapeptide DALDA (Tyr-D-Arg-Phe-Lys-NH$_2$; which carries a net positive charge of $+3$ at physiological plasma pH) was shown to be one of the most selective ligands towards μ-opioid receptors [39]. Another dermorphin analog, ADAMB (N-amidino-YrF-MeβAla-OH), exhibited high potency as a μ-receptor agonist and displayed *in vivo* analgesic activity fivefold stronger than that of morphine after oral administration [14]. The replacement of the Tyr residue of DALDA with Dmt (2′,6′-dimethyltyrosine) leads to the formation of the enzymatically stable compound [Dmt^1]DALDA [40]. It has been shown that insertion of the Dmt structure enhances the affinity and bioactivity of δ- and μ-receptor ligands [41]. In fact, [Dmt^1]DALDA exhibits a higher binding affinity for both δ- and μ-receptors than its parent compound, the selective μ-receptor agonist DALDA [40]. Furthermore, both *in vivo* and *in vitro* findings indicate that [Dmt^1] DALDA is capable of crossing the BBB better than DALDA. [Dmt^1]DALDA can readily translocate across *Caco-2* cells [42] and was also found to induce extraordinarily potent and long-lasting antinociceptive effects in the mouse tail-flick assay when given subcutaneously [43].

One possible strategy to develop new opioid-like compounds with improved potency and fewer side effects is via the simultaneous targeting of multiple opioid receptors.

Despite acting primarily at the μ-opioid receptor, morphine and the other clinically available opioids also have affinity for the other δ and κ-opioid receptors. It has been reported that the selective blockade of δ-opioid receptors with δ-antagonists greatly reduced the development of morphine tolerance and dependence in mice [44, 45]. Moreover, in δ-opioid receptor knockout mice no evidences of tolerance were observed upon chronic administration of morphine [46]. Therefore, the development of opioid ligands with mixed profile (i.e., μ-agonist/δ-antagonist) opens the possibility of having a potent analgesic with low propensity to produce tolerance and physical dependence [47]. The combination of Dmt and Tic (1,2,3,4-tetrahydroisoquinoline-3-carboxylic acid) moieties produces peptides with remarkable potency and unprecedented selectivity for μ- plus δ- opioid receptors [41]. The first *in vivo* application of such a bifunctional opioid peptide was reported in rats by Schiller and coworkers [48] with the synthetic compound DIPP-NH$_2$[ψ] (Dmt-Ticψ[CH$_2$NH]Phe-Phe-NH$_2$), which was shown to produce less tolerance, no physical dependence and a three-fold higher potency than morphine, but only when centrally delivered (i.e., i.c.v. administration). Efforts have been made to develop several other bifunctional compounds with mixed opioid agonist/opioid antagonist properties [47].

8.7
Kyotorphin – the Potential of an Endogenous Dipeptide

Kyotorphin (KTP) is an endogenous dipeptide (L-Tyr-L-Arg) first isolated from bovine brain [49] and subsequently found in the brains of other mammals [50]. In humans, a study using cerebrospinal fluid samples revealed that in patients with persistent pain, the KTP content is lower [51]. KTP acts as a neurotransmitter/ neuromodulator in nociceptive responses in the CNS, having an analgesic effect approximately 4.2-fold higher than endogenous opioid peptides, such as met-enkephalin [52]. Other activities have been proposed, such as inhibiting cell pro-liferation [53], an anti-hibernating regulation [54], and even an epilepsy seizure protection effect [55]. Kyotorphin owes its name to the city when it was discovered – Kyoto – and to its morphine-like effect. The similarities with opioid molecules go beyond the activity: structurally, both display a phenolic ring, considered essential for the interaction of morphine with receptors. Therefore, in the first decades following the discovery of KTP, researchers were essentially focused on the analgesic effect and on studying the mechanism of action, initially believed to be opioid-like. For that, they performed studies using a direct administration of KTP into different brain areas. Despite these efforts, the mode of action of KTP remains unclear. There is evidence suggesting that KTP does not bind to opioid receptors, but a specific receptor for KTP has not yet been identified. A direct binding to opioid receptors is indeed absent, but the naloxone reversible analgesia suggests that KTP activity is indirectly mediated by opioid receptors [56, 57]. An alternative mechanism is a fast degradation of KTP, resulting in L-Arg, a substrate for nitric oxide (NO) synthase [58]. Whatever the mechanism, a release of met-enkephalin is acknowledged by all the authors.

KTP clusters a very interesting set of biological activities. Moreover, being a dipeptide, its chemical synthesis is straightforward and relatively fast. Being aware of the biological potential of KTP and the appealing characteristics for pharma pipelines, researchers started to study its effect following systemic administration (intra-peritoneal, intra-venous, or oral). Disappointingly, KTP only showed a brief activity and at a high dose of 200 mg/kg when systemically administered to rodent animals [59]. The clear difference in activity when different administration routes are used (systemic vs. brain) was believed to be due to the most common reasons that prevent drugs reaching the CNS: limited capacity to cross the BBB and also susceptibility to various clearance mechanisms, such as lytic enzymes. Therefore, a logical strategy to target KTP to the brain is the chemical modification of KTP into lipophilic analogs [59–61], which can, in turn, make the molecules more resistant to enzyme degradation. However, while increasing lipid affinity, solubility in aqueous media, the most frequent formulation form for compounds, needs to be maintained at reasonable levels. This critical feature was the problem with a recent KTP derivative – the acylated KTP derivative, KTP-K-palmitoyl [61].

It is clear that KTP can only be turned into a valuable and marketable drug if modified to have an enhanced BBB-crossing ability, while preserving most of its structure and chemistry so that the end result can remain effective and nontoxic.

8.8
New KTP Derivatives

Taking the knowledge of structure–activity relationships into account, new KTP derivatives have been designed, such as KTP-amide (KTP-NH$_2$) and Ibuprofen-KTP-amide (IKTP-NH$_2$) (Figure 8.1). The amidation of KTP induced a change in the molecule net charge at physiological plasma pH, from neutral to positive. Cationization was once applied for other opioid peptides with success [28]. Since lipophilicity is the major concern for BBB-crossing ability, a lipophilic analgesic drug was further grafted to KTP-NH$_2$, forming an analgesic "tandem chimera." Ibuprofen (IBP) was selected to perform KTP-NH$_2$ hydrophobization. It not only meets the lipophilicity constraint but also is itself a well known analgesic molecule, whose pharmacology and toxicology have been extensively studied. However, regarding BBB-crossing, only limited information exists on the brain distribution of Ibuprofen. Although a few authors defend that it can get into the brain [62, 63],

Figure 8.1 Chemical structure of (a) endogenous KTP and KTP derivatives: (b) KTP-NH$_2$ and (c) IKTP-NH$_2$.

presenting a brain to blood concentration ratio of 0.90 [63], others reported a nearly nil permeability of BBB to IBP [64, 65]. IBP, a non-steroidal anti-inflammatory drug, acts by inhibiting enzymes ciclooxigenase 1 and 2 and, more recently, a new role of IBP as a neuroprotective agent has been described [63, 66, 67].

8.9
Assessing BBB Permeability with Peptide–Membrane Partition Studies

For a complete characterization on compounds analgesic activity, a study with model animals (mice and rats) and a set of *in vivo* anti-nociception tests (for detailed animal models of pain see reference [68]) is performed with different administration routes. Frequently, however, academic researchers limit their study to a direct injection into the brain to achieve proof of concept. This is not suitable when a pharmacological application is foreseen, for which systemic administrations should be performed. When a more mechanistic insight is needed, new players are added to this protocol and often a suspected agonist or antagonist is administered concomitantly with the molecule under study to prove the involvement of specific molecular pathways. While these methods relate directly to the animal response, they may fail at analyzing important molecular characteristics essential for activity, such as lipophilicity.

Molecular phenomena involving peptides at the cell membrane–blood interface play a fundamental role when assessing BBB permeability for those peptides. Typically, as a first evaluation of the BBB-crossing potential, industry uses a rather rudimentary, but nevertheless useful, parameter to account for lipophilicity, octanol/water partition [69, 70]. In the last decades other more realistic and reliable methods have arisen, namely, peptide–membrane partition studies [71, 72].

Sargent and Schwyzer [73, 74] proposed an active role of membranes, functioning as catalysts for peptide–receptor interactions. This hypothesis states that the membrane's role is to allow ligands to adopt the necessary docking constrains to bind cell receptors more efficiently. In addition, there is a so-called "concentration effect" which consists of the high local concentrations drugs achieve in some membrane domains favoring drug–target interactions; this effect is supported by experimental evidence [61, 75, 76]. As to neuropeptides, such as enkephalins, the tyrosine phenolic group location and orientation is a crucial factor for both interaction with cell surface receptors and biological activity.

8.10
Kyotorphins: Partition to the Membrane and Enhanced Analgesic Activity

Both KTP derivatives – KTP-NH$_2$ and IKTP-NH$_2$ were studied for their partition toward lipidic membranes. The Tyr residue of KTP peptides enables a study using fluorescence spectroscopy. Large unilamellar vesicles (LUVs) composed of the phospholipids 1-palmitoyl-2-oleyol-sn-glycero-3-phosphocoline (POPC) or POPC:POPG

(1-palmitoyl-2-oleyl-sn-glycero-3-(phosphor-rac-(1-glycerol))), were used to model the outer leaflet (neutral) and the inner leaflet (negatively charged) of mammals' biological membranes (Figure 8.2). In the presence of lipid bilayers, molecules with a tendency to interact with lipids leave the aqueous environment and insert in the lipid matrix. The extent of this "migration" depends on the concentration of the lipid and on the partition constant, K_p, a quantitative parameter of lipophilicity [71, 72] of the molecule under study. K_p can be calculated from the titration of the peptide with LUV, according to Eq. (8.1) [71]:

$$I = \frac{I_W + K_p\gamma_L[L]I_L}{1 + K_p\gamma_L[L]} \tag{8.1}$$

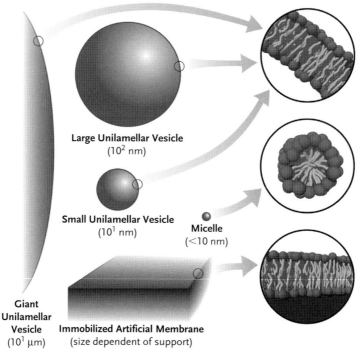

Large Unilamellar Vesicle
(10^2 nm)

Small Unilamellar Vesicle
(10^1 nm)

Micelle
(<10 nm)

Giant Unilamellar Vesicle
(10^1 μm)

Immobilized Artificial Membrane
(size dependent of support)

Figure 8.2 Different types of artificial phospholipid membranes (typical diameter magnitudes for each membrane model are indicated on the figure). Small unilamellar vesicles (SUVs), large unilamellar vesicles (LUVs), giant unilamellar vesicles (GUVs), micelles, and immobilized artificial membranes (IAMs) are all used as model membranes. LUVs, usually produced by extrusion techniques [84], are a commonly used model for K_p determination due to specific characteristics similar to biological membranes: being unilamellar vesicles they have free standing membranes with an aqueous environment on both sides, are large enough for their membrane to be considered locally plane at the molecular scale and their curvature resembles the curvature of biological membranes. (Reprinted from *Trends in Pharmacological Sciences*, **31**, Ribeiro MMB, Melo MN, Serrano ID, Santos NC and Castanho MARB, Drug–lipid interaction evaluation: why a 19th century solution?, 449–454, (2010), with permission from Elsevier).

where I_W and I_L are the limit fluorescence intensities in aqueous solution and in lipid, respectively, γ_L is the molar volume of the lipid and [L] is the lipid concentration.

The fluorescence of both peptides in the presence of lipidic vesicles increased, indicating interaction with model membranes. Amidation caused a significant increase in the K_p of KTP-NH$_2$, reaching a value of 2.5×10^3 for POPC vesicles. For IKTP-NH$_2$, K_p is 1.9×10^2 for the same lipidic mixture. As the molar fraction of the negatively charged lipid POPG in the POPC bilayer increases, K_p increases exponentially (Figure 8.3). Therefore, there is a clear effect of charge on the partition of IKTP-NH$_2$ toward the membrane, reaching a maximum when the membrane is 100% POPG (8.1×10^3). In the case of KTP-NH$_2$ it is difficult to define a specific pattern of interaction dependent on the anionic lipidic composition, with K_p varying over a small range of values. While interaction of unmodified KTP with lipids is nearly absent [61], both KTP-NH$_2$ and IKTP-NH$_2$ interact with lipid vesicles and preferably screen for liquid-crystal membranes. Thus, electrostatic attraction plays a fundamental role in the binding of IKTP-NH$_2$ to membranes, in a similar way as observed for enkephalin peptides [77].

In view of these promising results, the peptides' analgesic effects were evaluated following systemic administration to male Wistar rats. Acute pain models using thermal stimuli were applied: tail flick and hot plate tests [68]. Unlike the original KTP, a dose and time-dependent inhibition of painful behavior was detected in both tests (Figure 8.4). From these two peptides, IKTP-NH$_2$ showed the most remarkable analgesic performance – from 2.5 µM/100 g bw ($P = 0.0032$ – tail flick – and $P = 0.0005$ – hot plate, Friedman test), while for KTP-NH$_2$ twice this dose was needed to observe analgesia. IKTP-NH$_2$ potency was also strikingly higher than that of the combined injection of KTP-NH$_2$ and Ibuprofen. In fact, linking IBP to KTP-NH$_2$ increased two-fold the analgesic efficacy in relation to the control

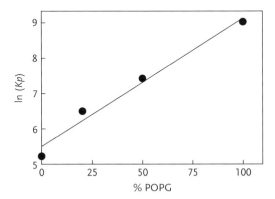

Figure 8.3 Partition coefficient (K_p) of IKTP-NH$_2$ (logarithmic scale) in LUVs with different molar ratios of POPC : POPG. For each lipidic mixture, partition is performed by successive additions of a concentrated LUV suspension to IKTP-NH$_2$ (153 µM) using 10 mM HEPES buffer pH 7.4 containing 150 mM NaCl. Data is fitted with Eq. (8.1) and the K_p value obtained.

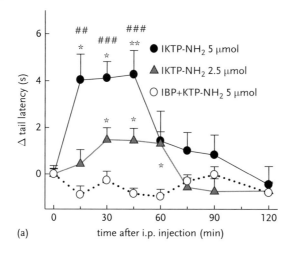

(a)

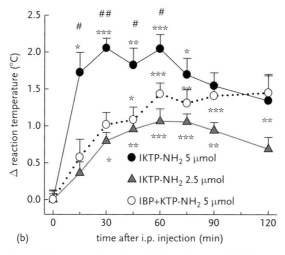

(b)

Figure 8.4 Analgesic profile of KTP derivatives. Inhibition of acute nociceptive responses in the Tail Flick (a) and Hot Plate (b) tests following KTP-derivatives systemic administration. For the sake of clarity, results are expressed as the variation of the behavioral responses at each evaluation time point in relation to baseline values (time 0) obtained immediately before injection. Doses represented for 100 g bw. In all experiments, $n \geq 6$. $*P < 0.05$; $**P < 0.01$; $***P < 0.001$ versus basal response, Friedman test, and $^{\#}P < 0.05$, $^{\#\#}P < 0.01$, $^{\#\#\#}P < 0.001$ versus IBP + KTP-NH$_2$ treated controls, Mann–Whitney test. Mean $\pm$ SEM for all groups.

IBP + KTP-NH$_2$ mixture. The analgesic effects were dose-dependent, starting at 15 min and lasting for at least 45 min.

Concomitantly with the biophysical results, which revealed IKTP-NH$_2$ as the peptide with highest affinity to lipid membranes, *in vivo* anti-nociception evaluation showed that this is the most effective analgesic compound. Additionally, there is evidence suggesting that both peptides can cross the BBB: not only lipophilicity

(IBP addition) but also amidation play an important role. Lipophilicity correlates to analgesic activity, hypothetically due to: (i) a more efficient BBB-translocation process, and/or (ii) a membrane-induced optimization of conformation for receptor docking, and/or (iii) a simple concentration effect in the vicinity of target receptors.

The negative charge associated with the presence of anionic phosphatidylserine (PS) in human BBB endothelial cells was shown to direct proteins with moderately positive charge to the endocytic pathway [78] – one of the major mechanisms of adsorption of peptides at the BBB level. In agreement, other authors [79] stated that optimal conditions of lipophilicity and cationic charge of the peptides are important for efficient transport across the BBB. In this situation, the amide group seems to confer to both peptides a more cationic charge that favors its interaction with BBB endothelial cells.

8.11
Academia and Pharmaceutical Industry: Friends or Foes?

The generation of new analgesic agents and/or the development of administration strategies, allowing their efficient delivery to the brain, are of major importance to address the social and clinical needs of patients suffering with pain.

Even if, through the last decades, considerable progress has been made towards designing improved therapeutic interventions, considerable efforts are still needed in the search for the most appropriate, safe, and effective strategies in the management of pain, thus allowing those patients to have a meaningful and productive life. Analgesics are mainly divided into two classes: opioid-like drugs and NSAIDS (non-steroidal anti-inflammatory drugs). Due to their interesting set of properties, peptides, (either opioid-like or not) have potential to be future pain-killers.

Nearly 90% of new drugs are discovered and developed by the pharmaceutical industry. That may explain why 70% of the funds for clinical drug trials in the United States of America, for instance, come from industry rather than from the National Institutes of Health [80]. While pharmaceutical companies invest more in drug Discovery and Development, academia tends to focus on basic biological research fundamental to the genesis of drug discovery. Several new drug hits arise from academia, but large pharmacodynamic and pharmakokinetic characterization is better performed by Pharma Companies. The scenario seems ideal for cooperation. However, despite sharing the ultimate goal – the discovery of a promising analgesic drug for social benefits – academic and pharma researchers rarely cooperate. Delays in academic labs, meaning the loss of huge amounts of money for pharma companies [80], and influence on the design of experiments, and even delay in publication when the results do not favor the companies [81] create a mutual distrust between academics and pharmaceutical companies. These dilemmas are still not resolved. Intellectual Property issues, fundamental for companies, do not fit the typical academic collaboration between labs. However, the development of KTP derivatives is an example of how molecules found and researched in academic labs may lead to academia–industry partnership programs [82] and enter industrial pipelines. Fortunately, this is just one example among many others. Partnerships are increasing and the benefits, such as the access to new technologies and the further development of drug candidates, are visible for both partners [80, 83].

Acknowledgements

Fundação para a Ciência e Tecnologia (Portugal) is acknowledged for funding (**Project PTDC/SAU-FCF/69493/2006** and grants: the **SFRH/BD/42158/2007** fellowship to M. Ribeiro, the **SFRH/BPD/37998/2007** fellowship to I. Serrano and the **SFRH/BI/51213/2010** fellowship associated to Marie Curie IAPP to S. Sá Santos). Marie Curie Industry-Academia Partnerships and Pathways (European Commission) is also acknowledged for funding (**FP7-PEOPLE-2007-3-1-IAPP. project 230654**).

References

1 World Health Organization. (2004) World Health Organization supports global effort to relieve chronic pain. http://www.who.int/mediacentre/news/releases/2004/pr70/en/index.html (30 August 2010)

2 Marx, V. (2005) Watching peptide drugs grow up. *Chem. Eng. News*, **83** (11), 17.

3 Bellmann-Sickert, K. and Beck-Sickinger, A.G. (2010) Peptide drugs to target G protein-coupled receptors. *Trends Pharmacol. Sci.*, **31** (9), 434–441.

4 Sewald, N. and Jakubke, H.-D. (2009) *Peptides: Chemistry and Biology*, WILEY-VCH verlag GmbH & Co. KGaA, Weinheim.

5 Egleton, R.D., Mitchell, S.A., Huber, J.D., Palian, M.M., Polt, R., and Davis, T.P. (2001) Improved blood–brain barrier penetration and enhanced analgesia of an opioid peptide by glycosylation. *J. Pharmacol. Exp. Ther.*, **299** (3), 967–972.

6 Egleton, R.D., Abbruscato, T.J., Thomas, S.A., and Davis, T.P. (1998) Transport of opioid peptides into the central nervous system. *J. Pharm. Sci.*, **87** (11), 1433–1439.

7 Eggen, I.F., Bakelaar, F.T., Petersen, A., Ten Kortenaar, P.B., Ankone, N.H., Bijsterveld, H.E., Bours, G.H., El Bellaj, F., Hartsuiker, M.J., Kuiper, G.J., and Ter Voert, E.J. (2005) A novel method for repetitive peptide synthesis in solution without isolation of intermediates. *J. Pept. Sci.*, **11** (10), 633–641.

8 Henriques, S.T. and Castanho, M.A. (2005) Environmental factors that enhance the action of the cell penetrating peptide pep-1 A spectroscopic study using lipidic vesicles. *Biochim. Biophys. Acta*, **1669** (2), 75–86.

9 Henriques, S.T., Quintas, A., Bagatolli, L.A., Homble, F., and Castanho, M.A. (2007) Energy-independent translocation of cell-penetrating peptides occurs without formation of pores. A biophysical study with pep-1. *Mol. Membr. Biol.*, **24** (4), 282–293.

10 Cupido, T., Tulla-Puche, J., Spengler, J., and Albericio, F. (2007) The synthesis of naturally occurring peptides and their analogs. *Curr. Opin. Drug Discov. Devel.*, **10** (6), 768–783.

11 Majumdar, S. and Siahaan, T.J. (2010) Peptide-mediated targeted drug delivery. *Med. Res. Rev.*, 1–22.

12 Myers, R.D. (1994) Neuroactive peptides: unique phases in research on

mammalian brain over three decades. *Peptides*, **15** (2), 367–381.

13 Janecka, A., Perlikowska, R., Gach, K., Wyrebska, A., and Fichna, J. (2010) Development of opioid peptide analogs for pain relief. *Curr. Pharm. Des.*, **16** (9), 1126–1135

14 Eguchi, M. (2004) Recent advances in selective opioid receptor agonists and antagonists. *Med. Res. Rev.*, **24** (2), 182–212.

15 Gentilucci, L. (2004) New trends in the development of opioid peptide analogues as advanced remedies for pain relief. *Curr. Top. Med. Chem.*, **4** (1), 19–38.

16 Stein, C., Schafer, M., and Machelska, H. (2003) Attacking pain at its source: new perspectives on opioids. *Nat. Med.*, **9** (8), 1003–1008.

17 Kieffer, B.L. and Gaveriaux-Ruff, C. (2002) Exploring the opioid system by gene knockout. *Prog. Neurobiol.*, **66** (5), 285–306.

18 Janecka, A., Staniszewska, R., and Fichna, J. (2007) Endomorphin analogs. *Curr. Med. Chem.*, **14** (30), 3201–3208.

19 Kieffer, B.L. (1999) Opioids: first lessons from knockout mice. *Trends Pharmacol. Sci.*, **20** (1), 19–26.

20 Zadina, J.E., Hackler, L., Ge, L.J., and Kastin, A.J. (1997) A potent and selective endogenous agonist for the mu-opiate receptor. *Nature*, **386** (6624), 499–502.

21 Hackler, L., Zadina, J.E., Ge, L.J., and Kastin, A.J. (1997) Isolation of relatively large amounts of endomorphin-1 and endomorphin-2 from human brain cortex. *Peptides*, **18** (10), 1635–1639.

22 Keresztes, A., Borics, A., and Toth, G. (2010) Recent advances in endomorphin engineering. *Chem. Med. Chem.*, **5** (8), 1176–1196.

23 Ribeiro, M.M., Cast anho, M.A., and Serrano, I. In vitro blood–brain barrier models – latest advances and therapeutic applications in a chronological perspective. *Mini. Rev. Med. Chem.*, **10** (3), 262–270.

24 Pardridge, W.M. (2002) Why is the global CNS pharmaceutical market so under-penetrated?. *Drug Discov. Today*, **7** (1), 5–7.

25 Ballet, S., Misicka, A., Kosson, P., Lemieux, C., Chung, N.N., Schiller, P.W., Lipkowski, A.W., and Tourwe, D. (2008) Blood–brain barrier penetration by two dermorphin tetrapeptide analogues: role of lipophilicity vs structural flexibility. *J. Med. Chem.*, **51** (8), 2571–2574.

26 Patel, M.M., Goyal, B.R., Bhadada, S.V., Bhatt, J.S., and Amin, A.F. (2009) Getting into the brain: approaches to enhance brain drug delivery. *CNS Drugs*, **23** (1), 35–58.

27 Rautio, J., Laine, K., Gynther, M., and Savolainen, J. (2008) Prodrug approaches for CNS delivery. *AAPS J.*, **10** (1), 92–102.

28 Witt, K.A. and Davis, T.P. (2006) CNS drug delivery: opioid peptides and the blood–brain barrier. *AAPS J.*, **8** (1), E76–88.

29 Egleton, R.D. and Davis, T.P. (2005) Development of neuropeptide drugs that cross the blood–brain barrier. *NeuroRx*, **2** (1), 44–53.

30 Fisher, J.F., Harrison, A.W., Bundy, G.L., Wilkinson, K.F., Rush, B.D., and Ruwart, M.J. (1991) Peptide to glycopeptide: glycosylated oligopeptide renin inhibitors with attenuated *in vivo* clearance properties. *J. Med. Chem.*, **34** (10), 3140–3143

31 Powell, M.F., Stewart, T., Otvos, L. Jr, Urge, L., Gaeta, F.C., Sette, A., Arrhenius, T., Thomson, D., Soda, K., and Colon, S.M. (1993) Peptide stability in drug development. II. Effect of single amino acid substitution and glycosylation on peptide reactivity in human serum. *Pharm. Res.*, **10** (9), 1268–1273.

32 Gourlay, G.K. (2002) Clinical pharmacology of opioids in the treatment of pain, in *Pain 2002: An Updated Review* (ed. M.A. Giamberardino), pp. 381–394, IASP Press, Seattle.

33 Knapp, R.J., Sharma, S.D., Toth, G., Duong, M.T., Fang, L., Bogert, C.L., Weber, S.J., Hunt, M., Davis, T.P., Wamsley, J.K. et al. (1991) [D-Pen2,4′-125I-Phe4,D-Pen5">D-Pen2,4′-125I-Phe4,D-Pen5]enkephalin: a selective high affinity radioligand for delta opioid receptors with exceptional specific activity. *J. Pharmacol. Exp. Ther.*, **258** (3), 1077–1083.

34 Lipkowski, A.W., Konecka, A.M., and Sroczynska, I. (1982) Double-enkephalins – synthesis, activity on guinea-pig ileum, and analgesic effect. *Peptides*, **3** (4), 697–700.

35 Horan, P.J., Mattia, A., Bilsky, E.J., Weber, S., Davis, T.P., Yamamura, H.I., Malatynska, E., Appleyard, S.M., Slaninova, J., Misicka, A. et al. (1993) Antinociceptive profile of biphalin, a dimeric enkephalin analog. *J. Pharmacol. Exp. Ther.*, **265** (3), 1446–1454.

36 Slaninova, J., Appleyard, S.M., Misicka, A., Lipkowski, A.W., Knapp, R.J., Weber, S.J., Davis, T.P., Yamamura, H.I., and Hruby, V.J. (1998) [125I-Tyr1]biphalin binding to opioid receptors of rat brain and NG108–15 cell membranes. *Life Sci.*, **62** (14), PL199–204.

37 Silbert, B.S., Lipkowski, A.W., Cepeda, M.S., Szyfelbein, S.K., Osgood, P.F., and Carr, D.B. (1991) Analgesic activity of a novel bivalent opioid peptide compared to morphine via different routes of administration. *Agents Actions*, **33** (3–4), 382–387.

38 Dietis, N., Guerrini, R., Calo, G., Salvadori, S., Rowbotham, D.J., and Lambert, D.G. (2009) Simultaneous targeting of multiple opioid receptors: a strategy to improve side-effect profile. *Br. J. Anaesth.*, **103** (1), 38–49.

39 Schiller, P.W., Nguyen, T.M., Chung, N.N., and Lemieux, C. (1989) Dermorphin analogues carrying an increased positive net charge in their "message" domain display extremely high mu opioid receptor selectivity. *J. Med. Chem.*, **32** (3), 698–703.

40 Schiller, P.W., Nguyen, T.M., Berezowska, I., Dupuis, S., Weltrowska, G., Chung, N.N., and Lemieux, C. (2000) Synthesis and *in vitro* opioid activity profiles of DALDA analogues. *Eur. J. Med. Chem.*, **35** (10), 895–901.

41 Bryant, S.D., Salvadori, S., Cooper, P.S., and Lazarus, L.H. (1998) New delta-opioid antagonists as pharmacological probes. *Trends Pharmacol. Sci.*, **19** (2), 42–46.

42 Zhao, K., Luo, G., Zhao, G.M., Schiller, P.W., and Szeto, H.H. (2003) Transcellular transport of a highly polar 3 + net charge opioid tetrapeptide. *J. Pharmacol. Exp. Ther.*, **304** (1), 425–432.

43 Zhao, G.M., Wu, D., Soong, Y., Shimoyama, M., Berezowska, I., Schiller, P.W., and Szeto, H.H. (2002) Profound spinal tolerance after repeated exposure to a highly selective mu-opioid peptide agonist: role of delta-opioid receptors. *J. Pharmacol. Exp. Ther.*, **302** (1), 188–196.

44 Abdelhamid, E.E., Sultana, M., Portoghese, P.S., and Takemori, A.E. (1991) Selective blockage of delta opioid receptors prevents the development of morphine tolerance and dependence in mice. *J. Pharmacol. Exp. Ther.*, **258** (1), 299–303.

45 Fundytus, M.E., Schiller, P.W., Shapiro, M., Weltrowska, G., and Coderre, T.J. (1995) Attenuation of morphine tolerance and dependence with the highly selective delta-opioid receptor antagonist TIPP[psi]. *Eur. J. Pharmacol.*, **286** (1), 105–108.

46 Zhu, Y., King, M.A., Schuller, A.G., Nitsche, J.F., Reidl, M., Elde, R.P., Unterwald, E., Pasternak, G.W., and Pintar, J.E. (1999) Retention of supraspinal delta-like analgesia and loss of morphine tolerance in delta opioid receptor knockout mice. *Neuron*, **24** (1), 243–252.

47 Schiller, P.W. (2010) Bi- or multifunctional opioid peptide drugs. *Life Sci.*, **86** (15–16), 598–603.

48 Schiller, P.W., Fundytus, M.E., Merovitz, L., Weltrowska, G., Nguyen, T.M., Lemieux, C., Chung, N.N., and Coderre, T.J. (1999) The opioid mu agonist/delta antagonist DIPP-NH(2)[Psi] produces a potent analgesic effect, no physical dependence, and less tolerance than morphine in rats. *J. Med. Chem.*, **42** (18), 3520–3526.

49 Takagi, H., Shiomi, H., Ueda, H., and Amano, H. (1979) A novel analgesic dipeptide from bovine brain is a possible Met-enkephalin releaser. *Nature*, **282** (5737), 410–412.

50 Kolaeva, S.G., Semenova, T.P., Santalova, I.M., Moshkov, D.A., Anoshkina, I.A., and Golozubova, V. (2000) Effects of L-thyrosyl – L-arginine (kyotorphin) on the behavior of rats and goldfish. *Peptides*, **21** (9), 1331–1336.

51 Nishimura, K., Kaya, K., Hazato, T., Ueda, H., Satoh, M., and Takagi, H. (1991) [Kyotorphin like substance in human cerebrospinal fluid of patients with persistent pain]. *Masui*, **40** (11), 1686–1690.

52 Shiomi, H., Ueda, H., and Takagi, H. (1981) Isolation and identification of an analgesic opioid dipeptide kyotorphin (Tyr-Arg) from bovine brain. *Neuropharmacology*, **20** (7), 633–638.

53 Bronnikov, G., Dolgacheva, L., Zhang, S.J., Galitovskaya, E., Kramarova, L., and Zinchenko, V. (1997) The effect of neuropeptides kyotorphin and neokyotorphin on proliferation of cultured brown preadipocytes. *FEBS Lett.*, **407** (1), 73–77.

54 Ignat'ev, D.A., Vorob'ev, V.V., and Ziganshin, R. (1998) Effects of a number of short peptides isolated from the brain of the hibernating ground squirrel on the EEG and behavior in rats. *Neurosci. Behav. Physiol.*, **28** (2), 158–166.

55 Godlevsky, L.S., Shandra, A.A., Mikhaleva, I.I., Vastyanov, R.S., and Mazarati, A.M. (1995) Seizure-protecting effects of kyotorphin and related peptides in an animal model of epilepsy. *Brain. Res. Bull.*, **37** (3), 223–226.

56 Rackham, A., Wood, P.L., and Hudgin, R.L. (1982) Kyotorphin (tyrosine-arginine): further evidence for indirect opiate receptor activation. *Life Sci.*, **30** (16), 1337–1342.

57 Stone, T.W. (1983) A comparison of the effects of morphine, enkephalin, kyotorphin and D-phenylalanine on rat central neurones. *Br. J. Pharmacol.* **79** (1), 305–312.

58 Arima, T., Kitamura, Y., Nishiya, T., Taniguchi, T., Takagi, H., and Nomura, Y. (1997) Effects of kyotorphin (L-tyrosyl-L-arginine) ON[3H]NG-nitro-L-arginine binding to neuronal nitric oxide synthase in rat brain. *Neurochem. Int.*, **30** (6), 605–611.

59 Chen, P., Bodor, N., Wu, W.M., and Prokai, L. (1998) Strategies to target kyotorphin analogues to the brain. *J. Med. Chem.*, **41** (20), 3773–3781.

60 Bodor, N., Prokai, L., Wu, W.M., Farag, H., Jonalagadda, S., Kawamura, M., and Simpkins, J. (1992) A strategy for delivering peptides into the central nervous system by sequential metabolism. *Science*, **257** (5077), 1698–1700.

61 Lopes, S.C., Soares, C.M., Baptista, A.M., Goormaghtigh, E., Cabral, B.J., and Castanho, M.A. (2006) Conformational and orientational guidance of the analgesic dipeptide kyotorphin induced by lipidic membranes: putative correlation toward receptor docking. *J. Phys. Chem. B* , **110** (7), 3385–3394.

62 Parepally, J.M., Mandula, H., and Smith, Q.R. (2006) Brain uptake of nonsteroidal anti-inflammatory drugs: ibuprofen, flurbiprofen, and indomethacin. *Pharm. Res.*, **23** (5), 873–881.

63 Prins, L.H., du Preez, J.L., van Dyk, S., and Malan, S.F. (2009) Polycyclic cage structures as carrier molecules for neuroprotective non-steroidal anti-inflammatory drugs. *Eur. J. Med. Chem.*, **44** (6), 2577–2582.

64 Chen, Q., Gong, T., Liu, J., Wang, X., Fu, H., and Zhang, Z. (2009) Synthesis, *in vitro* and *in vivo* characterization of glycosyl derivatives of ibuprofen as novel prodrugs for brain drug delivery. *J. Drug Target.*, **17** (4), 318–328.

65 Mannila, A., Rautio, J., Lehtonen, M., Jarvinen, T., and Savolainen, J. (2005) Inefficient central nervous system delivery limits the use of ibuprofen in neurodegenerative diseases. *Eur. J. Pharm. Sci.*, **24** (1), 101–105.

66 Asanuma, M., Nishibayashi-Asanuma, S., Miyazaki, I., Kohno, M., and Ogawa, N. (2001) Neuroprotective effects of non-steroidal anti-inflammatory drugs by direct scavenging of nitric oxide radicals. *J. Neurochem.*, **76** (6), 1895–1904.

67 Chen, H., Jacobs, E., Schwarzschild, M.A., McCullough, M.L., Calle, E.E., Thun, M.J., and Ascherio, A. (2005) Nonsteroidal antiinflammatory drug use

and the risk for Parkinson's disease. *Ann. Neurol.*, **58** (6), 963–967.

68 Le Bars, D., Gozariu, M., and Cadden, S.W. (2001) Animal models of nociception. *Pharmacol. Rev.*, **53** (4), 597–652.

69 Bodor, N. and Buchwald, P. (1999) Recent advances in the brain targeting of neuropharmaceuticals by chemical delivery systems. *Adv. Drug Deliv. Rev.*, **36** (2–3), 229–254.

70 Leo, A., Hansch, C., and Elkins, D. (1971) Partition coefficients and their uses. *Chem. Rev.*, **71** (6), 525–616.

71 Santos, N.C., Prieto, M., and Castanho, M.A. (2003) Quantifying molecular partition into model systems of biomembranes: an emphasis on optical spectroscopic methods. *Biochim. Biophys. Acta*, **1612** (2), 123–135.

72 Ribeiro, M.M., Melo, M.N., Serrano, I.D., Santos, N.C., and Castanho, M.A. Drug–lipid interaction evaluation: why a 19th century solution? *Trends Pharmacol. Sci.*, **31** (10), 449–454.

73 Sargent, D.F. and Schwyzer, R. (1986) Membrane lipid phase as catalyst for peptide–receptor interactions. *Proc. Natl. Acad. Sci. USA*, **83** (16), 5774–5778.

74 Castanho, M.A. and Fernandes, M.X. (2006) Lipid membrane-induced optimization for ligand-receptor docking: recent tools and insights for the "membrane catalysis" model. *Eur. Biophys. J*, **35** (2), 92–103.

75 Lopes, S.C., Fedorov, A., and Castanho, M.A. (2006) Chiral recognition of D-kyotorphin by lipidic membranes: relevance toward improved analgesic efficiency. *Chem. Med. Chem.*, **1** (7), 723–728.

76 Lopes, S.C., Fedorov, A., and Castanho, M.A. (2005) Lipidic membranes are potential "catalysts" in the ligand activity of the multifunctional pentapeptide neokyotorphin. *Chembiochem*, **6** (4), 697–702.

77 Romanowski, M., Zhu, X., Kim, K., Hruby, V.J., and O'Brien, D.F. (2002) Interaction of enkephalin peptides with anionic model membranes. *Biochim. Biophys. Acta*, **1558** (1), 45–53.

78 Yeung, T., Gilbert, G.E., Shi, J., Silvius, J., Kapus, A., and Grinstein, S. (2008) Membrane phosphatidylserine regulates surface charge and protein localization. *Science*, **319** (5860), 210–213.

79 Tamai, I., Sai, Y., Kobayashi, H., Kamata, M., Wakamiya, T., and Tsuji, A. (1997) Structure–internalization relationship for adsorptive-mediated endocytosis of basic peptides at the blood–brain barrier. *J. Pharmacol. Exp. Ther.*, **280** (1), 410–415.

80 Bodenheimer, T. (2000) Uneasy alliance – clinical investigators and the pharmaceutical industry. *N. Engl. J. Med.*, **342** (20), 1539–1544.

81 Chalmers, I. (1990) Underreporting research is scientific misconduct. *JAMA*, **263** (10), 1405–1408.

82 Ribeiro, M.M.B., Castanho, M.A.R.B., Melo, M., Bardaji, E., Heras, M., Pinto, M., Tavares, I., Calado, P., and Vieira, H. (2008) Compounds for treating pain. (0805912.3)

83 LaMattina, J.L. (2009) *Drug Truths: Dispelling the Myths about Pharma R&D*, John Wiley & Sons, Inc., Hoboken, New Jersey.

84 Mayer, L.D., Hope, M.J., and Cullis, P.R. (1986) Vesicles of variable sizes produced by a rapid extrusion procedure. *Biochim. Biophys. Acta*, **858** (1), 161–168.

9
The Development of Romiplostim – a Therapeutic Peptibody Used to Stimulate Platelet Production

Graham Molineux and Ping Wei

9.1
Introduction

Romiplostim (Nplate®) is the only peptibody approved for use in humans. It is a therapeutic protein comprising a peptide component that interacts with the cell surface receptor c-Mpl and a stabilizing carrier component that confers therapeutically appropriate residence time in the body. By binding to and activating c-Mpl, romiplostim provokes a cascade of intracellular events that ultimately lead to the formation of platelets. Platelets are essential for blood clotting and are also involved in other biological processes. Romiplostim has been approved for administration to patients with immune thrombocytopenic purpura (ITP), and is being investigated for a potential role in promoting platelet production in other types of thrombocytopenia.

9.2
Thrombopoietin and c-Mpl

Megakaryocytes represent one of several blood cell lineages all of which originate from hematopoietic stem cells under the influence of a range of hematopoietic cytokines. Megakaryocytes are very large cells containing multiple copies of the normal complement of DNA; so called polyploid cells. In the case of megakaryocytes the multiple copies of the genome derive from abortive mitoses (endomitoses) in which replication of the genetic payload is not followed by separation of the daughter cells. Instead, through successive rounds of endomitosis the DNA content increases from 2 to 4, 8, 16, and so on, up to perhaps 128n. Without cellular division this yields very large cells with extensive cytoplasm. Megakaryocyte cytoplasm can then form thread-like pseudopodia along which proplatelets are formed "like beads on a string." This structure protrudes from the marrow space into the blood stream, where shear forces are thought to break off the individual "beads" as platelets.

Peptide Drug Discovery and Development: Translational Research in Academia and Industry, First Edition.
Edited by Miguel Castanho and Nuno C. Santos.
© 2011 WILEY-VCH Verlag GmbH & Co. KGaA, Weinheim.
Published 2011 by WILEY-VCH Verlag GmbH & Co. KGaA

A normal human might have around 300 000 platelets in each microliter of blood or around 1.5×10^{12} in the whole blood volume (the total platelet number in the body is likely much larger than this since many platelets are sequestered in sites such as the spleen). Each platelet is expected to survive for around 10 days, suggesting that at least 1.5×10^{11} new ones need to be produced every day merely to maintain numbers; more if any platelets are consumed in clotting events or lost due to bleeding.

The question of how this process is controlled remained relatively mysterious until the work of Kelemen, published in successive papers in the 1950s, elegantly demonstrated the existence of what he called thrombopoietin – a heat labile activity, presumed to be either proteinaceous or protein associated. It was present in sera from thrombocytopenic patients and could cause an increase in platelet counts 3 days after being injected into normal mice [1]. It was many years later that this activity was purified to homogeneity, cloned, and produced by recombinant DNA technology [2–5]. Two of these recombinant forms entered clinical trials but development stopped around 1998 due to the paradoxical development of thrombocytopenia in a few patients who had been repeatedly exposed to one of them (PEGylated recombinant human megakaryocyte growth and development factor, PEG-rHuMGDF). This molecule was a semi-synthetic derivative of thrombopoietin (or TPO as it was known, and the recombinant version was referred to as rHuTPO) comprising the first 163 amino acids of the natural protein but attached covalently to a 20 kDa polyethylene glycol polymer. What had happened was that an immune reaction to PEGrHuMGDF had occurred in these patients and the antibodies produced not only recognized and neutralized the injected drug, but they also cross-reacted with and neutralized the patients' own TPO [6]. This left patients with a long-term lack of active TPO and a treatment refractory thrombocytopenia or even pancytopenia involving several blood cell lineages. It was apparent from this experience that a new derivative or mimic of TPO was needed, but it was also apparent that a lack of homology with any endogenous protein would be a desirable property in any successor molecule. It is also important to recognize that the potential relevance of the immunogenicity findings to other recombinant versions of naturally occurring proteins was not lost. Despite the fortunate absence of this issue with G-CSF and early EPO development (maybe because they were less modified then PEG-rHuMGDF) the issue of cross-neutralizing antibodies did arise later with reformulated epoetin alfa (Eprex® [7]) and could reasonably have been predicted to be a concern with, for example, PEG-epoetin beta (Mircera®) or pegfilgrastim (Neulasta®).

Despite this setback for first generation TPO-like molecules important knowledge was gained that offered indispensible guidance to teams formulating solutions to this newly emerging risk for recombinant TPO. The lessons included:

1. The expected pharmacological effect of agonizing c-Mpl was proven; in other words thrombopoietic agents specifically stimulated platelet production *in vivo*.

2. Platelet production kinetics were found to be relatively immutable and the delay between c-Mpl stimulation and a platelet response included an obligatory delay of several days. This outlined at least some dose and schedule guidance for next generation compounds.
3. Medical conditions which might be treated and offer substantial medical benefit and others where benefits might be minimal.

1. In patients treated with PEG-rHuMGDF the responses observed were confined to the platelet lineage. This was expected as c-Mpl (CD110) is the natural receptor for thrombopoietin and its expression is limited to blood-forming tissues, specifically the megakaryocytic lineage. To add strength to the argument for lineage fidelity of both c-Mpl expression and TPO effects, a mouse in which c-Mpl had been genetically deleted showed profound changes in platelet numbers but little else [8]. In addition, the TPO knockout mouse [9] looked similar, suggesting not only that there is a single ligand for c-Mpl, but also that there exists but a single receptor for TPO. There is known to be expression of c-Mpl on blood progenitor and stem cells [10, 11] perhaps presaging the pancytopenia seen in the patients discussed above and some mpl-mutant children[12], however, the relatively normal phenotype (outside of platelet numbers) of the knockout animals argues perhaps for a degree of redundancy in terms of the role of c-Mpl and TPO in regulating more primitive hematopoietic cells in the genetic mouse models.
2. The kinetics of platelet production illustrated by the administration of exogenous c-Mpl ligands include an obligatory delay between activation of the receptor and detection of its cellular products in the blood. In common with other hematopoietic cytokines, stimulation of progenitor cells can be separated by several days from seeing mature cells in the blood. This is particularly apparent for TPO/c-Mpl, since the majority of the effects of TPO are upon megakaryocyte development rather than platelet formation itself. The delay is 4–5 days in human and 2–3 days in mouse and presents an intriguing challenge in defining the optimum scheduling of treatment in settings such as the support of cancer chemotherapy delivered on a repeating cycle perhaps every 3 or 4 weeks[13].
3. Investigations in many settings were attempted with the first generation Mpl ligands, the most prominent of which were in support of (cancer) chemotherapy induced thrombocytopenia (CIT), bone marrow or stem cell transplant, myelodysplastic syndromes, idiopathic thrombocytopenic purpura and normal platelet donation. Of these, the deeper understanding obtained from real world experience (such as platelet response kinetics, degree of patient benefit, acceptable risk profile, etc.) suggested that the patient group who in the first instance were most likely to gain significant benefit were those suffering from thrombocytopenia due to the autoimmune destruction of platelets (ITP) [14]. In the other indications, more intricate development pathways would have to be followed to better account for scheduling, concurrent medications, and safety concerns.

9.3
Discovery and Optimization of Romiplostim

Romiplostim is the prototype of a novel class of therapeutics called "peptibodies." They are so called because they comprise one or several peptide "warheads" complexed with the Fc portion of an immunoglobulin molecule, yielding a structure with a superficial similarity to an antibody.

The peptide component was identified from recombinant peptide libraries expressed as either fusions to phage proteins or to *E. coli lac* repressor proteins [15]. The optimized peptide sequence Ile-Glu-Gly-Pro-Thr-Leu-Arg-Gln-Trp-Leu-Ala-Ala-Arg-Ala was shown to displace TPO in an ELISA-based assay platform. This peptide could also stimulate the proliferation of Ba/F3 cells engineered to express human c-Mpl. However, when administered as a bolus dose to mice it was modest at best in raising platelet counts (Figure 9.1a). Instability of the naked peptide was suspected as the cause of the limited response and so the same material was infused continuously for 7 days with markedly different effects (Figure 9.1b). The dose-dependent thrombocytosis noted in these mice in response to continual exposure prompted the question whether manipulating stability or clearance of the peptide may be a fruitful avenue of pursuit.

In parallel, work on the erythropoietin receptor (EpoR), a family member closely related to c-Mpl, showed that the erythropoietin ligand had upon its surface two interaction faces that formed the functional contact with the homodimeric receptor [16].

Two copies of the mimetic peptide were linked together with a spacer of eight glycine residues in order to maximally activate the receptor. The peptide dimer so formed was shown to be active *in vivo* (Figure 9.1c, TMP-TMP) but again the modest response was thought to arise from limited exposure due to instability or rapid clearance.

Several macromolecular conjugates had been used to manage the pharmaco-kinetic and immunogenic profiles of protein therapeutics, among them PEG, starch, human serum albumin, and components of immunoglobulin. A very similar peptide (AF15705 with the inclusion of two artificial amino acids; Ile-Glu-Gly-Pro-Thr-Leu-Arg-Gln-Npa-Leu-Ala-Ala-Arg-Sar) to that used in romiplostim was indeed developed as a PEG conjugate, GW395058 [17], but does not appear to have progressed beyond the preclinical stage of development. However, its half-life in dogs was improved.

Immunoglobulins persist in the body very much longer than would be expected simply from their constitution and molecular weight due to active recycling via the neonatal Fc receptor (FcRn). The half-life so conferred is one of the features that has led to the surge in popularity of therapeutic antibody development of late. Additionally, since this attribute of immunoglobulins is bestowed by the Fc component, therapeutics such as etanercept have been developed that benefit from the attachment of this component alone in order to extend the exposure of other therapeutic components of the drug in the case of etanercept, the soluble type 2 TNF-α receptor.

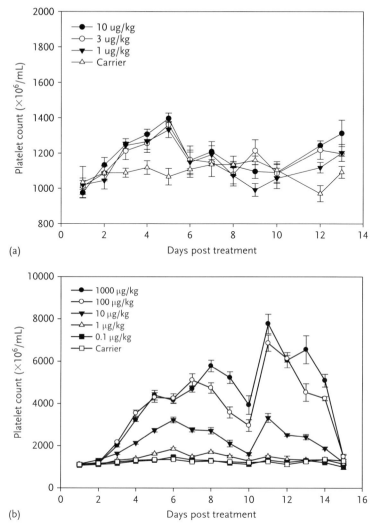

Figure 9.1 The pharmacodynamic effects at various stages of romiplostim construction. Platelet counts in mice in response to administration of: (a) a single subcutaneous (SC) dose of TMP (peptide only). Doses are μg of peptide per kg body weight and administration was on day 0; (b) various doses of TMP administered by continuous subcutaneous infusion. Pumps were implanted on day 0. Doses indicated are dose delivered per day and though the design life of the pump is 7 days, the reservoir of the pump contained enough material for up to 8.3 days delivery; (c) a single SC injection of each TMP construct, at 100 μg/kg on day 0. PEG-rHuMGDF was administered as a positive control. The naming convention is that TMP is the peptide, Fc preceding TMP indicates C-terminal conjugation, and succeeding TMP indicates N-terminal conjugation. TMP-TMP indicates TMP dimer spaced by polyglycine (see text for description). Carrier is phosphate-buffered saline supplemented with 0.1% bovine serum albumin as stabilizer. Platelet counts were measured daily post treatment on an ADVIA automated blood cell analyzer using species-appropriate software and presented as the mean platelet count and standard error of the mean (SEM) for five animals per group per time point.

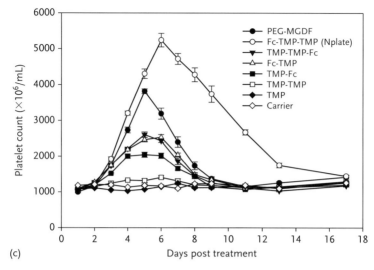

(c)

Figure 9.1 (Continued)

In considering Fc as a part of the drug molecule, an advantage of an amino acid based conjugation partner is that the entire molecule can be made from one construct using recombinant technology, in contrast to semi-synthetic protein therapeutics such as pegfilgrastim, pegasparaginase, or peg-interferon which require a separate chemical treatment to attach the two components. Candidate molecular constructs (Figure 9.2) were prepared with different orientations of Fc conjugated via a 5 glycine bridge with the tandem peptide dimer. These were assessed *in vivo* (Figure 9.1c) and, interestingly, though inexplicably, it was the C-terminally conjugated Fc-peptide-peptide (Fc-TMP-TMP) construct that out-performed the other candidates.

Romiplostim is expressed in *E. coli* as an insoluble protein comprising a 269 amino acid monomer that is then refolded into covalent homodimers of 50 096 Da molecular weight. The Fc fragment is derived from the human IgG1 heavy chain.

9.4
Pharmacodynamics (PD) and Pharmacokinetics (PK) of Romiplostim

The series of screening pharmacology studies introduced above (Figure 9.1a–c) give a basic impression of the pharmacodynamic response in rodents treated with romiplostim. Data illustrated in Table 9.1 and [18] show that romiplostim is a *bona fide* colony-stimulating factor for CFU-Mk, the lineage committed progenitor cell from which arise megakaryoctes. Romiplostim was shown to displace TPO from c-Mpl, to induce CFU-Mk growth and to increase the average ploidy of mega-karyocytes [18].

The data in Table 9.1 also show that the concentration of romiplostim required to stimulate colony formation from CFU-MK of human or non-human primate

TMP Mimetic: IEGPTLRQWLAARA

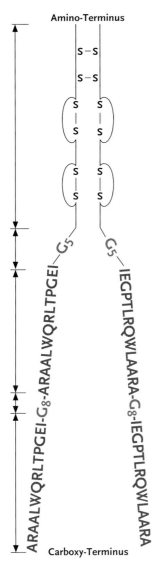

Figure 9.2 The structure of romiplostim [34]. The structure of romiplostim using single letter amino acid codes. S–S indicates a disulfide bond and G_x a polyglycine linker of length indicated by the suffix. Solid line indicates the Fc component of human IgG1.

(NHP) origin is broadly similar (0.2–0.5 nM EC50). However, *in vivo* NHP are relatively resistant to romiplostim, the dose required to double platelet counts being measured in hundreds of micrograms per kilogram (Figure 9.3). This compares with a dose in rodents of around 3 µg/kg to double platelet counts

Table 9.1 Effect of romiplostim or recombinant rHuMGDF on megakaryocyte colony formation (CFU-Mk) *in vitro*. CD34 + progenitor cells were purified from bone marrow of cynomolgus monkey or mobilized peripheral blood of human, and cultured in a collagen medium for 14 days. The culture media contained 10 ng/ml of stem cell factor (SCF), interleukin 3 (IL-3), and IL-6, and various concentrations of romiplostim or rHuMGDF (0–1000 ng/ml). Megakaryocyte colony-forming units (CFU-MK) were identified by anti-GPIIb/IIIa immunostaining and counted. EC50 and Confidence Intervals (CI) were determined using a GraphPad software.

	Cynomolgus CFU-MK EC50 in nM (95% CI)	Human CFU-MK EC50 in nM (95% CI)
Nplate® (romiplostim)	0.18 (0.060–0.57)	0.52 (0.07–4.21)
rHuMGDF	2.06 (0.91–4.66)	1.14 (0.35–3.76)

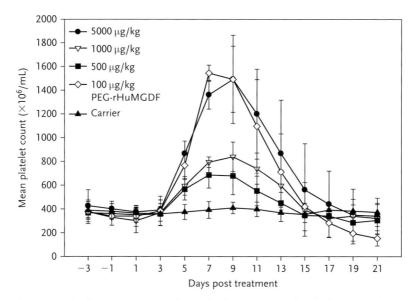

Figure 9.3 Platelet response in monkeys. Platelet response in female rhesus monkeys receiving a single romiplostim SC injection of 0, 500, 1000, and 5000 μg/kg. PEG-rHuMGDF, at 100 μg/kg, was administered as a positive control. Platelet counts were measured every other day post treatment on an ADVIA and presented as the mean platelet count and SEM for three animals per group per time point.

(Figure 9.1b) and perhaps 2 μg/kg for the same response in normal human volunteers [19]. This is not thought to result from reduced exposure in the NHP, and the CFU-Mk data would suggest that it is not driven by variation in the intrinsic sensitivity to the drug. The reason for this disparity remains unknown. An intriguing opportunity for investigation is presented by the recent development of the first antibody that is both specific and sensitive for c-Mpl [20], and with it not only can the true distribution of functional c-Mpl be determined, but the presence of soluble forms of the receptor that may act as a decoy can be investigated.

Intravenous and subcutaneous injection yield a similar PD response in rodents (Figure 9.4a) suggesting no issues with drug stability in the subcutaneous space. In addition, the platelet response pre- and post-splenectomy remained the same (Figure 9.4b). This is important as splenectomy is an accepted procedure for the treatment of refractory immune-mediated thrombocytopenia in humans. ITP is a complex disease and, even though results with first generation c-Mpl ligands had been encouraging, it remained important to show that romiplostim might work in a preclinical model of the disease. A generalized model of autoimmunity which features antibody-mediated destruction of platelets was used to show that romiplostim was effective in raising platelet counts in otherwise untreated animals. It was also possible to show that splenectomy in this model had a similar effect to what is observed in humans, and that romiplostim was effective not only pre-splenectomy, but also in splenectomy non-responders and in splenectomy responders who later relapsed (Figure 9.5).

Preclinical and clinical assessments of the PK/PD relationship of romiplostim have an important feature in general. This is end-cell mediated clearance and is common to a number of hematopoietic cytokines. First outlined for M-CSF [22], the general model suggests that the lineage restricted stimulator, once it has caused the production of its cellular target, will then be destroyed by those very target cells. Thus the highly specific cell surface receptor, in this case c-Mpl on megakaryocytes and platelets, is both the target of the mitogenic action of the cytokine and also a major clearance route for that same cytokine. This leads to a degree of self-regulation when stimulators such as these are administered in the absence of their target cells (cytopenias, e.g., thrombocytopenia). This has been more fully exploited with pegfilgrastim [23] but also occurs with romiplostim where modeling of the effects of the drug must take this into account [24].

The pharmacokinetic/pharmacodynamic relationship of romipostim was studied in normal human volunteers [19]. A single administration, whether administered SC or IV, produced a dose-dependent increase, up to sixfold, in platelet counts which occurred 12–16 days later. At the highest dose tested (10 µg/kg) the platelet increase was marked at $800–1800 \times 10^9$/L from a baseline value of around 300. By day 28 platelets had returned to baseline values. This response was driven by exposure to the drug which was non-linear with dose. Total AUC (0–∞) of romiplostim was 964 (pg.h/mL) at 0.3 µg/kg, 26 700 at 1 µg/kg, and 153 000 at 10µg/kg. A model [24] was developed to explain the relationship and relied upon the following components:

1. Initial distribution of the drug includes dissemination to the cells that bear the receptor c-Mpl – mainly platelets and megakaryocytes.
2. Drug levels in excess of the binding capacity of the c-Mpl+ cells remained in the circulation reliant upon the second slow process of elimination via non-c-Mpl mechanisms.
3. The pharmacodynamic response is to increase platelet and megakaryocyte mass, increasing the contribution of c-Mpl mediated clearance as the response mounts.

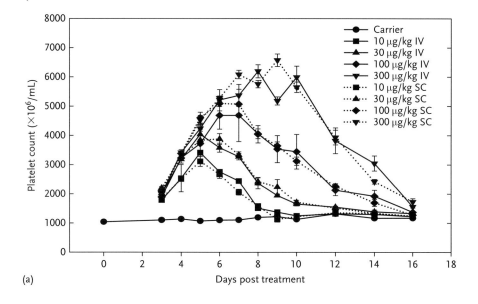

(a)

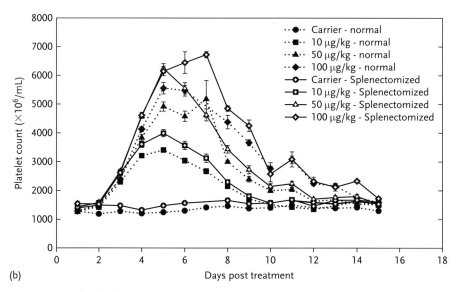

(b)

Figure 9.4 The platelet response to romiplostim in mice injected (a) SC or IV and (b) pre- or post-splenectomy. Platelet levels in mice treated with various doses of romiplostim given IV or SC. (b) Platelet response in romiplostim-treated normal and splenectomized mice. Data are not corrected for higher baseline platelet numbers in splenectomized mice. Doses are shown in μg romiplostim per kg body weight administered on day 0. All results are expressed as the mean and standard SEM for five mice at each time point. Some data adapted from Hartley *et al.* [21].

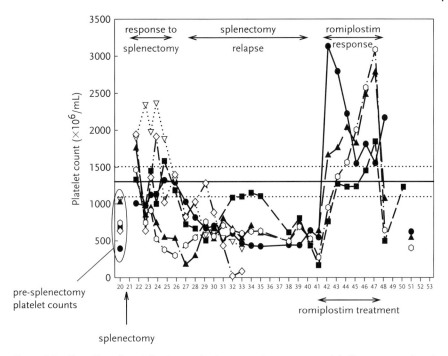

Figure 9.5 The effect of romiplostim on platelet counts in a mouse model of immune-mediated thrombocytopenia after relapse from splenectomy. Platelet count profile of ITP mice pre- and post-splenectomy, and in response to weekly romiplostim treatment. Each symbol-dotted line represents the profile of one mouse. Platelets were counted in WB/F1 mice at 20 weeks of age prior to surgical splenectomy. The majority of animals responded with increased platelet counts in the succeeding weeks. However, ultimately all animals relapsed and the resulting thrombocytopenia responded well to romiplostim at 100 μg/kg weekly. The solid horizontal line represents normal mice mean platelet counts ± standard deviation (SD) (dashed lines).

These steps account for the time-dependent nonlinear clearance of romiplostim and suggest that romiplostim acts very much like thrombopoietin, the endogenous ligand.

9.5
A Brief ITP Primer

9.5.1
Diagnosis and Treatment

ITP is an autoimimmune disease in which patients have abnormally low platelet counts ($<100\ 000 \times 10^9$). Manifestations of the disease depend upon the platelet count and include purpura, petechiae, or ecchymoses (patchy red or purple discoloration of the skin in ascending size order) and bleeding events which can be life-threatening. Both acute (<6 month duration) and chronic (>6 months) ITP are recognized, the former mainly in children, and often following a viral infection; the latter more frequently in adults, and more often in women than men, though with no known cause. The general aim of treatment is to protect against bleeding events by raising platelets into a safe zone for that patient (frequently only to >30 000 × 10⁹/L, accounting for severity, risk factors like dental surgery or childbirth, and lifestyle factors like level of physical activity), but not necessarily raising platelets into the normal range. Most of the available treatments for ITP aim to control the excessive platelet destruction which is a hallmark of the disease. A newly diagnosed patient (and often the diagnosis is one of exclusion) would first receive steroids like prednisone and perhaps 2/3 of patients might respond to this intervention. The consequences, even for those who respond, are manifold and may include hypertension, diabetes, and osteoporosis among other serious short- and long-term side effects. There are also more serious, life-threatening events associated with steroid-induced immune suppression, including infection which is a major cause of death in ITP. Intravenous immunoglobulin treatment is also effective in ITP but is often reserved for "rescue" scenarios, and alternative rescue treatments might include high dose steroids, WinRho® (IV anti-D), vincristine, denazol, azathioprine, cyclosporine, or anti-CD20 antibody (Rituxan®), although the latter is not approved for this use. Many of these treatments carry with them significant risks and a proportion of patients will still fail to respond. In such cases surgical splenectomy is often performed, though this too is often associated with a proportion of either non-response or short duration of response followed by relapse (for review see [14]).

Against this backdrop the need for a more effective therapy is obvious, but to suggest an intervention based upon the *production* end of the homeostatic control of platelet numbers would certainly require a paradigm shift in treating the disease; away from influencing destruction of platelets and focusing instead on the bone marrow progenitor pool and its ability to outpace the immune destruction of platelets.

9.5.2
Thrombopoietin and ITP

Thrombopoietin is normally produced by the liver constitutively; production is not regulated by any known mechanism. It has been shown that regulation of TPO levels is effected mainly by c-Mpl mediated destruction – and c-Mpl is present only on megakaryocytes and platelets. This results in an inverse relationship between platelet number and TPO levels in the plasma; a relationship that remains intact in most situations involving loss of platelets.

Hematologically normal humans have, on average, thrombopoietin levels of 81 ± 5 pg/mL of plasma. This was measured in the presence of a normal platelet count of 282 000 ± 5000 × 10⁹/L. Thrombocytopenic conditions such as aplastic anemia (AA) or (cancer) chemotherapy-induced thrombocytopenia (CIT) were found to have high TPO levels; 4552 ± 2090 and 870 ± 69 pg/mL, respectively, in association with platelet counts of $28\,000 \pm 3000$ and $15\,000 \pm 2000 \times 10^9$/L. ITP patients on the other hand had 121 ± 24 pg/mL thrombopoietin and platelet counts of $41\,000 \pm 7000$/L [25]. So in AA and CIT a 10–20-fold decrease in platelet count was associated with a 10–50-fold increase in thrombopoietin. In ITP an 8-fold decrease in platelets was associated with only a 1.5-fold increase in thrombopoietin – a relative shortfall. Though the reason for this is unknown, it may include the destruction of thrombopoietin along with platelets; in contrast to AA and CIT where it is likely the marrow simply cannot produce enough platelets to clear the thrombopoietin efficiently from the plasma. Nonetheless, it was surprising that romiplostim, as a replacement for thrombopoietin, was effective in raising platelet counts and managing some of the risks associated with ITP.

9.6
Romiplostim Clinical Data

The first clinical study of romiplostim was a normal volunteer single dose design in which four patients per dose level were given 0.3, 1, or 10 µg/kg IV or 0.1, 0.3, 1, or 2 µg/kg SC, in comparison with two placebo-treated volunteers per dose [19]. The results confirmed the promise of the preclinical data. Ultimately, four phase 1 or 2 trials were conducted with romiplostim in patients suffering from ITP. One of these was in Japanese subjects and was preceded by a further normal volunteer trial, again in Japanese subjects. As more knowledge was gained of the safety, PK profile, and PD response to romiplostim through these phase I/II trials it was possible to home in on the dose and schedule to be tested in two parallel phase III trials (Table 9.2).

Table 9.2 Clinical trials conducted with romiplostim. Relatively few people (just over 400) had received romiplostim prior to its approval for use in ITP, an orphan drug indication.

Phase	Subjects	Dose, schedule	Subjects enrolled
1	Healthy	0.3, 1.0, 10; IV, single dose	48
		0.1, 0.3, 1.0, 2.0; SC, single dose	
1	Healthy, Japanese	0.3, 1.0, 2.0, 3.0; SC, single dose	30
1–2	ITP	0.2, 0.5, 1.0, 3.0, 6.0, 10.0; SC, ≤2 doses	24
1–2	ITP	1.0, 3.0, 6.0; SC, weekly	21
1–2	ITP	30, 100, 300, 500; SC ≤2 doses	16
2	ITP, Japanese	1.0, 3.0, 6.0; SC, weekly	12
3	ITP, splenectomized	1.0–15.0 (dose adjusted); SC, weekly	63
3	ITP, non-splenectomized	1.0–15.0 (dose adjusted); SC, weekly	62
Open label extension	ITP	1.0–10.0 (dose adjusted); weekly	137

The total number of patients upon which the drug was approved for clinical use was relatively limited – as befits a rare disease designated "orphan" (fewer than 200 000 affected individuals) in the United States.

Two pivotal studies for romiplostim in adult chronic ITP were completed. Both were placebo-controlled, double-blind, and randomized trials, conducted in multiple centers internationally, one in patients who had an intact spleen, the other in splenectomized patients [26]. Patients enrolled had serious thrombocytopenia ($<30 \times 10^9$/L platelets) and were randomized 2 : 1 (test article : placebo) to receive romiplostim at a starting dose of 1 µg/kg weekly SC. Subsequent doses could be modified, depending upon response and according to the following alogorithm: dose was increased by 2 µg/kg/week if the platelet count was $<10 \times 10^9$/L and by the same dose every two weeks if the count was between 11 and 50×10^9/L. Once 50×10^9/L had been achieved a maintenance algorithm was used which allowed an increase in dose of 1 µg/kg/week if the platelet count was $\leq 10 \times 10^9$/L, an increase of 1 µg/kg every 2 weeks if the count was 11–50×10^9/L, and a reduction of 1 µg/kg after two consecutive weeks at 210–400×10^9/L. Dose was withheld if platelets exceeded 400×10^9/L and subsequent doses reduced by 1 µg/kg when resumed after the count had fallen to 200×10^9/L. The maximum dose allowed was 15 µg/kg. The primary endpoint was a platelet response maintained at $>50 \times 10^9$/L for 6 of the last 8 weeks of the 24 week study duration. Patients were classified as having a transient response where a platelet rise was seen for four or more weeks throughout the study period, during which they must not have received rescue medication. In total 125 patients enrolled with a median platelet count of 16×10^9/L, two thirds of whom had received some prior therapy and one third of whom were receiving concurrent treatment for ITP.

ITP was a long-term problem for most patients who entered the trial with a median duration of ITP of 2 years in non-splenectomized patients and 8 years in those who had undergone surgical splenectomy. Despite this, romiplostim achieved a durable response in 38% (16/42) of splenectomized and 61% (25/41) of non-splenectomized patients – impressive results considering the duration of the thrombocytopenia in many patients and their failure with multiple prior therapeutic interventions. If we include transient responders too, the numbers increase to 88% (36/41) of patients with a spleen and 79% (33/42) of those who had undergone splenectomy. Placebo-treated patients had 0/21 and 1/21 (splenectomized and non-splenectomized, respectively) responders which increased to 0/21 and 3/21 when transient response was included.

About a third of patients who entered the trial were taking concomitant medications such as corticosteroids, danazol or azathioprine. Of the romiplostim treated patients 87% were able to either discontinue these medicines or reduce the dose by more than 25%; in comparison 38% of placebo patients could do this too. In addition, romiplostim-treated patients required less frequent rescue medication (increased dosage steroids, IVIg or WinRho®); 26.2% versus 57.1% of splenectomized and 17.1% versus 61.9% of patients with an intact spleen. Adverse events were reported with high frequency in both arms – in 100% and 95% of patients receiving romiplostim or placebo, respectively. These were most likely related to the underlying disease.

Romiplostim-related events occurred infrequently, though in 2% of patients arterial embolism or reticulin deposition in the bone marrow was reported but only 3% discontinued use due to adverse events. Serious bleeding events were reduced in the romiplostim arms from 12% to 7%. Also, of great importance to the underlying philosophy behind romiplostim, no neutralizing antibodies to thrombopoietin were found.

Some patients who had completed a previous romiplostim study were enrolled into a long-term extension study so they could continue to receive the drug after completion of their initial participation [27]. Of patients treated for up to 3 years 60% had had a splenectomy and 87% had a durable response to romiplostim, defined as a doubling of their initial platelet count for 67% of the weekly blood counts in the absence of rescue medication.

About half of the patients were able to self-administer the drug and reductions in concurrent medication and rarity of rescue interventions were similar to those recorded in the twin phase 3 trials. Several patients (8 of 16 tested) had reticulin deposits in the bone marrow (see later discussion) and one had antibodies to romiplostim, but no antibodies to TPO were detected.

In parallel with these trials in ITP several studies were being conducted in cancer chemotherapy-induced thrombocytopenia [28] and myelodysplastic syndromes [29]. A group of European investigators also used romiplostim in cancer chemotherapy-induced thrombocytopenia [30]. Within the United States, romiplostim is subject to a Risk Evaluation and Mitigation Strategy, a so-called REMS. This is a relatively new yet increasingly complex set of rules stemming from new authority granted to the regulatory authorities in the United States under the FDA Amendment Act of 2007. Under the REMS for romiplostim, institutions where the drug is administered have to be registered, as do the prescribing physicians and the individual patients slated to receive the drug. This program should allow the tracing of individual patient-level data for tracking safety and other information around drug effects and will enable a heretofore impossible in-depth analysis of many aspects of a drug's performance.

9.7
Safety and Other Insights Gained from Romiplostim Design and Development

In the context of this volume the matters of greatest interest might be those that apply to drug design. Romiplostim is the first peptibody developed successfully as a therapeutic drug. As stated above it comprises two functional components – the peptide "warhead" and the IgG Fc "persistence" component. The design is more broadly applicable, as evidenced by AMG 386, a second peptibody in clinical development that, in this case, *inhibits* the interaction of a ligand pair (Ang-1 and -2) with their cognate receptor (Tie2) [31]. But what has been learned of drug design from the romiplostim experience?

First, with respect to the safety events observed with romiplostim can any be ascribed to the molecular structure? The disease setting of ITP is perhaps not ideal to study the issue of patient-reported events. As discussed above almost 100% of patients reported some adverse event in both the romiplostim and placebo groups of the romiplostim phase 3 trials. This perhaps reflects the nature of the disease and the extensive symptoms the patients suffer; such that health related quality of life for patients with ITP is worse than that associated with cancer and hypertension, similar to that of patients with diabetes, but better than that of patients with chronic heart failure or a missing limb. Confining the discussion to quantitative parameters of adverse events with romiplostim, the main issue observed was reticulin detection in the bone marrow. A similar observation had been made in transgenic mice over expressing TPO [32] and the effect is likely mediated by cytokines (PDGF or TGFβ perhaps) released from megakaryocytes, and is thus an indirect, but on-target, effect of romiplostim. There is, therefore, no evidence that peptibodies as a class of drugs might have this effect.

Immunogenicity is another concern and it was expected that the peptide sequence, being entirely unnatural, was likely to provoke an immune response. Indeed, mice treated with a single dose of romiplostim developed antibodies against the whole drug, the active peptide and the human Fc component. A single dose escalation was sufficient to dose-through the antibody effect in mice and there was no further induction of antibodies. Dogs treated for several months also saw reduced efficacy from administered romiplostim, but in no case in any preclinical species were antibodies to TPO encountered. In humans rare cases of romiplostim-binding antibodies were reported, and a single case of romiplostim-neutralizing antibodies was found, but the neutralizing activity was transient and 4 months later the patient tested negative for neutralizing activity. So the concerns of an antibody reaction to romiplostim were borne out, but the design of romiplostim was such that antibodies so created would be incapable of cross-neutralizing endogenous proteins – this design worked and by all available measures romiplostim specifically, and peptibodies generally, do not appear to be highly immunogenic constructs.

Did the Fc component function as planned? Romiplostim is a very potent molecule; the SC dose in humans is in the range of less than 5 µg/kg. Its PK is dose-dependent and nonlinear, as discussed above, but at a dose that likely saturates the c-Mpl binding capacity of platelets and megakaryocytes (10 µg/kg), and thus represents clearance through non-specific pathways, the half-life of romiplostim is an impressive 13.8 h [19], suggesting the Fc component is functioning as intended. In a further study to investigate this issue, romiplostim was admininstered to FcRn knockout mice and, in this case, the apparent half-life was significantly shorter than in FcRn wild type mice [33]. These data taken together suggest that the Fc component of romiplostim does function as was intended to prolong the exposure to the drug.

Another aspect of the serum stability of romiplostim is the potential for generation of fragments that may be active. Scrutiny of the data in Figure 9.1 would suggest that naked peptide and incomplete versions of the molecule are indeed active. Whether these fragments ever arise *in vivo* is unknown but the activity of the peptide is known to be confined to c-mpl as is the activity of the complete peptibody. It would seem unlikely that an intermediate metabolite would possess a different activity, but the formal possibility remains. The most effective construct in mice was the dual tandem dimer adopted for the final peptibody molecule. However, the lesser forms were also active. Other structures are obviously feasible and some, for instance "loop" peptides, have been made and tested [34], and shown to be effective preclinically.

References

1 Kelemen, E., Cserhati, I., and Tanos, B. (1958) Demonstration and some properties of human thrombopoietin in thrombocythaemic sera. *Acta Haematol.*, **20**, 350–355.

2 Bartley, T.D., Bogenberger, J., Hunt, P., Li, Y.S., Lu, H.S., Martin, F., Chang, M.S., Samal, B., and Nichol, J.L. (1994) Identification and cloning of a megakaryocyte growth and development factor that is a ligand for the cytokine receptor Mpl. *Cell*, **77**, 1117–1124.

3 Lok, S., Kaushansky, K., Holly, R.D., Kuijper, J.L., Lofton-Day, C.E., Oort, P.J., Grant, F.J., Heipel, M.D., Burkhead, S.K., and Kramer, J.M. (1994) Cloning and expression of murine thrombopoietin cDNA and stimulation of platelet production *in vivo*. *Nature*, **369**, 565–568.

4 Kuter, D.J., Beeler, D.L., and Rosenberg, R.D. (1994) The purification of megapoietin: a physiological regulator of megakaryocyte growth and platelet production. *Proc. Natl. Acad. Sci. USA*, **91**, 11104–11108.

5 De Sauvage, F.J., Hass, P.E., Spencer, S.D., Malloy, B.E., Gurney, A.L., Spencer, S.A., Darbonne, W.C., Henzel, W.J., Wong, S.C., Kuang, W.-J., Oles, K.J., Hultgren, B., and Solberg, L.A. Jr (1994) Stimulation of megakaryocytopoiesis and thrombopoiesis by the c-Mpl ligand. *Nature*, **369**, 533–538.

6 Basser, R.L., O'flaherty, E., Green, M., Edmonds, M., Nichol, J., Menchaca, D. M., Cohen, B., and Begley, C.G. (2002) Development of pancytopenia with neutralizing antibodies to thrombopoietin after multicycle chemotherapy supported by megakaryocyte growth and development factor. *Blood*, **99**, 2599–2602.

7 Casadevall, N., Nataf, J., Viron, B., Kolta, A., Kiladjian, J.J., Martin-Dupont, P., Michaud, P., Papo, T., Ugo, V., Teyssandier, I., Varet, B., and Mayeux, P. (2002) Pure red-cell aplasia and antierythropoietin antibodies in patients treated with recombinant erythropoietin. [see comments.]. *N. Eng. J. Med.*, **346**, 469–475.

8 Gurney, A.L., Carver-Moore, K., De Sauvage, F.J., and Moore, M.W. (1994) Thrombocytopenia in c-mpl-deficient mice. *Science*, **265** (5177), 1445–1447.

9 De Sauvage, F.J., Carver-Moore, K., Luoh, S.M., Ryan, A., Dowd, M., Eaton, D.L., and Moore, M.W. (1996) Physiological regulation of early and late stages of megakaryocytopoiesis by thrombopoietin. *J. Exp. Med.*, **183** (2), 651–656.

10 Sitnicka, E., Lin, N., Priestley, G.V., Fox, N., Broudy, V.C., Wolf, N.S., and Kaushansky, K. (1996) The effect of thrombopoietin on the proliferation and differentiation of murine hematopoietic stem cells. *Blood*, **87** (12), 4998–5005.

11 Ku, H., Yonemura, Y., Kaushansky, K., and Ogawa, M. (1996) Thrombopoietin, the ligand for the Mpl receptor, synergizes with steel factor and other early acting cytokines in supporting proliferation of primitive hematopoietic progenitors of mice. *Blood*, **87** (11), 4544–4551.

12 Ballmaier, M., Germeshausen, M., Schulze, H., Cherkaoui, K., Lang, S.,

Gaudig, A., Krukemeier, S., Eilers, M., Strauss, G., and Welte, K. (2001) c-mpl mutations are the cause of congenital amegakaryocytic thrombocytopenia. *Blood*, **97**, 139–146.

13 Basser, R.L., Underhill, C., Davis, I., Green, M.D., Cebon, J., Zalcberg, J., Macmillan, J., Cohen, B., Marty, J., Fox, R.M., and Begley, C.G. (2000) Enhancement of platelet recovery after myelosuppressive chemotherapy by recombinant human megakaryocyte growth and development factor in patients with advanced cancer. *J. Clin. Oncol.*, **18**, 2852–2861.

14 Molineux, G. and Newland, A. (2010) Development of romiplostim for the treatment of patients with chronic immune thrombocytopenia: from bench to bedside: review. *Br. J. Haematol.*, **150** (1), 9–20.

15 Cwirla, S.E., Balasubramanian, P., Duffin, D., Wagstrom, C.R., Gates, C.M., Singer, S.C., Davis, A.M., Tansik, R.L., Mattheakis, L.C., Boytos, C.M., Schatz, P.J., Baccanari, D.P., Wrighton, N.C., Barrett, R.W., and Dower, W.J. (1997) Peptide agonist of the thrombopoietin receptor as potent as the natural cytokine. *Science*, **276** (5319), 1696–1699.

16 Cheetham, J.C., Smith, D.M., Aoki, K. H., Stevenson, J.L., Hoeffel, T.J., Syed, R.S., Egrie, J., and Harvey, T.S. (1998) NMR structure of human erythropoietin and a comparison with its receptor bound conformation. *Nat. Struct. Biol.*, **5**, 861–866.

17 Case, B.C., Hauck, M.L., Yeager, R.L., Simkins, A.H., De Serres, M., Schmith, V.D., Dillberger, J.E., and Page, R.L. (2000) The pharmacokinetics and pharmacodynamics of GW395058, a peptide agonist of the thrombopoietin receptor, in the dog, a large-animal model of chemotherapy-induced thrombocytopenia. *Stem Cells*, **18**, 360–365.

18 Broudy, V.C. and Lin, N.L. (2004) AMG531 stimulates megakaryopoiesis in vitro by binding to Mpl. *Cytokine*, **25**, 52–60.

19 Wang, B., Nichol, J.L., and Sullivan, J.T. (2004) Pharmacodynamics and pharmacokinetics of AMG 531, a novel thrombopoietin receptor ligand. *Clin. Pharmacol. Ther.*, **76**, 628–638.

20 Abbott, C., Huang, G., Ellison, A.R., Chen, C., Arora, T., Szilvassy, S.J., and Wei, P. (2010) Mouse monoclonal antibodies against human c-Mpl and characterization for flow cytometry applications. *Hybridoma (Larchmt)*, **29**, 103–113.

21 Hartley, C.A., Wang, B., and Molineux, G. (2004) A novel platelet factor, AMG 531, elevates platelet counts in normal and thrombocytopenic mice in a dose-related manner. *Exp. Hematol.*, **1**, 93–94, JUL 04.

22 Bartocci, A., Mastrogiannis, D.S., Migliorati, G., Stockert, R.J., Wolkoff, A. W., and Stanley, E.R. (1987) Macrophages specifically regulate the concentration of their own growth factor in the circulation. *Proc. Natl. Acad. Sci. USA*, **84**, 6179–6183.

23 Molineux, G. (2004) The design and development of pegfilgrastim (PEG-rmetHuG-CSF, neulasta(R)). *Curr. Pharm. Des.*, **10**, 1235–1244.

24 Wang, Y.-M., Perez-Ruixo, J.J., Xiao, J., Doshi, S., Jaramilla, B., Chow, A., and Kryzyzanski, W. (2008) Pharmacokinetic and pharmacodynamic (PKPD) modeling of romiplostim, a novel thrombopoietic Fc-peptide fusion protein, in healthy subjects: a semi-mechanistic approach. *Exp. Hematol.*, **36**, S53–S54.

25 Nichol, J.L. (1997) Serum levels of thrombopoietin in health and disease, in *Thrombopoiesis and Thrombopoietins. Molecular, Cellular, Preclinical and Clinical Biology* (eds Kuter, D., Hunt, P., Sheridan, W., and Zucker-Franklin, D.), New Jersey, Humana Press.

26 Kuter, D.J., Bussel, J.B., Lyons, R.M., Pullarkat, V., Gernsheimer, T.B., Senecal, F.M., Aledort, L.M., George, J.N., Kessler, C.M., Sanz, M.A., Liebman, H.A., Slovick, F.T., De Wolf, J.T., Bourgeois, E., Guthrie, T.H., Jr, Newland, A., Wasser, J.S., Hamburg, S.I., Grande, C., Lefrere, F., Lichtin, A.E., Tarantino, M.D., Terebelo, H.R., Viallard, J.F., Cuevas, F.J., Go, R.S., Henry, D.H., Redner, R.L., Rice, L., Schipperus, M.R., Guo, D.M., and

Nichol, J.L. (2008) Efficacy of romiplostim in patients with chronic immune thrombocytopenic purpura: a double-blind randomised controlled trial. *Lancet*, **371**, 395–403.

27 Bussel, J.B., Kuter, D.J., Pullarkat, V., Lyons, R.M., Guo, M., and Nichol, J.L. (2009) Safety and efficacy of long-term treatment with romiplostim in thrombocytopenic patients with chronic ITP. *Blood*, **113**, 2161–2171.

28 Vadhan-Raj, S. (2009) Management of chemotherapy-induced thrombocytopenia: current status of thrombopoietic agents. *Semin. Hematol.*, **46**, S26–S32.

29 Kantarjian, H., Fenaux, P., Sekeres, M. A., Becker, P.S., Boruchov, A., Bowen, D., Hellstrom-Lindberg, E., Larson, R.A., Lyons, R.M., Muus, P., Shammo, J., Siegel, R., Hu, K., Franklin, J., and Berger, D.P. (2010) Safety and efficacy of romiplostim in patients with lower-risk myelodysplastic syndrome and thrombocytopenia. *J. Clin. Oncol.*, **28** (3), 437–444.

30 Demeter, J., Istenes, I., Fodor, A., Paksi, M., Dombi, P., Valasinyoszki, E., Csomor, J., Matolcsy, A., and Nagy, Z.G. (2010) Efficacy of romiplostim in the treatment of chemotherapy induced thrombocytopenia (CIT) in a patient with mantle cell lymphoma. *Pathol. Oncol. Res.*, **17** (1), 141–143.

31 Herbst, R.S., Hong, D., Chap, L., Kurzrock, R., Jackson, E., Silverman, J. M., Rasmussen, E., Sun, Y.N., Zhong, D., Hwang, Y.C., Evelhoch, J.L., Oliner, J.D., Le, N., and Rosen, L.S. (2009) Safety, pharmacokinetics, and antitumor activity of AMG 386, a selective angiopoietin inhibitor, in adult patients with advanced solid tumors. *J. Clin. Oncol.*, **27** (21), 3557–3565.

32 Kakumitsu, H., Kamezaki, K., Shimoda, K., Karube, K., Haro, T., Numata, A., Shide, K., Matsuda, T., Oshima, K., and Harada, M. (2005) Transgenic mice overexpressing murine thrombopoietin develop myelofibrosis and osteosclerosis. *Leukemia Res.*, **29** (7), 761–769.

33 Sun, Y.-N., Arends, R., Smithson, A., Watson, A., and Nichol, J.L. (2005) A novel thrombopoiesis-stimulating agent, AMG 531: pharmacokinetics and pharmacodynamics in FcRn knock-out and wild type mice. *Blood*, **106** (11, Part 1), 997 A.

34 Hall, M.P., Gegg, C., Walker, K., Spahr, C., Ortiz, R., Patel, V., Yu, S., Zhang, L., Lu, H., Desilva, B., and Lee, J.W. (2010) Ligand-binding mass spectrometry to study biotransformation of fusion protein drugs and guide immunoassay development: strategic approach and application to peptibodies targeting the thrombopoietin receptor. *AAPS J.*, **12** (4), 576–585.

10
HIV vs. HIV: Turning HIV-Derived Peptides into Drugs

Henri G. Franquelim, Pedro M. Matos, and A. Salomé Veiga

10.1
Introduction

Human immunodeficiency virus (HIV) is the causative agent of the acquired immunodeficiency syndrome (AIDS). There are two types of HIV: HIV-1 and HIV-2, HIV-1 being the most virulent [1]. HIV can be transmitted by blood and blood products, vertically (from mother to child), or through sexual activity. By the end of 2009, the United Nations Programme on AIDS (UNAIDS)/World Health Organization (WHO) epidemic update estimated 33.4 million (31.1–35.8 million) people worldwide living with HIV [2]. Despite much effort, no curative treatment or effective vaccine has yet been achieved.

The rational design of anti-HIV-1 therapeutics is based on detailed knowledge of the biology of the virus. Combination therapy with reverse transcriptase and protease inhibitors is the most common current treatment of HIV-1 infection [3]. Despite the success of this therapy, namely by reducing morbidity and mortality of HIV-1 infected patients [4], it has adverse effects and drug resistant HIV-1 strains have emerged [5]. This demands the development of new classes of drugs targeting different stages of the viral life cycle. A new class of antiviral agents in development, the entry inhibitors, exhibits promising inhibition profiles. Unlike reverse transcriptase and protease inhibitors, which target post-entry steps inside the host cells, entry inhibitors act extracellularly preventing viral entry into target cells [6].

10.2
HIV-1 Envelope Protein

HIV-1 is an enveloped virus that infects $CD4^+$ T cells, dendritic cells, and macrophages [1]. The HIV-1 envelope glycoprotein is the protein responsible for the viral entry into the target cells. It is expressed on the surface of the viral membrane as a trimer [7]. It is composed of two subunits noncovalently associated: the gp120 subunit, a globular-shaped subunit at the surface of the membrane that interacts

Peptide Drug Discovery and Development: Translational Research in Academia and Industry, First Edition.
Edited by Miguel Castanho and Nuno C. Santos.
© 2011 WILEY-VCH Verlag GmbH & Co. KGaA, Weinheim.
Published 2011 by WILEY-VCH Verlag GmbH & Co. KGaA

with cellular receptors, and the gp41 transmembrane subunit, responsible for the fusion between the viral and cellular membranes (reviewed in [6, 8, 9]).

gp41 is composed of an ectodomain (extracellular domain), a transmembrane domain (TM) and an endodomain (intracellular domain or cytoplasm tail (CT)). Several functional domains have been identified in the ectodomain. The fusion peptide (FP) is located at the ectodomain N-terminal. This region, hydrophobic and rich in glycine residues, interacts with the target cell membrane and plays an important role in membrane fusion (reviewed in [10]). Two heptad repeat regions ((HR(), with the tendency to form α-helical coiled-coils [11], are also present: the first (NHR or HR1) near the N-terminal is adjacent to the FP; the second (CHR or HR2) is located at the ectodomain C-terminal. Peptides derived from them are referred to as N- and C-peptides, respectively. The two HR are separated by a loop region (LR) that contains an intramolecular cysteine bridge. At the C-terminal between the CHR and the TM is located a Trp-rich domain (TRD), the membrane proximal external region (MPER), which also seems to play an important role during the viral membrane fusion [12]. As several monoclonal antibodies bind to this region, the MPER is seen as the major target for vaccine development (reviewed in [13]).

Protein dissection combined with biophysical analysis has demonstrated that the two HR regions within gp41 form a helical trimer of antiparallel dimers [14]. The crystal structures of portions of the ectodomain [15, 16] confirmed that the gp41 core tends to form a trimer of hairpins (also called trimeric coiled coil or six-helix bundle (6HB)). A central trimeric coiled coil formed by the N-peptide region is surrounded by three helical C-peptides that bind to conserved hydrophobic grooves on the coiled-coil surface in an antiparallel orientation. This structure represents the fusion-active conformation of gp41.

10.3
HIV Entry and Its Inhibition

HIV-1 entry into target cells is believed to be a multi-step and complex process (reviewed in [6, 8]). The first step is the binding of gp120 to the target cell surface molecule CD4, which serves as the main receptor for HIV-1 [17]. However, CD4 alone is not sufficient for HIV-1 to fuse with the cells [18, 19]. Two chemokine receptors, known as CCR5 and CXCR4, are the major HIV-1 coreceptors and all viral strains can use one (R5 and X4 viruses) or both (R5X4 viruses). The gp120-CD4 binding induces conformational changes in gp120 leading to the exposure or the formation of the coreceptor binding site. gp120 binding to the CD4 and coreceptor results in further conformational changes that lead to gp41 activation into its fusion-active state. The gp41 conformational changes lead to the insertion of its FP into the target cell membrane and the formation of an extended prehairpin intermediate that bridges the viral and cellular membranes. Subsequent changes within the gp41 ectodomain involve the interaction of CHR and NHR, and a 6HB structure is formed. The hairpin formation brings the viral and cell membrane into close proximity, allowing fusion of the membranes and then entry of the virus.

Each of the HIV-1 entry steps can be a target for entry inhibitors. The ones currently under development fall into one of three categories: gp120-CD4 binding inhibitors (or attachment inhibitors), gp120-coreceptors binding inhibitors (or chemokine coreceptors inhibitors), and fusion inhibitors (reviewed in [20, 21]). Several molecules that block gp120 binding to CD4 receptor and coreceptors have been identified and are reviewed elsewhere. This chapter reviews the molecular bases of fusion inhibition and the involvement of gp41. As such, the discussion will focus on peptide-based fusion inhibitors (Figure 10.1).

Fusion inhibitors, such as enfuvirtide (also known as DP-178, T-20, or Fuzeon) and T-1249 (Tifuvirtide), both from Trimeris, Inc. and Hoffmann-La Roche, Inc., are peptides whose mode of action involves binding to gp41. They interfere with the conformational changes that lead to the 6HB formation and membrane fusion. These kinds of inhibitors are the leading compounds, enfuvirtide being approved by the FDA since 2003 [23, 24]. Enfuvirtide remains the standard in HIV fusion inhibitor peptides as the only drug to complete the whole development track up to clinical use.

10.4
HIV-1 Fusion Inhibitors: from Bench to Clinical Administration

The initial development of HIV-1 fusion inhibitors was based on peptides that were derived from the HR regions of gp41, mainly obtained by protein dissection strategies. Some synthetic C-peptides, such as C34 and enfuvirtide, are highly potent inhibitors of HIV-1 infection at low nanomolar range [25, 26]. It has been proposed that these C-peptides act by interfering with the formation of the 6HB in a dominant negative fashion, by binding to the NHR region of gp41 exposed in the prehairpin intermediate [8, 14, 27].

Synthetic N-peptides also exhibit inhibitory activity against HIV. They are less potent inhibitors (micromole range) than the C-peptides [14, 28, 29]. It was proposed that one of the main reasons for this behavior is their tendency to aggregate in solution [14]. N36 and DP107 are examples of N-peptide inhibitors. In their mode of action, N-peptides may either target the CHR region [14] or intercalate with the NHR region [30].

A critical aspect of the inhibition by HR-derived peptides is the propensity of the central NHR core to form a highly stable helical 6HB complex with CHR peptides. Structural analysis of gp41 indicated that the NHR core formed deep hydrophobic pockets. A complementary specific region of CHR, named the pocket binding domain (PBD), packs into those domains on the NHR core faces enabling effective interactions within the helical complex [31].

C34, a 34 amino acid residues peptide, was the C-peptide used to discover the trimeric coiled coil structure of gp41 [15]. It can be used as a fusion inhibitor and is one of the most potent early-discovered fusion inhibitors. This peptide overlaps the

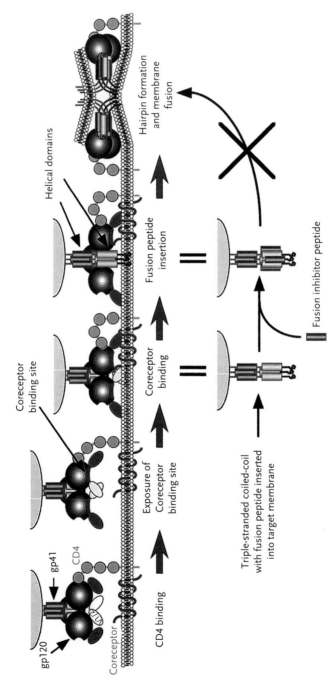

Figure 10.1 HIV-1 entry and its inhibition by peptides. Schematic representation of the steps required for the envelope glycoprotein mediated viral fusion with the target cell membrane (CD4$^+$ cells). Peptides based on CHR region of gp41 interact with the respective NHR region inhibiting the formation of the hairpin-like structure of 6-helix bundle (6HB) that is essential for membrane fusion. Adapted from [22].

CHR region, including the PBD region, which is essential for its antiviral effectiveness [31]. In terms of activity, it showed an increased *in vitro* activity. At a molecular level, C34 forms highly stable helical complexes with N-peptides, such as N36 [29]. Considering the mode of action, evidence (using the C34-like 36 residues inhibitor T649) suggests that the hydrophobic pocket domain and the LLSGIV sequence of the NHR are both preferential docking sites for this peptide, explaining its increased inhibition efficacy [32]. Nevertheless, despite being more potent, C34 is not a good drug candidate due to its low solubility [33].

Enfuvirtide is a 36 amino acid residues peptide that was developed as a novel anti-HIV drug [26, 34]. It is currently the more advanced fusion inhibitor drug approved for clinical application. Since 2003, enfuvirtide has been licensed by the FDA for the treatment of HIV patients who failed to respond to current antiretroviral therapeutics [23].

Enfuvirtide shares 24 identical residues with C34, but lacks the PBD at the N-terminal. In terms of molecular interaction, unlike C34, enfuvirtide does not form stable helical complexes with N36 [35]. Despite the reduced helicity, it possesses high antiretroviral activity. Crucial for this inhibitory effect are the C-terminal residues not included in C34 [36]. Mutations and deletions of the C-terminal domain have been shown to impair the antiretroviral activity of enfuvirtide [35]. This region overlaps the TRD and is responsible for efficient lipid membrane binding [37, 38]. Lipid membranes play an important role during HIV inhibition, since the fusion process must occur in extreme confinement between the viral envelope and the cellular plasma membrane [39]. Membranes participate in enfuvirtide's action, by increasing its concentration at its site of action. It was demonstrated that enfuvirtide incorporates extensively into neutral liquid-crystal lipid membranes and occupies a shallow position in the lipid membrane [40] (Figure 10.2).

The mode of action by which enfuvirtide inhibits viral fusion is still not completely clear and is rather complex. Several proposals have been presented involving different target sites in gp41, gp120, and at the membrane level. The most currently accepted mechanism is the one proposed for C-peptides in general, involving interaction with the gp41 NHR region, thus preventing the conformational changes that lead to the fusion-active arrangement [26, 41, 42].

However, accumulated evidence suggests that this assumption may be too simplistic. Due to the lack of the PBD region, it was suggested that enfuvirtide binding affinity to the NHR region cannot justify its strong inhibitory activity and the peptide should have at least two different interactions modes with gp41 [43].

In addition, Kliger *et al.* [44] showed that enfuvirtide can bind to membranes and oligomerize on their surface. The involvement of lipids in the mechanism of interaction of enfuvirtide, by contrast with C34, has also been reported by Jiang and coworkers [37]. Therefore, two possible enfuvirtide target sites in gp41 can be proposed, both contributing to fusion inhibition: interaction with the NHR region in aqueous solution prevents the formation of the 6HB structure, while interaction with gp41 in the membrane environment inhibits fusion pore formation [43–45].

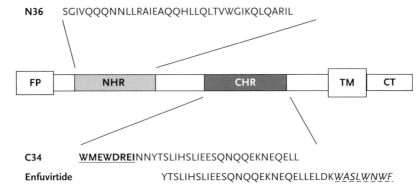

Figure 10.2 Peptide fusion inhibitors and respective gp41 domains. Schematic representation of the location of the N- and C-terminal heptad repeats domains (NHR and CHR, respectively) on gp41 and the sequences from which three first-generation fusion inhibitors are derived: N-peptide N36 (residues 546–581) and C-peptides C34 (residues 628–661) and enfuvirtide (residues 638–673). The underlined and bold sequence in C34 represents the pocket-binding domain (PBD), whereas the underlined and italic sequence in enfuvirtide represents the Trp-rich domains (TRD). FP – fusion peptide, TM – transmembrane domain, CT – cytoplasmic tail.

Less accepted, but also proposed modes of action for enfuvirtide involve its binding to the gp41 FP, preventing the insertion of the latter into the target cell membrane and thus membrane fusion [46], and binding to the gp120 subunit, as an additional target site contributing to its inhibitory activity [47].

During pre-clinical and clinical trial phases, enfuvirtide was demonstrated to be effective against a broad spectrum of HIV-1 strains. Maximum efficacy and safety were achieved with a dose of 90 mg injected subcutaneously twice daily [48]. Though it possess potent anti-HIV activity, enfuvirtide has several pitfalls, such as a short half-life *in vivo*, local side effects and induction of drug-resistant strains.

Based on the knowledge gathered on the structure, activity, and function of fusion inhibitors such as enfuvirtide or C34, several modified peptides have been created, in an attempt to achieve better antiretroviral activity *in vivo* (reviewed in [35]).

One of these new molecules is the rationally designed second generation fusion inhibitor T-1249. This 39 amino acid residues peptide is composed of sequences derived from HIV-1, HIV-2, and simian immunodeficiency virus (SIV) [49], and incorporates both PBD and TRD regions, which explains the efficacy enhancement. Despite the need for clarification, it is believed that, in its mechanism of action, T-1249 acts like most C-peptides, interacting with the NHR region and preventing 6HB formation [23]. It is also able to concentrate on lipid membranes. At variance with enfuvirtide, T-1249 adsorbs on the surface of raft-like platforms in lipid membranes, this difference being one possible explanation for its improved activity. Pre-clinical and clinical studies have demonstrated that this peptide is more potent (2 to 100-fold increase in activity *in vitro* [35]) and has a higher half-life than enfuvirtide, thus enabling a once-daily subcutaneous dose. Furthermore,

T-1249 has been demonstrated to be active against enfuvirtide resistant HIV-1 isolates [50]. Nevertheless, in spite of these optimistic results, the clinical development of T-1249 was discontinued due to formulation difficulties [35, 48].

Another peptide that has recently completed phase IIb clinical trials (http://www.fusogen.com/en/news.asp?id=146) is Sifuvirtide. This 36 aa peptide designed by FusoGen Pharmaceuticals Inc. has been engineered using 3D structure information of HIV-1 gp41 and computer modeling analysis [51]. Sifuvirtide has 16 different residues compared to C34 and 22 compared to enfuvirtide. Like C34, it maintains the PBD region and lacks the TRD region important for membrane binding [52]. Its mode of action is believed to be similar to C34. Nevertheless, it was demonstrated that this peptide adsorbs selectively on the surface of rigid phosphatidylcholine membranes [53, 54]. Sifuvirtide can form a stable 6HB structure with the N-peptide N36 and has potent inhibitory activity against enfuvirtide-resistant strains. Phase Ia clinical studies demonstrated that this peptide has a better safety profile, tolerability, and pharmacokinetic properties than enfuvirtide [52, 55]. This peptide presents low injection side reactions, a longer half-life *in vivo* and a 20-fold higher potency *in vitro*, which enables the administration of a lower once-daily dose compared to enfuvirtide [52, 55]. This peptide was modified by introducing several salt bridges, which favored its solubility, α-helicity, durability and antiviral potency [52]. In the next section new modifications of the C- and N-peptides, as those applied in Sifuvirtide, will be discussed in more detail.

10.5
New Strategies for Creating New HIV Fusion Inhibitor Peptides

Understanding the trimeric gp41 structure and the putative interaction of the CHR and NHR explained why peptides derived from sequences of gp41 inhibited HIV infection of cells. This unlocked a new wave of research that aimed to discover new peptide drugs that target gp41-mediated fusion. In fact, the peptide nature of these drugs gives the researcher a particularly flexible framework with defined rules, which can be played in a myriad of ways. Also, exploring these diverse combinations gives important information on the factors that are most important for the effectiveness of these drugs. In this setting, and not surprisingly, the majority of the fusion inhibitor peptides that were or will be described did not proceed to clinical trials nor were intended to. Hence, many of the peptides were created for research purposes only, as intermediates or precursors for possible future drugs.

In this section we will describe new fusion inhibitor peptides and the strategies behind their design to improve their activity. The starting point is always the wild type (wt) sequence of gp41 (HXB2) or an already modified gp41-based peptide. The rational design of new sequences for these types of drugs usually takes into account factors such as binding to native gp41, secondary structure (helicity), solubility, oligomerization, isomerism, or even lipophilicity.

10.5.1
Increasing Helicity and Binding to gp41

One of the first practical rationalizations in order to improve enfuvirtide activity was to increase the helicity of the peptide in solution [56]. Enfuvirtide does not have a defined secondary structure in solution [26], but assumes an α-helical structure when bundled with a corresponding gp41 N-terminal peptide [14]. Hence, forcing a helical conformation in solution could reduce the energy necessary for the interaction to occur. For this, HIV35, a shorter derivative of enfuvirtide in which the hydrophobic C-terminal TRD (KWASLWNWF) is absent, was used. Ablation of this domain actually results in a peptide with substantially decreased antiviral activity. Covalent crosslinks between aminoacids at positions i and $i+7$ were used to lock the α-helical conformation. Peptides derived from HIV35 with one (HIV24) or two (HIV31) cross-links were prepared, and circular dichroism studies confirmed the increased helicity of these forms. The crosslinking in HIV24 partially restored the activity of the truncated peptide, while in HIV31 it increased it to levels similar to enfuvirtide. This proved the importance of the secondary structure in determining the binding with gp41, even when an important domain for activity is ablated.

A similar approach was used with other short C-peptides that were targeted to the hydrophobic pocket region [57]. The α-helix was stabilized via chemical crosslinking with a diaminoalkane group linking two Glu residues at i and $i+7$ and with the use of an unnatural aminoacid that favors helicity (α-aminoisobutyric acid). The sequence C14wt (gp160 HXB2 626–639) showed very weak antiviral activity, measured by cell–cell fusion assay. The highest antiviral activity was obtained for the version of the peptide cross-linked in the middle at positions 629 and 636 (C14linkmid) followed by an unlinked version but with those positions substituted by α-aminoisobutyric acid (C14Aib). For this case, an important binding site, targeting the hydrophobic pocket, was maintained, and the short sequences used proved to be sufficient for inhibition but modifications to achieve helical constrain were mandatory.

A possible disadvantage of this kind of approach is that cross-linking strategies are not favorable to large scale manufacturing, if a peptide of this kind is able to reach broad clinical use.

Besides these two examples of peculiar use of chemical crosslinking, the majority of the approaches for modifying this kind of peptide involves aminoacid residue changes, rearrangements, and shortening/elongation.

A good example of rational design by modifying the aminoacid sequence was done for C34. It is less soluble than enfuvirtide which is one of the reasons why C34 never progressed in a clinical setting. Otaka *et al.* [33] modified C34 with the following rationale: (i) maintenance of the aminoacids responsible for the interaction with gp41, when represented in a helical-wheel diagram against a trimer of N36; (ii) substitution of non-conserved aminoacids of the solvent accessible site by Glu and Lys that should form ions pairs at positions i and $i+4$. This would enhance solubility and helicity due to formation of intrahelical salt bridges [58].

Two main peptides were derived, SC34 and SC34EK, with the latter neglecting the maintenance of some conserved aminoacids in favor of more salt bridges to stabilize the helix. These two peptides had significantly higher antiviral activity *in vitro* than enfuvirtide, SC34EK being a little more potent than SC34. An extreme version of these peptides (SC35EK) was also synthesized in the form Z-EE-ZZ-KK (with Z representing an arbitrary aminoacid), maintaining the interactive site while the solvent accessible was exclusively Glu and Lys, with activity still comparable with the other peptides. The stable structure of SC34EK with N36 was later confirmed by X-ray crystallography [59]. This shows that increasing helicity by aminoacid substitution while maintaining the residues that interact with gp41 NHR is a successful strategy to increase the activity of fusion inhibitor peptides (Figure 10.3).

The same approach was taken for enfuvirtide, by introducing the same motif Z-EE-ZZ-KK resulting in an increase in the antiviral activity [60]. Shorter versions of SC35EK were also produced with 29 (SC29EK) and 22 (SC22EK) aminoacids by truncation at the C-terminal region [61]. Only SC29EK maintained activity similar to SC34EK and also inhibited enfuvirtide-resistant strains of HIV.

In an effort to screen for the next generation fusion inhibitor that would follow enfuvirtide and T-1249, scientists from Trimeris designed a new set of peptides to improve helical propensity and affinity to gp41 NHR that self-associate to stable

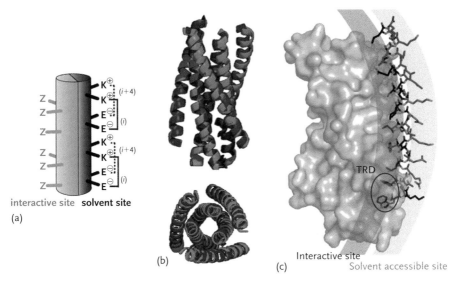

Figure 10.3 Design and structure of SC34EK. (a) The C34 sequence was modified by introducing EK (*i*, *i* + 4) motif in the solvent accessible site, while maintaining the aminoacid residues (Z) of the interactive site. (b) Side and top views of the structure of the 6HB formed by N36/SC34EK (gray), superimposed by the gp41 native core structure (black). (c) Stick model representation of SC34EK modeled in interaction with part of a N36/SC34EK bundle (gray structure). The location of the N-terminal Trp rich domain is indicated by a circle (TRD). Adapted from [59].

oligomers in solution and are active against enfuvirtide-resistant strains [62]. The starting peptide was named T-2410, a wt sequence from gp41 CHR that included the hydrophobic pocket binding sequence. Residues that could be changed without compromising antiviral activity and 6HB stability were selected by Ala scanning. Charged aminoacids Glu and Arg were introduced in spaced positions i and $i+4$ in order to favor formation of salt bridges. To further increase helicity, some noncritical aminoacids not participating in salt bridges were substituted by Ala, an aminoacid with high helical propensity. Up to 15 peptides were obtained with this rational design, from which we will highlight T-2635. This peptide was found, by circular dichroism, to be 75% helical, compared with the starting point of only 7% for T-2410 (enfuvirtide is 12%). It oligomerizes in solution, being a trimer in the concentration range from 50 to 1000 μM and a mixture of trimer and monomer below 50 μM. Its *in vitro* activity can be up to >3600-fold greater than enfuvirtide in certain strains. Importantly, it takes much longer for the virus to aquires mutations to resist these peptides than with enfuvirtide and they have improved pharmacokinetics in cynomolgus monkeys, including extended half-life. Besides the usual structural refinements, this work also emphasizes the role of the oligomerization state in the antiviral activity.

Although the majority of the peptides described here contain the pocket binding sequence and/or the TRD lipid binding domain, He *et al.* identified a new motif upstream of the pocket binding domain important for the stabilization of gp41 6HB (621QIWNNMT627) [63]. A series of peptides containing this sequence was obtained, from which we will highlight CP621–652. This peptide was able to interact with a counterpart NHR peptide in a more stable way than C34. Moreover, improved activity was observed compared to enfuvirtide and the peptide also inhibited strains resistant to enfuvirtide and C34. Based on CP621–652, a new peptide was designed by introducing Lys and Glu in order to create ion pairs, and the first residue at the C-terminal was changed to Val to enhance hydrophobic interaction with the NHR counterpart [64]. This new peptide, CP32M, had improved characteristics over its predecessor and we can emphasize the high potency in low picomolar amounts against enfuvirtide- and C42-resistant strains. These peptides do not rely on the 547GIV549 motif to interact with NHR, a sequence previously shown to be a major determinant of resistance to enfuvirtide and C34 [65].

However, creating peptides that are effective against resistant strains should not be more difficult. Single aminoacid residue modification of enfuvirtide or C34 can overcome such resistance. Izumi *et al.* [66] took into account that the CHR mutations S138A and N126K enhance resistance to enfuvirtide and C34, respectively, and created a peptide with modified aminoacids on those positions. For enfuvirtide, substitution with all natural aminoacids was tried, resulting in the fact that only T-20S138A inhibited replication of enfuvirtide-resistant virus as efficiently as the wt clone. Other efficient substitutions were for smaller hydrophobic residues (Ala, Leu, Ile) or more flexible ones (Met, Thr). The same happened for a C34 modified through the mutation N126K, which became active against the respective resistant strain. This case highlights the importance of having resistance information in order to specifically tailor the peptides to overcome such barrier.

Another example of an innovative approach comes from the creation of C34coil, a derivative of C34 grafted into a GCN4 Leu zipper [67]. In this case, residues of C34 critical for binding to NHR are transferred to a GCN4 sequence, functioning as a scaffold. After that, the C34-GCN4 peptide was disulfide linked to a GCN4 peptide only in order to form a coiled coil dimer. This resulted in a more stable and structurally defined peptide, with enhanced solubility and helicity. Importantly, C34coil was 1000 times more resistant to proteolytic degradation than C34 itself. This new peptide is not more potent than C34; however, IC50 values for cell–cell fusion and infectivity assays are within an order of magnitude.

We should also not forget that computational biology is nowadays a major tool to design new drugs tailored to a specific molecular target. The computation power available makes the simulation of structures and interactions increasingly accessible and informative. A series of 10 variants of C34 (KYK01 to 10) was designed based on molecular dynamics simulations of 6HB stability to increase the binding to the gp41 NHR region [68]. KYK01, KYK02, and KYK03 were more efficient in inhibiting virus replications than the original C34; however, they were inactive against enfuvirtide-resistant viruses. To overcome this, KYK02 was modified to carry the previously mentioned S138A substitution. For this case more than one strategy was applied in order to design a truly efficient drug.

10.5.2
Isomeric Peptides and Resistance to Proteolysis

To specifically tackle the problem of the oral bioavailability of these drug peptides, due to rapid preoteolytic degradation in the gastrointestinal tract, the main strategy that emerged was to design peptides with different chirality from the natural ones: D-peptides. Using once again the pocket binding site as a target, a D-peptide IQN17 was designed to properly present this target to serve as a template for the new peptides [69]. Using mirror-image phage display, several D-peptides were identified (D10-p1 through D10-p12). They presented a 10 residues consensus sequence to the binding of the pocket region. Cys flanking the consensus sequence generated an intramolecular disulfide bond to yield a cyclic peptide. Lys were added at the N-terminus to increase solubility. These peptides were capable of inhibiting HIV-1 entry into cells in the micromolar concentration range. This kind of approach was refined in a later study [70] in which the authors locked the consensus residues and randomized the other ones in the phage-display rounds. The new peptides were more potent than those obtained in the first studies and were active against laboratory-adapted strains (HXB2) and primary isolates.

In another attempt to create proteolysis resistant fusion inhibitors, the C34 sequence was modified by introducing D-aminoacid point substitutions at sites not directly involved in 6HB integrity [71]. These modifications were able to create stable and helical peptides with similar activity to C34.

10.5.3
Bacterially Expressed Peptides

From the pharmaceutical point of view, even if a peptide is very potent, it may not be feasible for commercialization if its manufacturing is difficult and costly. To address the problem of large scale manufacturing, Deng *et al.* tried, for the first time, to express a fusion inhibitor peptide, C52L in *E. coli* [72]. This peptide spans the sequence of enfuvirtide and C34, containing at the C-terminus a heptad register of three residues from the N-terminus of GCN4-pII isoleucine trimer to enhance helicity. The peptide was produced by extraction from insoluble bacterial inclusion bodies. It possessed broad activity, inhibiting infection of all clades of HIV-1 group M and also enfuvirtide resistant variants. This was the first and only time that this kind of production was tried, aiming at a solution for getting more affordable drugs of this type.

10.5.4
Modification of Peptides by Derivatization with Lipids or Proteins

In the constant search for ways to optimize and increase the effectiveness of HIV fusion inhibitor peptides, sometimes it takes more than just residue substitutions to achieve a better result. In this section we will describe how HIV fusion inhibitor peptides can be modified by covalently attaching another molecular entity to increase potency.

An unconventional approach was taken by Hildinger *et al.* by expressing a membrane-anchored version of enfuvirtide [73]. In this case enfuvirtide was expressed fused with a membrane protein, so that the peptide was displayed at the surface of a T-helper cell line. In this way, the peptide potently inhibited viral replication in these transduced cell lines. In contrast, a construct that attached enfuvirtide to a secreted protein instead of a membrane spanning one, did not inhibit the replication. This indicates that attachment of the drug to the cell membrane, where viral fusion occurs, increases the efficacy of the drug.

Following different observations of the enhanced efficacy of membrane associated peptides, Peisajovich *et al.* [74] synthesized SIV-derived enfuvirtide peptides acylated at their C-terminus. Octylation of enfuvirtide rendered the peptide significantly more potent than the peptide itself. The same did not happen for propyl and hexyl variations and for N-terminal acylation. Moreover, an inactive enfuvirtide mutant in which part of the TRD, GNWF, was substituted by ANAA, was rescued when octylated. The acylation seemed to mimic the role of the hydrophobic C-terminal region of the peptide. This C-terminal modification to the peptide could direct the peptide to the cell membranes in order to be readily available if the virus infects the cell, and with the favorable orientation to interact with gp41 NHR. This membrane association effect is similar to the previously presented case of enfuvirtide covalently attached to a membrane spanning protein.

A series of enfuvirtide peptides was truncated at this region to arrive at a minimal inhibitory sequence, named DP [75]. In this version, the entire region containing the three C-terminal Trp residues was removed. This peptide was then attached to fatty acids of 8, 12, or 16 carbons to assess the effect of chain length. Indeed, the higher the length the more potent was the conjugate in inhibiting viral fusion. N-terminal conjugation did not lead to similar improved efficacy, hence the importance of the orientation of the peptide. The hydrophobic anchor of these modified peptides permitted higher potency, presumably due to membrane targeting and concentration effects.

Trimeris, the company behind enfuvirtide and T-1249, also developed a peptide conjugated with fatty-acid. TRI-999 is a peptide that includes the pocket binding domain regions but not the C-terminal hydrophobic tail. Instead, a C18 fatty acid is attached to the only Lys residue near the C-terminus through a PEG3 linker [76]. This peptide was more potent than enfuvirtide, having an IC50 up to 250-fold lower. Importantly, the pharmacokinetics clearance values were up to sixfold slower than enfuvirtide, showing a slow and steady release of the drug [77].

In an effort by scientists of Merck Research Laboratories to increase the efficacy of C34, a new type of conjugate was synthesized with a cholesteryl moiety attached [78]. The rationale for the use of cholesterol instead of a fatty acid was the higher affinity towards membranes and targeting of the drug to the receptor-rich membrane microdomains (lipid rafts) where HIV-cell fusion is likely to occur. This modification increases the antiviral activity from 15-fold to 300-fold compared to enfuvirtide and T-1249, and increases significantly the half-life of the peptide *in vivo*. Moreover, the activity is retained *in vitro* if pre-treated host cells are washed. Contrary to C34, the addition of cholesterol to enfuvirtide does not have the same effects of enhancing potency, probably due to the existence of the lipid binding domain already. Interestingly, this cholesterol tagging strategy was also later used for fusion inhibitor peptides of paramoxyvirus [79].

Beside these lipopeptide conjugates that turned out to be quite successful, protein conjugates were recently considered. The C34 fusion inhibitor peptide was conjugated with human serum albumin and tested for *in vitro* and *in vivo* action [80]. A maleimido-C34 derivative was reacted with cysteine 34 of HSA, the only cysteine of this protein, resulting in a 1 : 1 complex, named PC-1505. The potency of this conjugate was still similar to C34 and enfuvirtide, indicating that the accessory protein did not prevent the peptide from reaching gp41 in the pre-fusion state. More importantly, the PC-1505 activity *in vivo* was 3 times higher than the unconjugated form and was more sustained, resulting in an improved pharmacokinetic profile. A similar approach was taken by Xie *et al.* [81], where they modified a C34 peptide in order to carry a maleimido group in Lys 13 (FB006M). When injecting this modified peptide in SCID/hu mouse model the peptide reacted with Cys 34 of albumin in the blood, generating a 1 : 1 complex which prolonged the half-life of the drug while maintaining its efficacy.

Another interesting approach was taken by Ji *et al.* [82]. They created a construct CD4-BFFI which consists of two HIV-1 fusion inhibitor peptides T-651 [62] fused to the Fc (fragment, crystallizable) end of a humanized anti-CD4 monoclonal antibody. This antibody part would direct the conjugate to the CD4 receptor making the peptides available at the exact site of viral attachment. CD4-BFFI presented improved antiviral activities over nonconjugated T-651, as well as improved serum stability and pharmacokinetics, with a half-life of several days. This demonstrates once again the utility of using peptide conjugates to improve the pharmacological profiles of these kinds of peptide drugs.

10.6
Drug-Resistance and Combination Therapy

The emergence of drug-resistant HIV-1 variants in patients under fusion inhibitor therapy is one of the aspects that should be taken into consideration in the development of novel compounds. Resistance to enfuvirtide has been observed both *in vitro* and during clinical studies and is governed by changes in the NHR region, especially in and around the GIV motif (amino acids 35–45 of gp41) (reviewed in [83]). Those mutations have been shown to reduce the level of enfuvirtide binding and sensitivity, but at a fitness cost. These mutations interfere in the interaction between the viral NHR and CHR domains, thus decreasing viral bundle stability, which may alter fusion kinetics, pathogenicity, replicative fitness, and other aspects of the viral fusion process. Nevertheless, the virus may further evolve to repair its fitness loss by introducing a compensatory mutation, normally in the CHR domain. For instance, Baldwin and Berkhout reported that, for the V38A mutated virus, the compensatory mutation N126K promoted a drug-dependent phenotype [83]. Alternatively, Bai *et al.* [84] and Tolstrup *et al.* [85] reported the E137K mutation that partially compensated the loss of stability at the helical bundle level for N43D-mutated viruses and further increased its resistance to enfuvirtide.

A way to delay the emergence of drug resistance and/or take advantage of the loss of replicative fitness of drug-resistant strains could be the use of combination therapy. The simultaneous use of antiretroviral drugs with different targets is able to increase the antiviral potency because of the synergistic effect resulting from the combination. For instance, strong synergistic activity was reported when entry inhibitors targeting gp120 (e.g., PRO 542), gp41 (e.g., enfuvirtide), and the cor-eceptor, CXCR4 (e.g., AMD3100) or CCR5 (e.g., SCH-C), were used in combination [86–88]. Additionally, some studies demonstrated that combination of fusion inhibitors targeting different sites would also result in a similar phenomenon. Hrin *et al.* demonstrated that a combination of enfuvirtide and (CCIZN17)$_3$, a trimer of N-peptides targeting the CHR domain, worked synergistically in inhibiting the entry of primary HIV-1 isolates in an *in vitro* infectivity assay [89]. The combinations of enfuvirtide with other C-peptides have also demonstrated potent synergistic effects. For instance, the combination of enfuvirtide (which possesses the TRD) and Sifuvirtide (which presents the PBD) exhibited strong synergic activity against laboratory-adapted and primary HIV-1 strains [90]. More recently,

Pan *et al.* tested the combination of enfuvirtide with both second-generation T-1249 and next-generation fusion inhibitor T-1144 (drug similar to T-2635) against HIV-1 induced cell–cell fusion [91]. The double combination exhibited strong synergism, leading to two orders of dose reduction. Exceptional synergistic activity was retrieved using the triple combination, where a three-order dose reduction was demonstrated. Furthermore, combination therapy with enfuvirtide, T-1249 and T-1144 led also to strong synergism against enfuvirtide- and T-1249-resistant HIV-1 variants. Enfuvirtide, T-1249 and T-1144, and also Sifuvirtide, contain different functional domains and present distinct primary binding sites. The binding of one of those C-peptides to the viral gp41 NHR domain may extend the temporal window period of the already transient fusion intermediate, which would then become more accessible to the other C-peptides, resulting in a potent synergism [51].

To conclude, synergistic strategies may provide higher efficacy with lower antiretroviral doses, overcoming limitations of a one-drug therapy to patients, such as ineffectiveness against resistant-strains, requirement of high doses per injection and serious injection side effects. In the end, the use of a combination of fusion inhibitors may result in lower costs and lower rejection of the antiretroviral therapy.

10.7
Concluding Remarks

The notions underlying the HIV-1 membrane fusion process and the contribution of gp41 fusion intermediate are nowadays well accepted among the scientific community. The discovery of the structure of the gp41 hairpin, prior and after gp41 NHR and CHR reorganization, contributed significantly to the development of new strategies to inhibit HIV-1. To ensure a competent viral and plasma membrane fusion, the CHR and NHR domains of the viral protein gp41 must interact to form a trimeric hairpin structure. The inhibition of this viral process is the basis of the mode of action, potency, efficacy and selectivity of fusion inhibitors. Since the early 1990s, when the first peptide inhibitors were discovered, major advances have occurred in the way we understand and design these peptidic compounds. The development of more potent and novel fusion inhibitors is being addressed, understanding the contribution of structural features and specific domains that are needed for a stronger and efficient interaction with gp41. Enfuvirtide is still the only licensed and FDA-approved drug of the fusion inhibitor class, but other drugs are now in pre-clinical or clinical development. Moreover, new insights on the mechanism of resistance and tolerance of these compounds have been discovered and several strategies involving synergistic approaches are being tested. Therefore, we can expect better outcomes and more compounds to appear in the near future, thus providing new hope for the treatment not only of AIDS but also of other viral diseases.

References

1 Janeway, C.A., Travers, P., Walport, M., and Shlomchik, M. (2005) *Immunobiology: The Immune System in Health and Disease*, Garland Science, New York, NY.

2 UNAIDS/WHO. (2009) AIDS epidemic update 2009. http://data.unaids.org/pub/Report/2009/JC1700_Epi_Update_2009_en.pdf (7 October 2010).

3 De Clercq, E. (2002) New developments in anti-HIV chemotherapy. *Biochim. Biophys. Acta*, **1587** (2–3), 258–275.

4 Palella, F. J. Jr, Delaney, K.M., Moorman, A.C., Loveless, M.O., Fuhrer, J., Satten, G.A., Aschman, D.J., and Holmberg, S.D. (1998) Declining morbidity and mortality among patients with advanced human immunodeficiency virus infection. HIV outpatient study investigators. *N. Engl. J. Med.*, **338** (13), 853–860.

5 Carr, A. (2003) Toxicity of antiretroviral therapy and implications for drug development. *Nat. Rev. Drug Discov.*, **2** (8), 624–634.

6 Eckert, D.M. and Kim, P.S. (2001) Mechanisms of viral membrane fusion and its inhibition. *Annu. Rev. Biochem.*, **70**, 777–810.

7 Center, R.J., Leapman, R.D., Lebowitz, J., Arthur, L.O., Earl, P.L., and Moss, B. (2002) Oligomeric structure of the human immunodeficiency virus type 1 envelope protein on the virion surface. *J. Virol.*, **76** (15), 7863–7867.

8 Chan, D.C. and Kim, P.S. (1998) HIV entry and its inhibition. *Cell*, **93** (5), 681–684.

9 Wyatt, R. and Sodroski, J. (1998) The HIV-1 envelope glycoproteins: fusogens, antigens, and immunogens. *Science*, **280** (5371), 1884–1888.

10 Tamm, L.K. and Han, X. (2000) Viral fusion peptides: a tool set to disrupt and connect biological membranes. *Biosci. Rep.*, **20** (6), 501–518.

11 Chambers, P., Pringle, C.R., and Easton, A.J. (1990) Heptad repeat sequences are located adjacent to hydrophobic regions in several types of virus fusion glycoproteins. *J. Gen. Virol.*, **71** (Pt 12), 3075–3080.

12 Lorizate, M., Huarte, N., Saez-Cirion, A., and Nieva, J.L. (2008) Interfacial pre-transmembrane domains in viral proteins promoting membrane fusion and fission. *Biochim. Biophys. Acta*, **1778** (7–8), 1624–1639.

13 Montero, M., van Houten, N.E., Wang, X., and Scott, J.K. (2008) The membrane-proximal external region of the human immunodeficiency virus type 1 envelope: dominant site of antibody neutralization and target for vaccine design. *Microbiol. Mol. Biol. Rev.*, **72** (1), 54–84, table of contents

14 Lu, M., Blacklow, S.C., and Kim, P.S. (1995) A trimeric structural domain of the HIV-1 transmembrane glycoprotein. *Nat. Struct. Biol.*, **2** (12), 1075–1082.

15 Chan, D.C., Fass, D., Berger, J.M., and Kim, P.S. (1997) Core structure of gp41 from the HIV envelope glycoprotein. *Cell*, **89** (2), 263–273.

16 Weissenhorn, W., Dessen, A., Harrison, S.C., Skehel, J.J., and Wiley, D.C. (1997) Atomic structure of the ectodomain from HIV-1 gp41. *Nature*, **387** (6631), 426–430.

17 Maddon, P.J., Dalgleish, A.G., McDougal, J.S., Clapham, P.R., Weiss, R.A., and Axel, R. (1986) The T4 gene encodes the AIDS virus receptor and is expressed in the immune system and the brain. *Cell*, **47** (3), 333–348.

18 Chesebro, B., Buller, R., Portis, J., and Wehrly, K. (1990) Failure of human immunodeficiency virus entry and infection in CD4-positive human brain and skin cells. *J. Virol.*, **64** (1), 215–221.

19 Clapham, P.R., Blanc, D., and Weiss, R.A. (1991) Specific cell surface requirements for the infection of CD4-positive cells by human immunodeficiency virus types 1 and 2 and by Simian immunodeficiency virus. *Virology*, **181** (2), 703–715

20 Briz, V., Poveda, E., and Soriano, V. (2006) HIV entry inhibitors: mechanisms of action and resistance

pathways. *J. Antimicrob. Chemother.*, **57** (4), 619–627.

21 De Clercq, E. (2009) Anti-HIV drugs: 25 compounds approved within 25 years after the discovery of HIV. *Int. J. Antimicrob. Agents*, **33** (4), 307–320.

22 Doms, R.W. and Trono, D. (2000) The plasma membrane as a combat zone in the HIV battlefield. *Genes Dev.*, **14** (21), 2677–2688.

23 Kilby, J.M. and Eron, J.J. (2003) Novel therapies based on mechanisms of HIV-1 cell entry. *N. Engl. J. Med.*, **348** (22), 2228–2238.

24 Robertson, D. (2003) US FDA approves new class of HIV therapeutics. *Nat. Biotechnol.*, **21** (5), 470–471.

25 Kilby, J.M., Hopkins, S., Venetta, T.M., DiMassimo, B., Cloud, G.A., Lee, J.Y., Alldredge, L., Hunter, E., Lambert, D., Bolognesi, D., Matthews, T., Johnson, M.R., Nowak, M.A., Shaw, G.M., and Saag, M.S. (1998) Potent suppression of HIV-1 replication in humans by T-20, a peptide inhibitor of gp41-mediated virus entry. *Nat. Med.*, **4** (11), 1302–1307.

26 Wild, C.T., Shugars, D.C., Greenwell, T. K., McDanal, C.B., and Matthews, T.J. (1994) Peptides corresponding to a predictive alpha-helical domain of human immunodeficiency virus type 1 gp41 are potent inhibitors of virus infection. *Proc. Natl. Acad. Sci. U. S. A.*, **91** (21), 9770–9774.

27 Kilgore, N.R., Salzwedel, K., Reddick, M., Allaway, G.P., and Wild, C.T. (2003) Direct evidence that C-peptide inhibitors of human immunodeficiency virus type 1 entry bind to the gp41 N-helical domain in receptor-activated viral envelope. *J. Virol.*, **77** (13), 7669–7672.

28 Eckert, D.M. and Kim, P.S. (2001) Design of potent inhibitors of HIV-1 entry from the gp41 N-peptide region. *Proc. Natl. Acad. Sci. U. S. A.*, **98** (20), 11187–11192.

29 Naider, F. and Anglister, J. (2009) Peptides in the treatment of AIDS. *Curr. Opin. Struct. Biol.*, **19** (4), 473–482.

30 Wild, C., Dubay, J.W., Greenwell, T., Baird, T. Jr, Oas, T.G., McDanal, C., Hunter, E., and Matthews, T. (1994) Propensity for a leucine zipper-like domain of human immunodeficiency virus type 1 gp41 to form oligomers correlates with a role in virus-induced fusion rather than assembly of the glycoprotein complex. *Proc. Natl. Acad. Sci. U. S. A.*, **91** (26), 12676–12680.

31 Chan, D.C., Chutkowski, C.T., and Kim, P.S. (1998) Evidence that a prominent cavity in the coiled coil of HIV type 1 gp41 is an attractive drug target. *Proc. Natl. Acad. Sci. U. S. A.*, **95** (26), 15613–15617.

32 Chang, D.K. and Hsu, C.S. (2007) Biophysical evidence of two docking sites of the carboxyl heptad repeat region within the amino heptad repeat region of gp41 of human immunodeficiency virus type 1. *Antiviral Res.*, **74** (1), 51–58

33 Otaka, A., Nakamura, M., Nameki, D., Kodama, E., Uchiyama, S., Nakamura, S., Nakano, H., Tamamura, H., Kobayashi, Y., Matsuoka, M., and Fujii, N. (2002) Remodeling of gp41-C34 peptide leads to highly effective inhibitors of the fusion of HIV-1 with target cells. *Angew. Chem. Int. Ed. Engl.*, **41** (16), 2937–2940.

34 Wild, C., Greenwell, T., and Matthews, T. (1993) A synthetic peptide from HIV-1 gp41 is a potent inhibitor of virus-mediated cell-cell fusion. *AIDS Res. Hum. Retroviruses*, **9** (11), 1051–1053.

35 Liu, S., Wu, S., and Jiang, S. (2007) HIV entry inhibitors targeting gp41: from polypeptides to small-molecule compounds. *Curr. Pharm. Des.*, **13** (2), 143–162.

36 Jiang, S., Zhao, Q., and Debnath, A.K. (2002) Peptide and non-peptide HIV fusion inhibitors. *Curr. Pharm. Des.*, **8** (8), 563–580.

37 Liu, S., Jing, W., Cheung, B., Lu, H., Sun, J., Yan, X., Niu, J., Farmar, J., Wu, S., and Jiang, S. (2007) HIV gp41 C-terminal heptad repeat contains multifunctional domains. Relation to mechanisms of action of anti-HIV peptides. *J. Biol. Chem.*, **282** (13), 9612–9620.

38 Liu, S., Lu, H., Niu, J., Xu, Y., Wu, S., and Jiang, S. (2005) Different from the HIV fusion inhibitor C34, the anti-HIV drug Fuzeon (T-20) inhibits HIV-1 entry by targeting multiple sites in gp41 and gp120. *J. Biol. Chem.*, **280** (12), 11259–11273.

39 Bar, S. and Alizon, M. (2004) Role of the ectodomain of the gp41 transmembrane envelope protein of human immunodeficiency virus type 1 in late steps of the membrane fusion process. *J. Virol.*, **78** (2), 811–820.

40 Veiga, S., Henriques, S., Santos, N.C. and Castanho, M. (2004) Putative role of membranes in the HIV fusion inhibitor enfuvirtide mode of action at the molecular level. *Biochem. J.*, **377** (Pt 1), 107–110

41 Kliger, Y. and Shai, Y. (2000) Inhibition of HIV-1 entry before gp41 folds into its fusion-active conformation. *J. Mol. Biol.*, **295** (2), 163–168.

42 Rimsky, L.T., Shugars, D.C., and Matthews, T.J. (1998) Determinants of human immunodeficiency virus type 1 resistance to gp41-derived inhibitory peptides. *J. Virol.*, **72** (2), 986–993.

43 Ryu, J.R., Jin, B.S., Suh, M.J., Yoo, Y.S., Yoon, S.H., Woo, E.R., and Yu, Y.G. (1999) Two interaction modes of the gp41-derived peptides with gp41 and their correlation with antimembrane fusion activity. *Biochem. Biophys. Res. Commun.*, **265** (3), 625–629.

44 Kliger, Y., Gallo, S.A., Peisajovich, S.G., Munoz-Barroso, I., Avkin, S., Blumenthal, R., and Shai, Y. (2001) Mode of action of an antiviral peptide from HIV-1 Inhibition at a post-lipid mixing stage. *J. Biol. Chem.*, **276** (2), 1391–1397.

45 Munoz-Barroso, I., Salzwedel, K., Hunter, E., and Blumenthal, R. (1999) Role of the membrane-proximal domain in the initial stages of human immunodeficiency virus type 1 envelope glycoprotein-mediated membrane fusion. *J. Virol.*, **73** (7), 6089–6092.

46 Mobley, P.W., Pilpa, R., Brown, C., Waring, A.J., and Gordon, L.M. (2001) Membrane-perturbing domains of HIV type 1 glycoprotein 41. *AIDS Res. Hum. Retroviruses.*, **17** (4), 311–327.

47 Alam, S.M., Paleos, C.A., Liao, H.X., Scearce, R., Robinson, J., and Haynes, B.F. (2004) An inducible HIV type 1 gp41 HR-2 peptide-binding site on HIV type 1 envelope gp120. *AIDS Res. Hum. Retroviruses.*, **20** (8), 836–845.

48 Veiga, A.S., Santos, N.C., and Castanho, M.A. (2006) An insight on the leading HIV entry inhibitors. *Recent. Pat. Antiinfect. Drug Discov.*, **1** (1), 67–73.

49 Eron, J.J., Gulick, R.M., Bartlett, J.A., Merigan, T., Arduino, R., Kilby, J.M., Yangco, B., Diers, A., Drobnes, C., DeMasi, R., Greenberg, M., Melby, T., Raskino, C., Rusnak, P., Zhang, Y., Spence, R., and Miralles, G.D. (2004) Short-term safety and antiretroviral activity of T-1249, a second-generation fusion inhibitor of HIV. *J. Infect. Dis.*, **189** (6), 1075–1083.

50 Lalezari, J.P., Bellos, N.C., Sathasivam, K., Richmond, G.J., Cohen, C.J., Myers, R.A. Jr, Henry, D.H., Raskino, C., Melby, T., Murchison, H., Zhang, Y., Spence, R., Greenberg, M.L., Demasi, R. A., and Miralles, G.D. (2005) T-1249 retains potent antiretroviral activity in patients who had experienced virological failure while on an enfuvirtide-containing treatment regimen. *J. Infect. Dis.*, **191** (7), 1155–1163.

51 Pan, C., Liu, S., and Jiang, S. (2010) HIV-1 gp41 fusion intermediate: a target for HIV therapeutics. *J. Formos. Med. Assoc.*, **109** (2), 94–105.

52 He, Y., Xiao, Y., Song, H., Liang, Q., Ju, D., Chen, X., Lu, H., Jing, W., Jiang, S., and Zhang, L. (2008) Design and evaluation of Sifuvirtide, a novel HIV-1 fusion inhibitor. *J. Biol. Chem.*, **283** (17), 11126–11134.

53 Franquelim, H.G., Loura, L.M., Santos, N.C., and Castanho, M.A. (2008) Sifuvirtide screens rigid membrane surfaces. Establishment of a correlation between efficacy and membrane domain selectivity among HIV fusion inhibitor peptides. *J. Am. Chem. Soc.*, **130** (19), 6215–6223.

54 Franquelim, H.G., Veiga, A.S., Weissmuller, G., Santos, N.C., and Castanho, M.A. (2010) Unravelling the molecular basis of the selectivity of the HIV-1 fusion inhibitor Sifuvirtide towards phosphatidylcholine-rich rigid

membranes. *Biochim. Biophys. Acta*, **1798** (6), 1234–1243.

55 Wang, R.R., Yang, L.M., Wang, Y.H., Pang, W., Tam, S.C., Tien, P., and Zheng, Y.T. (2009) Sifuvirtide, a potent HIV fusion inhibitor peptide. *Biochem. Biophys. Res. Commun.*, **382** (3), 540–544.

56 Judice, J.K., Tom, J.Y., Huang, W., Wrin, T., Vennari, J., Petropoulos, C.J., and McDowell, R.S. (1997) Inhibition of HIV type 1 infectivity by constrained alpha-helical peptides: implications for the viral fusion mechanism. *Proc. Natl. Acad. Sci. U. S. A.*, **94** (25), 13426–13430.

57 Sia, S.K., Carr, P.A., Cochran, A.G., Malashkevich, V.N., and Kim, P.S. (2002) Short constrained peptides that inhibit HIV-1 entry. *Proc. Natl. Acad. Sci. U. S. A.*, **99** (23), 14664–14669.

58 Marqusee, S. and Baldwin, R.L. (1987) Helix stabilization by Glu-... Lys + salt bridges in short peptides of de novo design. *Proc. Natl. Acad. Sci. U. S. A.*, **84** (24), 8898–8902.

59 Nishikawa, H., Nakamura, S., Kodama, E., Ito, S., Kajiwara, K., Izumi, K., Sakagami, Y., Oishi, S., Ohkubo, T., Kobayashi, Y., Otaka, A., Fujii, N., and Matsuoka, M. (2009) Electrostatically constrained alpha-helical peptide inhibits replication of HIV-1 resistant to enfuvirtide. *Int. J. Biochem. Cell Biol.*, **41** (4), 891–899.

60 Oishi, S., Ito, S., Nishikawa, H., Watanabe, K., Tanaka, M., Ohno, H., Izumi, K., Sakagami, Y., Kodama, E., Matsuoka, M., and Fujii, N. (2008) Design of a novel HIV-1 fusion inhibitor that displays a minimal interface for binding affinity. *J. Med. Chem.*, **51** (3), 388–391.

61 Naito, T., Izumi, K., Kodama, E., Sakagami, Y., Kajiwara, K., Nishikawa, H., Watanabe, K., Sarafianos, S.G., Oishi, S., Fujii, N., and Matsuoka, M. (2009) SC29EK, a peptide fusion inhibitor with enhanced alpha-helicity, inhibits replication of human immunodeficiency virus type 1 mutants resistant to enfuvirtide. *Antimicrob. Agents Chemother.*, **53** (3), 1013–1018.

62 Dwyer, J.J., Wilson, K.L., Davison, D.K., Freel, S.A., Seedorff, J.E., Wring, S.A., Tvermoes, N.A., Matthews, T.J., Greenberg, M.L., and Delmedico, M.K. (2007) Design of helical, oligomeric HIV-1 fusion inhibitor peptides with potent activity against enfuvirtide-resistant virus. *Proc. Natl. Acad. Sci. U. S. A.*, **104** (31), 12772–12777.

63 He, Y., Cheng, J., Li, J., Qi, Z., Lu, H., Dong, M., Jiang, S., and Dai, Q. (2008) Identification of a critical motif for the human immunodeficiency virus type 1 (HIV-1) gp41 core structure: implications for designing novel anti-HIV fusion inhibitors. *J. Virol.*, **82** (13), 6349–6358.

64 He, Y., Cheng, J., Lu, H., Li, J., Hu, J., Qi, Z., Liu, Z., Jiang, S., and Dai, Q. (2008) Potent HIV fusion inhibitors against enfuvirtide-resistant HIV-1 strains. *Proc. Natl. Acad. Sci. U. S. A.*, **105** (42), 16332–16337.

65 Trivedi, V.D., Cheng, S.F., Wu, C.W., Karthikeyan, R., Chen, C.J., and Chang, D.K. (2003) The LLSGIV stretch of the N-terminal region of HIV-1 gp41 is critical for binding to a model peptide, T20. *Protein Eng.*, **16** (4), 311–317.

66 Izumi, K., Kodama, E., Shimura, K., Sakagami, Y., Watanabe, K., Ito, S., Watabe, T., Terakawa, Y., Nishikawa, H., Sarafianos, S.G., Kitaura, K., Oishi, S., Fujii, N., and Matsuoka, M. (2009) Design of peptide-based inhibitors for human immunodeficiency virus type 1 strains resistant to T-20. *J. Biol. Chem.*, **284** (8), 4914–4920.

67 Sia, S.K. and Kim, P.S. (2003) Protein grafting of an HIV-1-inhibiting epitope. *Proc. Natl. Acad. Sci. U. S. A.*, **100** (17), 9756–9761.

68 Soonthornsata, B., Tian, Y.S., Utachee, P., Sapsutthipas, S., Isarangkura-na-Ayuthaya, P., Auwanit, W., Takagi, T., Ikuta, K., Sawanpanyalert, P., Kawashita, N., and Kameoka, M. (2010) Design and evaluation of antiretroviral peptides corresponding to the C-terminal heptad repeat region (C-HR) of human immunodeficiency virus type 1 envelope glycoprotein gp41. *Virology*, **405** (1), 157–164.

69 Eckert, D.M., Malashkevich, V.N., Hong, L.H., Carr, P.A., and Kim, P.S. (1999) Inhibiting HIV-1 entry: discovery of D-peptide inhibitors that target the gp41 coiled-coil pocket. *Cell*, **99** (1), 103–115.

70 Welch, B.D., VanDemark, A.P., Heroux, A., Hill, C.P., and Kay, M.S. (2007) Potent D-peptide inhibitors of HIV-1 entry. *Proc. Natl. Acad. Sci. U. S. A.*, **104** (43), 16828–16833.

71 Gaston, F., Granados, G.C., Madurga, S., Rabanal, F., Lakhdar-Ghazal, F., Giralt, E., and Bahraoui, E. (2009) Development and characterization of peptidic fusion inhibitors derived from HIV-1 gp41 with partial D-amino acid substitutions. *ChemMedChem.*, **4** (4), 570–581.

72 Deng, Y., Zheng, Q., Ketas, T.J., Moore, J.P., and Lu, M. (2007) Protein design of a bacterially expressed HIV-1 gp41 fusion inhibitor. *Biochemistry (Mosc.)*., **46** (14), 4360–4369.

73 Hildinger, M., Dittmar, M.T., Schult-Dietrich, P., Fehse, B., Schnierle, B.S., Thaler, S., Stiegler, G., Welker, R., and von Laer, D. (2001) Membrane-anchored peptide inhibits human immunodeficiency virus entry. *J. Virol.*, **75** (6), 3038–3042.

74 Peisajovich, S.G., Gallo, S.A., Blumenthal, R., and Shai, Y. (2003) C-terminal octylation rescues an inactive T20 mutant: implications for the mechanism of HIV/SIMIAN immunodeficiency virus-induced membrane fusion. *J. Biol. Chem.*, **278** (23), 21012–21017.

75 Wexler-Cohen, Y. and Shai, Y. (2007) Demonstrating the C-terminal boundary of the HIV 1 fusion conformation in a dynamic ongoing fusion process and implication for fusion inhibition. *FASEB J.*, **21** (13), 3677–3684.

76 Zhang, H.Y., Schneider, S.E., Bray, B.L., Friedrich, P.E., Tvermoes, N.A., Mader, C.J., Whight, S.R., Niemi, T.E., Silinski, P., Picking, T., Warren, M., and Wrings, S.A. (2008) Process development of TRI-999, a fatty-acid-modified HIV fusion inhibitory peptide. *Org. Process Res. Dev.*, **12** (1), 101–110

77 Stanfield-Oakley, S.A., Mosier, S.M., Davison, D.K., Medinas, R.J., Jin, L., Delmedico, M.K., Dwyer, J.J., Heilek-Snyder, G., and Greenberg, M.L. (2006) Next generation HIV peptide fusion inhibitors TRI-999 and TRI-1144 display enhanced activity against enfuvirtide sensitive and resistant viruses. *Antivir. Ther.*, **11** (5), S25–S25.

78 Ingallinella, P., Bianchi, E., Ladwa, N.A., Wang, Y.J., Hrin, R., Veneziano, M., Bonelli, F., Ketas, T.J., Moore, J.P., Miller, M.D., and Pessi, A. (2009) Addition of a cholesterol group to an HIV-1 peptide fusion inhibitor dramatically increases its antiviral potency. *Proc. Natl. Acad. Sci. U. S. A.*, **106** (14), 5801–5806.

79 Porotto, M., Yokoyama, C.C., Palermo, L.M., Mungall, B., Aljofan, M., Cortese, R., Pessi, A., and Moscona, A. (2010) Viral entry inhibitors targeted to the membrane site of action. *J. Virol.*, **84** (13), 6760–6768.

80 Stoddart, C.A., Nault, G., Galkina, S.A., Thibaudeau, K., Bakis, P., Bousquet-Gagnon, N., Robitaille, M., Bellomo, M., Paradis, V., Liscourt, P., Lobach, A., Rivard, M.E., Ptak, R.G., Mankowski, M.K., Bridon, D., and Quraishi, O. (2008) Albumin-conjugated C34 peptide HIV-1 fusion inhibitor: equipotent to C34 and T-20 *in vitro* with sustained activity in SCID-hu Thy/Liv mice. *J. Biol. Chem.*, **283** (49), 34045–34052.

81 Xie, D., Yao, C., Wang, L., Min, W., Xu, J., Xiao, J., Huang, M., Chen, B., Liu, B., Li, X., and Jiang, H. (2010) An albumin-conjugated peptide exhibits potent anti-HIV activity and long *in vivo* half-life. *Antimicrob. Agents Chemother.*, **54** (1), 191–196.

82 Ji, C., Kopetzki, E., Jekle, A., Stubenrauch, K.G., Liu, X., Zhang, J., Rao, E., Schlothauer, T., Fischer, S., Cammack, N., Heilek, G., Ries, S., and Sankuratri, S. (2009) CD4-anchoring HIV-1 fusion inhibitor with enhanced potency and *in vivo* stability. *J. Biol. Chem.*, **284** (8), 5175–5185.

83 Baldwin, C. and Berkhout, B. (2007) HIV-1 drug-resistance and drug-dependence. *Retrovirology*, **4**, 78.

84 Bai, X., Wilson, K.L., Seedorff, J.E., Ahrens, D., Green, J., Davison, D.K., Jin, L., Stanfield-Oakley, S.A., Mosier, S.M., Melby, T.E., Cammack, N., Wang, Z., Greenberg, M.L., and Dwyer, J.J. (2008) Impact of the enfuvirtide resistance mutation N43D and the associated baseline polymorphism E137K on peptide sensitivity and six-helix bundle structure. *Biochemistry (Mosc.)*, **47** (25), 6662–6670.

85 Tolstrup, M., Selzer-Plon, J., Laursen, A. L., Bertelsen, L., Gerstoft, J., Duch, M., Pedersen, F.S., and Ostergaard, L. (2007) Full fusion competence rescue of the enfuvirtide resistant HIV-1 gp41 genotype (43D) by a prevalent polymorphism (137K). *AIDS*, **21** (4), 519–521.

86 Nagashima, K.A., Thompson, D.A., Rosenfield, S.I., Maddon, P.J., Dragic, T., and Olson, W.C. (2001) Human immunodeficiency virus type 1 entry inhibitors PRO 542 and T-20 are potently synergistic in blocking virus-cell and cell-cell fusion. *J. Infect. Dis.*, **183** (7), 1121–1125.

87 Tremblay, C.L., Giguel, F., Kollmann, C., Guan, Y., Chou, T.C., Baroudy, B.M., and Hirsch, M.S. (2002) Anti-human immunodeficiency virus interactions of SCH-C (SCH 351125), a CCR5 antagonist, with other antiretroviral agents *in vitro*. *Antimicrob. Agents Chemother.*, **46** (5), 1336–1339.

88 Tremblay, C.L., Kollmann, C., Giguel, F., Chou, T.C., and Hirsch, M.S. (2000) Strong *in vitro* synergy between the fusion inhibitor T-20 and the CXCR4 blocker AMD-3100. *J. Acquir. Immune Defic. Syndr.*, **25** (2), 99–102.

89 Hrin, R., Montgomery, D.L., Wang, F., Condra, J.H., An, Z., Strohl, W.R., Bianchi, E., Pessi, A., Joyce, J.G., and Wang, Y.J. (2008) Short communication: *in vitro* synergy between peptides or neutralizing antibodies targeting the N- and C-terminal heptad repeats of HIV type 1 gp41. *AIDS Res. Hum. Retroviruses*, **24** (12), 1537–1544.

90 Pan, C., Lu, H., Qi, Z., and Jiang, S. (2009) Synergistic efficacy of combination of enfuvirtide and sifuvirtide, the first- and next-generation HIV-fusion inhibitors. *AIDS*, **23** (5), 639–641.

91 Pan, C., Cai, L., Lu, H., Qi, Z., and Jiang, S. (2009) Combinations of the first and next generations of human immunodeficiency virus (HIV) fusion inhibitors exhibit a highly potent synergistic effect against enfuvirtide-sensitive and -resistant HIV type 1 strains. *J. Virol.*, **83** (16), 7862–7872.

11
Sifuvirtide, A Novel HIV-1 Fusion Inhibitor

Xiaobin Zhang, Hao Wu, and Fengshan Wang

11.1
Ideal Drug Target HIV-1 gp41

Advances in the understanding and treatment of the human immunodeficiency virus type 1 infection, HIV-1, have dramatically decreased the morbidity and mortality associated with HIV-1 [1]. More than 30 antiretroviral drugs have been approved for the treatment of HIV-1 infections, including reverse transcriptase inhibitors, protease inhibitors, an integrase inhibitor, a CCR5 inhibitor, and a fusion inhibitor [2]. Although several combination therapies are potent [3–5], the durability of the current therapies is often limited due to adverse effects [6] and drug resistance [7–9].

The HIV-1 life cycle includes the following steps: (i) its binding to CD4 and coreceptor, followed by fusion with the host cell and release of viral RNA into the cell; (ii) reverse transcription of single-stranded HIV-1 RNA to double-stranded HIV-1 DNA; (iii) integration of HIV-1 DNA into host DNA; (iv) transcription to mRNA as a blueprint to produce long chains of HIV-1 proteins; (v) assembly of new virus using protease-treated small proteins; (vi) release by budding from the host cell and infection of new cells. All existing anti-HIV-1 drugs aim to block one of the above steps to inhibit viral replication.

The mutation rates, which cause drug resistance, are very high for the active sites of HIV-1 reverse transcriptase, integrase, and protease, while low for the CCR5/CXCR4 and gp41 active sites. The side effects are very severe for drugs targeting CCR5/CXCR4 because the target is human protein, and serious for drugs targeting reverse transcriptase, integrase, and protease, because there are many human proteins similar to these targets. However, the side effects for drugs targeting gp41 are very mild, because gp41 is a unique viral protein; no human proteins are similar to it. The inhibition actions are, in the early stages, outside cells in the HIV-1 life cycle for CCR5/CXCR4 and gp41, while those inside cells are in the middle or late stages for reverse transcriptase, integrase, and protease (Table 11.1).

As a key protein in the first step of HIV-1 infection, gp41 is an ideal and effective drug target for anti-HIV-1 drug development. In comparison with other

Peptide Drug Discovery and Development: Translational Research in Academia and Industry, First Edition.
Edited by Miguel Castanho and Nuno C. Santos.
© 2011 WILEY-VCH Verlag GmbH & Co. KGaA, Weinheim.
Published 2011 by WILEY-VCH Verlag GmbH & Co. KGaA

Table 11.1 HIV/AIDS drug targets.

Drug target	CCR5/ CXCR4	Gp41	Reverse transcriptase	Integrase	Protease
Mutation rate	Low	Low	High	High	High
Side effect	Severe	Mild	Medium	Medium	Medium
Action stage	Early	Early	Middle	Middle	Late
Position	Extracellular	Extracellular	Intracellular	Intracellular	Intracellular

anti-HIV-1 therapies, HIV-1 fusion inhibitors have the potential advantages of lower side effects, less drug resistance, and inhibition of HIV infection at the early stage outside cells. HIV-1 fusion inhibitors are a relatively new class of drugs distinguished by targeting the fusion of the viral envelope and the cellular membrane. The entry of HIV-1 into host cells mainly involves three critical steps: First, HIV-1 gp120 recognizes and binds to CD4 molecules on the surface of the target cell, and then binds to chemokine receptors. Then, a cascade of conformational changes of gp41 is triggered. The hydrophobic N-terminal heptad repeat of gp41 is exposed, which allows embedding of the C-terminal heptad repeat. Sequentially, N-terminal heptad repeat and C-terminal heptad repeat fold into a stabilized six-helix trimer, which brings approximation of the virus and target cell and results in the completion of the fusion process [10–16]. The increased understanding of the HIV-1 entry allowed the design and discovery of HIV-1 fusion inhibitors, including peptide-based and small molecules [17–25]. T20 (enfuvirtide) is the first FDA-approved fusion inhibitor for the treatment of HIV-1 infections in treatment-experienced patients with evidence of HIV-1 replication despite ongoing anti-retroviral therapy [26, 27]. However, its use is restricted by high dosage and injection site reactions.

The successful clinical application of T20 clearly indicated that fusion inhibitors could be highly effective in the inhibition of HIV-1 replication. However, when T20 was screened and discovered, the three-dimensional structure of gp41 had not yet been solved, so that T20 covered only about two-thirds of the C-terminal heptad repeat sequence and missed the deep pocket of gp41. This may ultimately attenuate the efficiency of the drug as a fusion inhibitor. High dosage and frequent injection with 90 mg twice daily were required during T20 long term treatment, Injection site reactions were experienced in 98% of patients [26, 27]. The development of better fusion inhibitors with lower dosage and much less injection site reaction would be highly desirable.

11.2
Structure-Based Drug Design of Sifuvirtide

Sifuvirtide is a 36 amino acid peptide fusion inhibitor, and was designed based on the three-dimensional structure of the HIV-1 gp41 fusogenic core conformation.

Sifuvirtide covers the deep hydrophobic pocket which was missed by T20. Based on the three-dimensional structural information of HIV-1 gp41 and computer modeling analysis, amino acid substitutions were introduced to further improve the affinity of Sifuvirtide to the inner core of gp41, leading to improvement in stability, pharmacokinetics, and antiviral potency compared with T20. Several negatively charged glutamic acid and positively charged arginine residues were introduced for the formation of salt bridges at the i and $i+4$ positions of the helical conformation. Glu119 was substituted by threonine to cover the hydrophobic pocket. Furthermore, a serine was added to the N-terminus of the peptide, because its location at the N-terminal of an -helix is expected to increase its stability (Figure 11.1a and b).

As shown in Figure 11.1c, Sifuvirtide, shown in blue, mimics the HIV-1 gp41 C-terminal heptad repeat, shown in red, better than T20, shown in yellow and red,

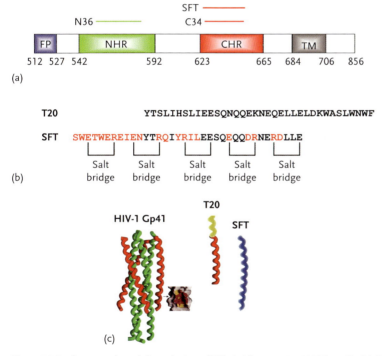

Figure 11.1 Structure-based drug design of Sifuvirtide targeting HIV-1 gp41. (a) Schematic view of HIV-1 gp41 functional regions. The residue numbers of each region correspond to their positions in gp160 of HIV-1$_{HXB2}$. FP, fusion peptide; NHR, N-terminal heptad repeat; CHR, C-terminal heptad repeat; TM, transmembrane domain; N36, part of N-terminal heptad repeat; C34, part of C-terminal heptad repeat; SFT, Sifuvirtide; T20, Enfuvirtide. (b) Sequence comparison of SFT and T20; the salt bridges in SFT are formed between negatively charged glutamic acid and positively charged arginine. (c) Comparison of sequence coverage between SFT and T20 over the C-terminal heptad repeat.

and thereby binds to thegp41 N-terminal heptad repeat, shown in green, more precisely and tightly. This is the structural basis for the prolonged half-life and improved efficacy of Sifuvirtide.

According to CD spectroscopic studies [28], Sifuvirtide can tightly bind to N36, a peptide containing 36 amino acids derived from the N-terminal heptad repeat, to form a very stable α-helix, while the binding between T20 and N36 is very weak. Even the binding between SFT and N36 is more stable than the native type N36 with C34, a peptide containing 34 amino acids derived from the C-terminal heptad repeat. It has been shown, in thermal denaturation experiments, that the melting temperature T_m of SFT/N36 complex is ~72 °C, whereas T_m of the C34/N36 complex is ~62 °C.

11.3
High Potency of Sifuvirtide

The inhibition activity of the structure-based designed peptide, Sifuvirtide, was confirmed by cell-based assay. According to cell–cell fusion assay, as shown in Figure 11.2, the 50% effective concentration for Sifuvirtide is 1.2 ± 0.2 nM, compared to 23 ± 6 nM for T20. Sifuvirtide has 20-fold better inhibitory activity than the first marketed fusion inhibitor, T20.

It has been demonstrated in cell-mediated viral infections that Sifuvirtide also has much higher potency than T20 in a wide range of primary and laboratory-adapted HIV-1 isolates from multiple genotypes with CCR5 or CXCR4 phenotypes, and in different cell types [28]. It has also been shown, by means of p24 antigen or syncytia detection assay, that Sifuvirtide has better potency than T20 against HIV-1 and HIV-2 [29].

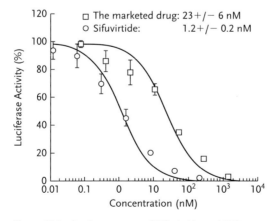

Figure 11.2 *In vitro* potency of Sifuvirtide and T20.

11.4
Limited Drug Resistance

According to studies on the mechanisms of action for Sifuvirtide and T20, Sifuvirtide binds to the inner core of gp41 only, while T20 not only binds to gp41, but also has another binding target with its C-terminus part [30]. The difference in the mechanisms of action and the binding capability to gp41 between Sifuvirtide and T20 could lead to different drug resistance profiles. It has been shown that Sifuvirtide is still sensitive against T20-resistant strains [31]. Sifuvirtide showed strong inhibitory activities against all T20-resistant strains with EC_{50} from 2.68 to ∼47.78 nM, whereas T20 showed much less potency with EC_{50} higher than 2000 nM (Table 11.2) [28].

When mutations that were selected at low frequency and/or reside outside the T20 target region, position 36–45 in the N-terminal heptad repeat of gp41, were introduced, such as mutants N43D, N43D/A50V, N43T/V38M, N43T/V38M/A50V, the inhibitory activity of T20 against these mutants was dramatically decreased. However, Sifuvirtide still shows very strong inhibition activity against these mutants (Table 11.3) [32].

It is well known that combinations of two or three drugs with different target sites or mechanisms of action may exhibit synergistic efficacy [33]. According to a series of studies on the combination of Sifuvirtide and T20 to identify their synergistic anti-HIV-1 effect [34], combination of Sifuvirtide and T20 resulted in strong synergism in blocking HIV-1-mediated membrane fusion with a combination index of 0.182 and potency increase of more than 600%. Moreover, the combination of Sifuvirtide and T20 also exhibited significant synergism in inhibiting infection by HIV-1 CCR5, CXCR4, and T20-resistant strains, compared with their potency when separately tested. These results implied a potential strategy with combination of two peptide fusion inhibitors for HIV/AIDS therapy, especially for patients who have failed to respond to T20.

Table 11.2 Inhibitory activities of Sifuvirtide against T20 resistant strains.

Mutations (NL4–3)	Phenotype[a]	EC_{50} (Mean ± SD, nM)	
		SFT	T20
Parental	S	12.56 ± 1.18	22.04 ± 1.19
N42S	S	2.68 ± 0.87	26.95 ± 12.98
V38A	R	3.44 ± 0.23	> 2000
V38A/N42D	R	47.78 ± 4.70	> 2000
V38A/N42T	R	30.42 ± 4.36	> 2000
V38E/N42S	R	43.47 ± 3.36	> 2000
N42T/N43K	R	37.79 ± 15.55	> 2000

[a]S, sensitive; R, resistant to T20.

Table 11.3 Inhibitory activities of Sifuvirtide against mutants in the N-terminal heptad repeat of gp41.

Mutations	Fold change of EC_{50}[a]	
	SFT	**T20**
N42S	0.28	0.38
N42G	0.63	0.07
A50V	0.83	1.21
D36G	0.40	8.11
D36G + A50V	0.32	10.88
V38M	0.63	10.74
V38M + A50V	0.50	7.40
N43T	0.32	1.60
N43T + A50V	0.37	3.10
N43D	0.76	31.43
N43D + A50V	0.36	41.56
V38M + N43T	0.35	34.81
V38M + N43T + A50V	0.40	84.59

[a]Fold change of EC_{50} value of the mutant virus compared to that of the wild-type virus.

11.5
Enhancement of the Efficiency of Sifuvirtide by Biomembrane Selectivity

To further investigate the correlation between efficacy and membrane domain selectivity, Franquelim *et al.* adopted fluorescence spectroscopy-based methodologies to reveal a unique selectivity of Sifuvirtide to gel-phase membranes. T20 presented a high affinity for POPC fluid membranes [35], and T-1249 (an improved but terminated drug candidate after T20), in addition to its affinity to POPC fluid membranes, adsorbed at the surface of cholesterol-rich domains [36]. Sifuvirtide is remarkably efficient in selecting and adsorbing only to the rigid lipid platforms, as seen in the quenching and Förster resonance energy transfer (FRET) experiments. On the other hand, it does not have a significant interaction with either POPC fluid membranes or cholesterol-rich membranes. This was compatible with its lower hydrophobicity compared to both T20 and T-1249 [37].

Subsequently, intensive biophysical studies were carried out to reveal the molecular basis of the selectivity of Sifuvirtide towards phosphatidylcholine (PC)-rich rigid membranes. As shown in Figure 11.3a, no significant changes in the fluorescence intensity or spectral shifts (data not shown) were observed for the fluid phase POPC and DLPC vesicles. Nonetheless, for the gel phase DPPC and DSPC bilayers, a significant increase in the fluorescence intensity, as well a significant blue-shift of the emission spectra (7 nm), was observed. This indicated that Sifuvirtide binds specifically to gel phase PC bilayers, such as DPPC or DSPC, but not to PC with saturated acyl chains presenting a fluid phase organization, such as DLPC. Furthermore, quenching experiments were performed to elucidate and quantify this interaction. Findings revealed that for all the studied lipid

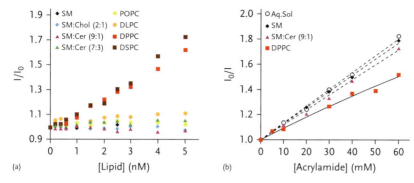

Figure 11.3 Sifuvirtide interaction with lipid membranes. (a) Titration of Sifuvirtide with LUV. (b) Fluorescence quenching of Sifuvirtide in the presence of lipid vesicles.

compositions, except DPPC, a linear quenching profile similar to the peptide in the absence of lipid was obtained (Figure 11.3b) [38].

In conclusion, Sifuvirtide's ability to screen the more-rigid domains of the membranes provided a locally increased concentration of the drug at the fusion site. Consequently, this finding may help to explain the improved clinical efficacy of this peptide compared to that of other drugs from the same class.

11.6
Pharmacokinetics of Sifuvirtide with Long Half-Life

A phase Ia clinical trial was performed in healthy volunteers to evaluate the safety and pharmacokinetic profiles of Sifuvirtide with single dose and multiple doses [28]. The safety and pharmacokinetic studies of multiple doses of Sifuvirtide were conducted in 12 volunteers with repeated subcutaneous injections of 30 mg of Sifuvirtide once daily for 7 days. The mean half-life was 26.0 ± 7.9 h, which was consistent with that of single dose administration. In conclusion, this dose level in consecutive administration was safe and also had a satisfactory pharmacokinetics profile (Table 11.4).

To further investigate the pharmacokinetic profiles in HIV-infected patients, a phase IIa trial was carried out. Twenty-four treatment-naïve subjects with HIV-1

Table 11.4 Pharmacokinetic parameters of Sifuvirtide in healthy and HIV-infected subjects.

Parameter	Healthy subjects (Ia-30 mg)	HIV-infected subjects (IIa-20 mg)
$AUC_{(0-t)}$ (ng h/mL)	5169 ± 1251	$20{,}313 \pm 5152$
$AUC_{(0-\infty)}$ (ng h/mL)	6120 ± 1752	$23{,}009 \pm 5297$
$T_{1/2}$ (h)	26.0 ± 7.9	39.0 ± 3.5
C_{max} (ng/mL)	394 ± 102	897 ± 136
T_{max} (h)	2.5 ± 1.0	2.9 ± 0.3
C_{min} (ng/mL)	40 ± 11	307 ± 90

infection were enrolled into the study and received 10 or 20 mg of subcutaneous Sifuvirtide once daily for 28 consecutive days. Blood samples were taken from the subjects in both dose groups. The plasma concentration of Sifuvirtide was determined utilizing liquid chromatography-tandem mass spectrometry (LC-MS/MS) [39]. It was shown that Sifuvirtide has a predictable pharmacokinetic response in HIV-infected subjects. After the Day 28 injection, Sifuvirtide in plasma was detectable for 120 h at a 20 mg dose level. The plasma drug concentration reached steady-state in the subjects after five consecutive doses of Sifuvirtide. There was no significant difference in either the pharmacokinetic parameters or plasma concentration of Sifuvirtide on Day 1 and Day 28, suggesting that there was no accumulative effect for Sifuvirtide when continuously administered. At a 20 mg dose level, the steady-state trough concentration C_{ss} of 307 ± 90 ng/mL and the average concentration C_{av} of 445 ± 111 ng/mL were all remarkably higher than the *in vitro* cell fusion inhibitory concentration EC_{90} of less than 4 ng/mL. The terminal elimination half-life for Sifuvirtide at 20 mg dose level was 39.0 ± 3.5 h, compared to the 3.8 h for T20 (Table 11.4).

11.7
Stratification of Monotherapy

For untreated HIV/AIDS patients, the infection usually advances from the HIV latent stage to the AIDS symptomatic stage (Figure 11.4) [40]. At the latent stage, the plasma HIV-1 viral load increases slowly and linearly with time till the transition point at about eight years after primary infection. After this point, the viral load quickly increases non-linearly with time, which is called the symptomatic stage. The viral load value at the transition point is around 10^4 copies/ml. The dynamic mechanisms of HIV-1 infection and immune response at the latent stage and symptomatic stage should be different.

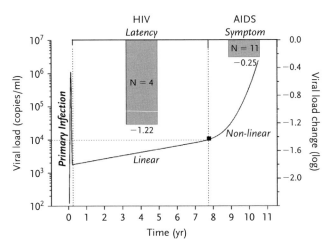

Figure 11.4 Treatment stratification for infection stage transition from HIV to AIDS with monotherapy.

The combined data analysis of Phase Ib and IIa studies of the fusion inhibitor Sifuvirtide has shown that higher efficacy was achieved at 20 mg dose level in patients at the HIV latent stage than those at the AIDS symptomatic stage. The median change in plasma viral load from baseline for each dose level was determined in Phase Ib and Phase IIa. If the HIV-1 infection stages were not separated, there was no clear dose-dependent relationship observed. If the HIV-1 infection stages were analyzed separately, the treatment stratification of fusion inhibitor Sifuvirtide has shown up at the 20 mg dose level for the infection stage transition from HIV to AIDS. At 20 mg dose level, the median viral load reduction for patients was 1.22 log with baseline lower than the transition point, compared with 0.25 log with baseline higher than the transition point (Figure 11.4).

11.8
20 mg Sifuvirtide Once Daily vs. 100 mg T20 Twice Daily

As described above, 20 mg of Sifuvirtide could achieve a viral load reduction of 1.22 log for the patients with baseline viral load of less than 10^4 copies/mL, compared with 0.25 log of reduction for those with higher viral load. Data from the marketed fusion inhibitor T20 twice daily at 100 mg dose level showed very similar monotherapeutic effectiveness compared to Sifuvirtide once daily at 20 mg dose level [24]. The median baseline for the T20 at 100 mg dose group twice daily was 3.83 log, which was comparable with 3.86 log for the Sifuvirtide at 20 mg dose group once daily. The viral load reduction was also very similar for both T20 and Sifuvirtide with 1.14 log and 1.22 log, respectively (Table 11.5). For patients with baseline higher than the transition point, monotherapy of Sifuvirtide showed limited efficacy. However, there was no data available for T20 monotherapy for naïve patients with baseline higher than the transition point. Such comparable treatment effect has indicated that the efficacy of 20 mg Sifuvirtide once daily is equivalent to that of 100 mg T20 twice daily with monotherapy (Figure 11.5).

Table 11.5 Comparison of monotherapy between SFT and T20.

	Items	SFT	T20
Similarities	N	4	4
	Median baseline($\log_{10}$ copies/mL)	3.86	3.83
	Viral load change($\log_{10}$ copies/mL)	−1.22	−1.14
	C_{min} (ng/mL)	307	89×20
Differences	Daily dose (mg)	20	100×2
	Half-life (h)	39.0 ± 3.5	3.8 ± 0.6
	EC_{50} (nM)	1.2 ± 0.2	23.0 ± 6.0
	Target	gp41	Partly gp41
	Sequence	Designed	Wild-type

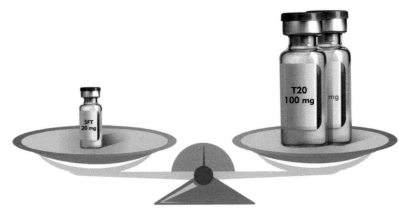

Figure 11.5 Graphic comparison of monotherapy between Sifuvirtide and T20. To achieve similar efficacy in monotherapy, 20 mg Sifuvirtide once daily was equivalent to 100 mg T20 twice daily.

11.9
Conclusions and Discussion

HIV-1 gp41 is an ideal target for drug development because gp41 has a very conserved active site that leads to limited drug resistance, and it is a unique viral protein; no similar human protein was found thus leading to milder side effects. In contrast, HIV-1 reverse transcriptase, integrase, and protease, as drug targets, have the tendency to develop drug resistance due to high mutation rates and have serious side effects due to similarities with human proteins. Although drug resistance is not an issue for the human protein CCR5 or CXCR4 as a drug target, severe side effects of any targeted drugs would limit their applications.

Sifuvirtide, a 36 amino acid peptide fusion inhibitor, was designed based on the 3D structure of gp41. It has a higher binding capability to gp41 than T20, the first fusion inhibitor, by covering a different fragment of the C-terminal heptad repeat and introducing substitution of several amino acids to form salt bridges. The inhibitory activity of Sifuvirtide is 20-fold better than that of T20, based on the cell–cell fusion assay. The inhibition superiority of Sifuvirtide was confirmed in other assays, with different cells, and in different viral strains. T20-resistant strains are still sensitive to Sifuvirtide. The selectivity of biomembrane by Sifuvirtide could enhance the efficiency by increasing the local peptide concentration, while a similar phenomenon was not observed for T20. The terminal half-life of Sifuvirtide as monotherapy for HIV-1 patients is 39 h compared with 3.8 h for T20.

At the 20 mg dose level, a median viral load reduction of 1.22 log was observed with a baseline lower than the transition point at the viral load of 10^4 copies/ml, which was significantly better than 0.25 log reduction with a baseline higher than the transition point. It is thus assumed that when used as a monotherapy, fusion inhibitors, including Sifuvirtide and T20, might be more effective during the clinical latent stage than the symptomatic stage. The effective dose at an early treatment should be much lower than that at a late stage. This lower drug dosage may lead to fewer side effects and less financial burden. For patients with a baseline higher than the transition point, combination therapy may be needed for fusion inhibitors. Indeed, T20 has shown strong effectiveness when used with other HIV-1 drugs in patients with high baselines [26, 27].

To achieve similar efficacy as monotherapy, 20 mg Sifuvirtide once daily is equivalent to 100 mg T20 twice daily. The significant reduction in dosage for Sifuvirtide over T20 would overcome the limitation of T20 as a HIV/AIDS treatment. The clinical treatment of HIV/AIDS patients with T20 combined with other antiretroviral drugs is very efficient; however, the application of T20 is limited by its high dosage, presenting 98% patients with injection site reactions. Sifuvirtide at 20 mg once daily has the potential to substantially reduce injection site reactions.

References

1 Palella, F.J. Jr, Delaney, K.M., Moorman, A.C., Loveless, M.O., Fuhrer, J., Satten, G.A., Aschman, D.J., and Holmberg, S. D. (1998) Declining morbidity and mortality among patients with advanced human immunodeficiency virus infection. HIV outpatient study investigators. *N. Engl. J. Med.*, **338** (13), 853–860.

2 Flexner, C. (2007) HIV drug development: the next 25 years. *Nat. Rev. Drug Discov.*, **6** (12), 959–966.

3 Eron, J.J., Benoit, S.L., Jemsek, J., MacArthur, R.D., Santana, J., Quinn, J. B., Kuritzkes, D.R., Fallon, M.A., and Rubin, M. (1995) Treatment with lamivudine, zidovudine, or both in HIV-positive patients with 200 to 500 CD4+ cells per cubic millimeter. North American HIV Working Party. *N. Engl. J. Med.*, **333** (25), 1662–1669.

4 Markowitz, M., Saag, M., Powderly, W. G., Hurley, A.M., Hsu, A., Valdes, J.M., Henry, D., Sattler, F., Marca, A.L., Leonard, J.M., and Ho, D.D. (1995) A preliminary study of ritonavir, an inhibitor of HIV-1 protease, to treat HIV-1 infection. *N. Engl. J. Med.*, **333** (23), 1534–1540.

5 Hammer, S.M., Squires, K.E., Hughes, M.D., Grimes, J.M., Demeter, L.M., Currier, J.S., Eron, J.J., Jr, Feinberg, J.E., Balfour, H.H., Jr, Deyton, L.R., Chodakewitz, J.A., and Fischl, M.A.

(1997) A controlled trial of two nucleoside analogues plus indinavir in persons with human immunodeficiency virus infection and CD4 cell counts of 200 per cubic millimeter or less. AIDS clinical trials group 320 study team. *N. Engl. J. Med.*, **337** (11), 725–733.

6 O'Brien, M.E., Clark, R.A., Besch, C.L., Myers, L., and Kissinger, P. (2003) Patterns and correlates of discontinuation of the initial HAART regimen in an urban outpatient cohort. *J. Acquir. Immune Defic. Syndr.*, **34** (4), 407–414.

7 Condra, J.H., Schleif, W.A., Blahy, O.M., Gabryelski, L.J., Graham, D.J., Quintero, J.C., Rhodes, A., Robbins, H.L., Roth, E. Shivaprakash, M. *et al.* (1995) *In vivo* emergence of HIV-1 variants resistant to multiple protease inhibitors. *Nature*, **374** (6522), 569–571.

8 Zhang, F.J., Maria, A., Haberer, J., and Zhao, Y. (2006) Overview of HIV drug resistance and its implications for China. *Chin. Med. J. (Engl.)*, **119** (23), 1999–2004.

9 Clavel, F. and Hance, A.J. (2004) HIV drug resistance. *N. Engl. J. Med.*, **350** (10), 1023–1035.

10 Weissenhorn, W., Dessen, A., Harrison, S.C., Skehel, J.J., and Wiley, D.C. (1997) Atomic structure of the ectodomain from HIV-1 gp41. *Nature*, **387** (6631), 426–430.

11 Chan, D.C., Fass, D., Berger, J.M., and Kim, P.S. (1997) Core structure of gp41 from the HIV envelope glycoprotein. *Cell*, **89** (2), 263–273.

12 Chan, D.C. and Kim, P.S. (1998) HIV entry and its inhibition. *Cell*, **93** (5), 681–684.

13 Moore, J.P. and Stevenson, M. (2000) New targets for inhibitors of HIV-1 replication. *Nat. Rev. Mol. Cell Biol.*, **1** (1), 40–49.

14 Eckert, D.M. and Kim, P.S. (2001) Mechanisms of viral membrane fusion and its inhibition. *Annu. Rev. Biochem.*, **70**, 777–810.

15 LaBranche, C.C., Galasso, G., Moore, J.P., Bolognesi, D.P., Hirsch, M.S., and Hammer, S.M. (2001) HIV fusion and its inhibition. *Antiviral Res.*, **50** (2), 95–115.

16 Weiss, C.D. (2003) HIV-1 gp41: mediator of fusion and target for inhibition. *AIDS Rev.*, **5** (4), 214–221.

17 Ferrer, M., Kapoor, T.M., Strassmaier, T., Weissenhorn, W., Skehel, J.J., Oprian, D., Schreiber, S.L., Wiley, D.C., and Harrison, S.C. (1999) Selection of gp41-mediated HIV-1 cell entry inhibitors from biased combinatorial libraries of non-natural binding elements. *Nat. Struct. Biol.*, **6** (10), 953–960.

18 Zhou, G., Ferrer, M., Chopra, R., Kapoor, T.M., Strassmaier, T., Weissenhorn, W., Skehel, J.J., Oprian, D., Schreiber, S.L., Harrison, S.C., and Wiley, D.C. (2000) The structure of an HIV-1 specific cell entry inhibitor in complex with the HIV-1 gp41 trimeric core. *Bioorg. Med. Chem.*, **8** (9), 2219–2227.

19 Root, M.J., Kay, M.S., and Kim, P.S. (2001) Protein design of an HIV-1 entry inhibitor. *Science*, **291** (5505), 884–888.

20 Jiang, S., Zhao, Q., and Debnath, A.K. (2002) Peptide and non-peptide HIV fusion inhibitors. *Curr. Pharm. Des.*, **8** (8), 563–580.

21 Liu, S., Wu, S., and Jiang, S. (2007) HIV entry inhibitors targeting gp41: from polypeptides to small-molecule compounds. *Curr. Pharm. Des.*, **13** (2), 143–162.

22 Rusconi, S., Scozzafava, A., Mastrolorenzo, A., and Supuran, C.T.

(2007) An update in the development of HIV entry inhibitors. *Curr. Top. Med. Chem.*, **7** (13), 1273–1289.

23 Schneider, S.E., Bray, B.L., Mader, C.J., Friedrich, P.E., Anderson, M.W., Taylor, T.S., Boshernitzan, N., Niemi, T.E., Fulcher, B.C., Whight, S.R., White, J.M., Greene, R.J., Stoltenberg, L.E., and Lichty, M. (2005) Development of HIV fusion inhibitors. *J. Pept. Sci.*, **11** (11), 744–753.

24 Kilby, J.M., Hopkins, S., Venetta, T.M., DiMassimo, B., Cloud, G.A., Lee, J.Y., Alldredge, L., Hunter, E., Lambert, D., Bolognesi, D., Matthews, T., Johnson, M.R., Nowak, M.A., Shaw, G.M., and Saag, M.S. (1998) Potent suppression of HIV-1 replication in humans by T-20, a peptide inhibitor of gp41-mediated virus entry. *Nat. Med.*, **4** (11), 1302–1307.

25 He, Y., Xiao, Y., Song, H., Liang, Q., Ju, D., Chen, X., Lu, H., Jing, W., Jiang, S., and Zhang, L. (2008) Design and evaluation of sifuvirtide, a novel HIV-1 fusion inhibitor. *J. Biol. Chem.*, **283** (17), 11126–11134.

26 Lalezari, J.P., Henry, K., O'Hearn, M., Montaner, J.S., Piliero, P.J., Trottier, B., Walmsley, S., Cohen, C., Kuritzkes, D.R., Eron, J.J. Jr, Chung, J., DeMasi, R., Donatacci, L., Drobnes, C., Delehanty, J., and Salgo, M. (2003) Enfuvirtide, an HIV-1 fusion inhibitor, for drug-resistant HIV infection in North and South America. *N. Engl. J. Med.*, **348** (22), 2175–2185.

27 Lazzarin, A., Clotet, B., Cooper, D., Reynes, J., Arasteh, K., Nelson, M., Katlama, C., Stellbrink, H.J., Delfraissy, J.F., Lange, J., Huson, L., DeMasi, R., Wat, C., Delehanty, J., Drobnes, C., and Salgo, M. (2003) Efficacy of enfuvirtide in patients infected with drug-resistant HIV-1 in Europe and Australia. *N. Engl. J. Med.*, **348** (22), 2186–2195.

28 He, Y., Xiao, Y., Song, H., Liang, Q., Ju, D., Chen, X., Lu, H., Jing, W., Jiang, S., and Zhang, L. (2008) Design and evaluation of sifuvirtide, a novel HIV-1 fusion inhibitor. *J. Biol. Chem.*, **283** (17), 11126–11134.

29 Wang, R.R., Yang, L.M., Wang, Y.H., Pang, W., Tam, S.C., Tien, P., and

Zheng, Y.T. (2009) Sifuvirtide, a potent HIV fusion inhibitor peptide. *Biochem. Biophys. Res. Commun.*, **382** (3), 540–544.

30 Liu, S., Lu, H., Niu, J., Xu, Y., Wu, S., and Jiang, S. (2005) Different from the HIV fusion inhibitor C34, the anti-HIV drug Fuzeon (T-20) inhibits HIV-1 entry by targeting multiple sites in gp41 and gp120. *J. Biol. Chem.*, **280** (12), 11259–11273.

31 Rimsky, L.T., Shugars, D.C., and Matthews, T.J. (1998) Determinants of human immunodeficiency virus type 1 resistance to gp41-derived inhibitory peptides. *J. Virol.*, **72** (2), 986–993.

32 Covens, K., Megens, S., Dekeersmaeker, N., Kabeya, K., Balzarini, J., De Wit, S., Vandamme, A.M., and Van Laethem, K. (2010) The rare HIV-1 gp41 mutations 43T and 50V elevate enfuvirtide resistance levels of common enfuvirtide resistance mutations that did not impact susceptibility to sifuvirtide. *Antiviral Res.*, **86** (3), 253–260.

33 Chou, T.C. (2006) Theoretical basis, experimental design, and computerized simulation of synergism and antagonism in drug combination studies. *Pharmacol. Rev.*, **58** (3), 621–681.

34 Pan, C., Lu, H., Qi, Z., and Jiang, S. (2009) Synergistic efficacy of combination of enfuvirtide and sifuvirtide, the first- and next-generation HIV-fusion inhibitors. *AIDS*, **23** (5), 639–641.

35 Veiga, S., Henriques, S., Santos, N.C., and Castanho, M. (2004) Putative role of membranes in the HIV fusion inhibitor enfuvirtide mode of action at the molecular level. *Biochem. J.*, **377** (Pt 1), 107–110.

36 Veiga, A.S., Santos, N.C., Loura, L.M., Fedorov, A., and Castanho, M.A. (2004) HIV fusion inhibitor peptide T-1249 is able to insert or adsorb to lipidic bilayers. Putative correlation with improved efficiency. *J. Am. Chem. Soc.*, **126** (45), 14758–14763.

37 Franquelim, H.G., Loura, L.M., Santos, N.C., and Castanho, M.A. (2008) Sifuvirtide screens rigid membrane surfaces. Establishment of a correlation between efficacy and membrane domain selectivity among HIV fusion inhibitor peptides. *J. Am. Chem. Soc.*, **130** (19), 6215–6223.

38 Franquelim, H.G., Veiga, A.S., Weissmuller, G., Santos, N.C., and Castanho, M.A. (2010) Unravelling the molecular basis of the selectivity of the HIV-1 fusion inhibitor sifuvirtide towards phosphatidylcholine-rich rigid membranes. *Biochim. Biophys. Acta*, **1798** (6), 1234–1243.

39 Che, J., Meng, Q., Chen, Z., Hou, Y., Shan, C., and Cheng, Y. (2010) Quantitative analysis of a novel HIV fusion inhibitor (sifuvirtide) in HIV infected human plasma using high-performance liquid chromatography-electrospray ionization tandem mass spectrometry. *J. Pharm. Biomed. Anal.*, **51** (4), 927–933.

40 Fauci, A.S., Pantaleo, G., Stanley, S., and Weissman, D. (1996) Immunopathogenic mechanisms of HIV Infection. *Ann. Intern. Med.*, **124** (7), 654–663.

Part III
Whither Peptide Drugs? Peptides Shaping the Future of Drug Development

Peptide Drug Discovery and Development: Translational Research in Academia and Industry, First Edition.
Edited by Miguel Castanho and Nuno C. Santos.
© 2011 WILEY-VCH Verlag GmbH & Co. KGaA, Weinheim.
Published 2011 by WILEY-VCH Verlag GmbH & Co. KGaA

12

Endogenous Peptides and Their Receptors as Drug Discovery Targets for the Treatment of Metabolic Disease

Mary Ann Pelleymounter, Yuren Wang, and Ning Lee

The maintenance of body mass is a function of energy intake and energy expenditure, as dictated by the first law of thermodynamics. Obesity occurs when energy intake exceeds energy expenditure, resulting in increased energy stored in the form of adipose tissue [1]. Obesity is commonly defined by a body mass index (BMI) $>30 \, \mathrm{kg \, m}^{-2}$ [2]. Obesity has been shown to increase the risk of type II diabetes 3.5–23.4-fold, depending upon BMI [3] and to increase the risk of heart disease by 1.4–2.2-fold, again depending upon BMI [3, 4]. In the United States, it is estimated that 30% of adults and 17.6% of youths 12–19 years of age are clinically obese [5, 6].

Since it is difficult to perturb energy expenditure physiologically (exercise accounts for only ∼15% of total energy expenditure) [7], changes in food intake are more likely to produce significant alterations in energy balance. Food intake is tightly controlled by a complex network of peripheral and central nervous system signals which are integrated and processed into responses by the brain. Organs involved in digestion and metabolism release neuroactive peptides and hormones in response to changes in nutrient status [8]. These substances act as nutrient sensors in the brain, which integrates these signals with other information about the current environment and implements a response which restores energy balance. Nutrient sensors released from peripheral organs are received by areas in the brain with a semi-permeable blood–brain barrier, such as the area postrema (AP) in the brainstem and areas of the hypothalamus such as the median eminance [9]. Signals received in the hypothalamus and the brainstem are then transmitted through a complex neural network composed of neuropeptide, biogenic amine and amino acid neural pathways to brain areas associated with reward, memory and sensory pathways. The integrated information is then processed into either voluntary motor or autonomic nervous system responses (Figure 12.1) [9–11]. Neuropeptides play important roles in all aspects of this signaling process. There are more than 50 neuroactive peptides known to be released by neurons in the mammalian brain, many having quite distinct functions depending upon where they are expressed [12]. Neuropeptides are often co-localized with conventional neurotransmitters such as the biogenic amines or acetylcholine and released from

Peptide Drug Discovery and Development: Translational Research in Academia and Industry, First Edition.
Edited by Miguel Castanho and Nuno C. Santos.
© 2011 WILEY-VCH Verlag GmbH & Co. KGaA, Weinheim.
Published 2011 by WILEY-VCH Verlag GmbH & Co. KGaA

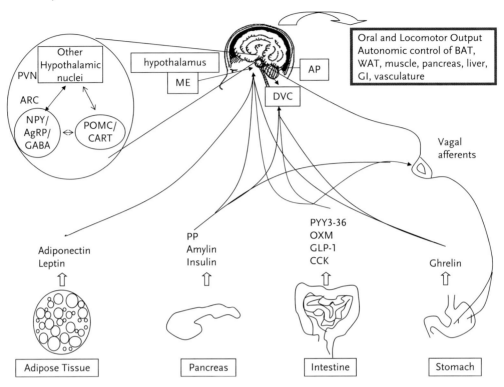

Figure 12.1 Hypothesized nutrient sensing pathways. Nutrient sensors released from peripheral organs are received by areas in the brain with a semi-permeable blood–brain barrier, such as the area postrema in the brainstem and areas of the hypothalamus such as the median eminance. The integrated information is then processed into either voluntary motor or autonomic nervous system responses. PVN = paraventricular nucleus, ARC = arcuate nucleus, NPY = neuropeptide Y, AgRP = agouti-related protein, GABA = gamma amino butyric acid, POMC = pro-opiomelanocortin, CART = cocaine amphetamine related transcript, DVC = dorsal vagal complex, AP = area postrema, ME = median eminance, PP = pancreatic polypeptide, OXM = oxyntomodulin, GLP-1 = glucagon-like peptide 1, CCK = choleycystokinin, BAT = brown adipose tissue, WAT = white adipose tissue, GI-gastrointestinal.

large dense-core vesicles. Release of these peptides can affect not only membrane polarization, but also gene expression, synaptogenesis, and local blood flow [12]. This chapter will focus on the major classes of peripherally and centrally secreted neuropeptides which are thought to play primary roles in energy homeostasis.

12.1
Centrally Secreted Neuropeptide Systems

12.1.1
Corticotropin Releasing Factor (CRF) Peptides

CRF is a 41 amino acid peptide which is best known for its primary role in basal and stress-induced activation of the pituitary-adrenal axis [13]. It is produced in neurons of the hypothalamic PVN and is released at nerve endings in the median eminance, resulting in the stimulation of corticotrophs in the anterior pituitary and the secretion of ACTH [14]. CRF is also expressed in many other brain areas, as well as in peripheral tissues. In addition to its role in the stress response, CRF is a potent anorexic agent. Central administration of CRF activates the sympathetic nervous system (SNS) and inhibits the parasympathetic nervous system (PNS), which may explain its general arousal properties and its ability to stimulate cardiorespiratory responses and brown fat thermogenesis while inhibiting digestive and reproductive activity [14]. The urocortins (urocortin I, urocortin II, and urocortin III) (UCN I, UCN II, UCN III) are homologous to CRF and have similar anorectic properties, suggesting that the CRF family may play a physiological role in energy homeostasis. UCN I is a 40 amino acid peptide, has a 45% sequence homology to CRF and is expressed in brain and peripheral tissues [15]. UCN II and UCN III are both 38 amino acid peptides with 58% and 32% homology to human CRF, respectively. UCN II is expressed in the PVN, ARC, and locus coruleus, while UCN III is expressed in the median preoptic nucleus, the lateral septum, the amygdala, the bed nucleus of the stria terminalis (BNST), and other areas. Both of these peptides are also expressed in the small intestine, colon, skin, and adrenal glands [16, 17]. While none of the urocortin peptides appear to have the same role as CRF in stress-induced activation of the HPA axis, all of them have been shown to modulate digestive processes, blood pressure, anxiety, and food intake. All of these peptides bind to two CRF receptors, which are Class B GPCRs, signaling through the Gs subunit and activating adenyl cyclase. CRF and UCN I are most potent at the CRF1 receptor, which is widely expressed throughout the brain and periphery. UCN II and UCN III are much more selective for the CRF 2 receptor, which has a more restricted expression pattern than CRF1, localized primarily in certain brain areas (NTS, PVN, lateral septum, BNST, hippocampus, and olfactory bulb) and in the intestine, skeletal muscle, heart, and myocardial vasculature [16, 17]. Work with selective CRF receptor antagonists has suggested that the CRF2 receptor may be more primarily involved in the anorectic effects of CRF than the CRF1 receptor, whereas the role of this receptor in the SNS activating and thermogenic properties of CRF is not as clear [14]. The potential of the CRF system as a target for metabolic disease therapeutics has been explored by some researchers, but has been hampered by the lack of orally available CRF2 modulators and by the potential for cardiovascular side effects of the peptides themselves. To date, there are no CRF agonists or antagonists in clinical development for the treatment of metabolic disorders.

12.1.2
Melanin Concentrating Hormone (MCH)

Mammalian MCH is a cyclic 19 amino acid peptide which is synthesized in the magnocellular neurons of the lateral hypothalamus and in the zona incerta. Cell bodies expressing this peptide project to many brain areas, including the cortex, amygdala, nucleus accumbens, olfactory tubercle, and brainstem nuclei [18, 19]. The effects of MCH are mediated by two G protein-coupled receptors (GPCR), MCHR1, and MCHR2. MCHR1 is a 353 amino acid Class A GPCR with highest

homology to the somatostatin receptor family. MCHR1 couples to several G proteins, including G_i, G_o, and G_q, with the apparent strongest affinity to G_i, based
upon a comparison of EC_{50} values for cAMP and Ca^{+2} responses [18]. MCHR1 is
most densely expressed in brain, with some expression in muscle, eye, tongue, and
adipose tissue. In brain, it is widely distributed, with particularly high levels of
expression in areas involved in the processing of olfactory information and in the
nucleus accumbens. MCHR2 is a 340 amino acid GPCR with low homology to
MCHR1 (38%) and has a very similar expression pattern to that of MCHR1.
MCHR2 is not functionally expressed in rodents, guinea pigs, or rabbits, but is
expressed in ferrets, dogs, non-human primates and humans. MCHR2 appears to
signal exclusively through G_q [18, 19]. MCH expression is increased in the leptin-
deficient ob/ob mouse and increases food intake when administered centrally.
Deletion of MCH during development results in a lean phenotype with slight
increases in energy expenditure and reduced food intake, whereas overexpression
on a high fat diet results in an obese, insulin-resistant phenotype. Deletion of the
MCHR1 receptor results in resistance to diet-induced obesity, increased locomotor
activity, and increased food intake during the light cycle [18]. The impact of these
genetic manipulations on body mass are generally recapitulated with chronic
administration of MCH or MCHR1 antagonists [19]. Whether or not MCHR1
antagonism will be an effective therapeutic for obesity is unknown at this time, but
should become apparent within the next 5 years. At least two companies have
candidates in early development at this time [5] (Table 12.1).

12.1.3
Melanocortins

The melanocortins comprise a very complex system of pituitary hormones,
regulatory proteins, and pro-peptides. All of the melanocortin hormones [α-mel-
anocyte stimulating hormone (α-MSH), β- melanocyte stimulating hormone
(β-MSH), γ-melanocyte stimulating hormone (γ-MSH) and adrenocorticotropic
hormone (ACTH)] are derived from pro-opiomelanocortin (POMC), which is a
31–36 kDa protein expressed in the pituitary and the brain [20]. POMC is associated
with energy balance for several reasons: (i) it is expressed in brain areas which are
thought to regulate energy homeostasis and food intake, such as the arcuate
nucleus of the hypothalamus and the nucleus tractus solitaris of the brainstem;
(ii) genetic deletion of POMC in mice results in an obese, hyperphagic animal with
increased linear growth, metabolic defects and altered fur pigmentation; and (iii)
genetic defects in humans result in similar characteristics, such as obesity, ACTH
insufficiency, and red hair [21]. The melanocortin peptides produce their activity
through melanocortin receptors, which are all Class A GPCRs. All of them couple
primarily to the Gs protein subunit and stimulate cAMP production. Only two of
them are associated with energy balance; the MC3 and MC4 receptors. The MC3
receptor is primarily localized in the brain, particularly in areas of the hypothalamus such as the arcuate nucleus (ARC) and ventromedial hypothalamus (VMH), as
well as in other areas, such as the central grey, lateral septum, and olfactory

Table 12.1 Endogenous peptides/receptors in clinical trials for obesity/metabolic disease indication.

Candidate(s)	Modality	Pharmacology	Developers	Status
Naltrexone + Bupropin (Contrave)	Small Molecule	Opioid receptor antagonist/NE reuptake inhibitor	Orexigen	Pre-Registration
Liraglutide (Victoza)	Peptide	GLP-1 agonist	Novo Nordisk	Launched for Type 2 diabetes; Phase III on-going for obesity
Pramlintide + metreleptin	Peptide	Amylin receptor agonist/Leptin agonist	Amylin/Takeda	Phase II completed
Davalintide	Peptide	Amylin receptor agonist	Amylin	Phase II/Discontinued
MK-0493	Small Molecule	MC4R agonist	Merck	Discontinued
TM-30339	Peptide	Y4 receptor agonist	7TM Pharma A/S	Phase I/II
Obinepitide	Peptide	Y2/Y4 dual-acting agonist	7TM Pharma A/S	Phase I/II
TTP-435	Small Molecule	AgRP inhibitor	TransTech Pharma	Phase II
GSKI-181771X	Small Molecule	CCK-1 agonist	GlaxoSmithKline	Phase II
BMS-830216	Small Molecule	MCHR1 antagonist	Bristol-Myers Squibb	Phase I/II
ALB-127158	Small Molecule	MCHR-1 antagonist	Albany Molecular Research Inc.	Phase I
GSK-1521498	Small Molecule	μ-opioid receptor inverse agonist	GSK	Phase I
Peptide YY 3-36/GLP-1	Peptide	Y2 receptor agonist/GLP-1 agonist	Emisphere	Phase I
S-234462	Small Molecule	Y5 antagonist	Shionogi	Phase I

tubercle. γ-MSH has a higher affinity for MC3R than for other MC receptors. Genetic deletion of MC3R in mice results in a phenotype characterized by mild obesity, an atypical metabolic adaptation to a high fat diet and increased feed efficiency [20, 22]. The MC4 receptor has a much more diffuse distribution in both the brain and periphery than the MC3 receptor. Its distribution in brain is similar to that of dopamine receptors and is found in adipose tissue, the gut, and in the genital organs. α-MSH has a higher affinity for the MC4 receptor than other endogenous melanocortins. Genetic deletion of this receptor in mice results in severe, adult onset obesity accompanied by hyperphagia, hyperinsulimemia, hyperglycemia, and increased body length. These characteristics are also found in humans with genetic defects in the MC4R gene; indeed, alterations in the MC4R gene are the basis of one of the most common forms of monogenetic obesity in humans, accounting for up to 5% of the incidence in adults and children [21, 22]. Finally, there are two natural antagonists of the melanocortin system: agouti-signaling protein (ASIP) and agouti-related protein (AGRP). ASIP is expressed in hair follicles and acts as a functional antagonist of the MC1 receptor, inhibiting melanin synthesis and lightening skin and fur [20]. AGRP is the centrally located counterpart to ASIP, acting as a functional antagonist of the MC3 and MC4 receptors. It is expressed in the ARC and PVN, as well as in the adrenal gland. In addition, AGRP is co-localized in the ARC with NPY on GABAergic neurons, making synaptic connections with neurons containing POMC and cocaine-amphetamine-related transcript (CART). Both AGRP and NPY are powerful appetite stimulants, whereas POMC and CART are equally powerful appetite suppressants, providing a "microcircuit" in the arcuate nucleus which has the capacity to regulate food intake [21, 23]. Transgenic overexpression of AGRP in mice results in severe obesity, hyperphagia, and hyperinsulinemia, as does chronic administration of synthetic AGRP. Taken together, the melanocortin system appears to play a pivotal role in the development of obesity, accounting for three of the six known monogenetic forms of obesity in humans (proconvertase 1, which catalyzes the initial cleavage of POMC, POMC, and MC4R) [20]. For this reason, MC4R has been the target of intense drug discovery research for >20 years. Merck Pharmaceuticals tested the hypothesis that agonism of the MC4 receptor would reduce appetite and body weight with MK-0493. Unfortunately, the compound did not produce sufficient efficacy in multiple phase II trials to support further development [24] (Table 12.1). In addition, this mechanism has now been associated with hemodynamic and erectile dysfunction side effects, which may be related to the role of the melanocortins in general autonomic control [23].

12.1.4
Neuropeptide Y (NPY)

The large number of tyrosines (designated "Y") are the basis for the term, neuropeptide "Y". NPY belongs to the PP-fold peptide superfamily, which is characterized by its U-shaped structure, composed of an N-terminal polyproline helix, followed by a β-turn, and a C-terminal α-helix. NPY and two other members of this superfamily, including pancreatic polypeptide (PP) and peptide YY (PYY), all consist of 36 amino acids with C-terminal amidations. NPY is one of the most abundant neuropeptides, in both central and peripheral nervous systems. In human brain, it is mainly expressed in the hypothalamus, amygdala, and hippocampus. In the periphery, NPY is primarily expressed in sympathetic neurons. The NPY peptide sequence is highly conserved, with only 2 amino acids variable across species. NPY has been implicated in numerous physiological functions, including stress responses, blood pressure, circadian rhythms, pain, hormone secretion, reproduction, and alcohol consumption. The most well characterized role, however, is the regulation of food intake. NPY is the most potent endogenous stimulator of feeding in mammals. Hypothalamic NPY levels increase after fasting, and return to normal levels after feeding. Chronic central infusion of NPY in rodents results in a syndrome similar to that of some genetic obese/diabetic models [25].

The role of NPY in feeding is also confirmed by several genetically modified mouse models [26]. Ablation of NPY/AgRP neurons in adult mice causes a complete loss of feeding behavior. The gremlin NPY knock out mice have normal body weight and food intake, but display an attenuated orexigenic response to fasting. In addition, a well-characterized L7P polymorphism which results in elevated NPY release, (possibly acting to stimulate the sympathetic nervous system), is associated with high triglycerides, carotid atherosclerosis, diabetes, and obesity [27].

Six mammalian NPY receptor subtypes, designated Y1 through Y7 (Y3 is inferred from pharmacological experiments and does not exist as a separate gene), have been identified. Among those, only Y1, Y2, Y4, and Y5 exist in human. Although only a moderate 30–50% amino acid identity is shared between subfamilies, Y1, Y2, and Y5 all show equally high affinity to NPY, whereas Y4 is selectively activated by PP. NPY receptors all belong to the Class A GPCR subfamily, mainly signaling through the $G_{i/o}$ pathway. The central orexigenic effect of NPY is primarily mediated through the Y1 and Y5 receptors. Y1 is the most abundant among all NPY receptor subtypes and is primarily a postsynaptic receptor. The Y2 receptor, in contrast, is primarily an inhibitory presynaptic receptor. The Y5 receptor is mostly expressed in brain, with highest density in the arcuate nucleus POMC neurons [28].

Both Y1 and Y5 receptors have been popular targets for obesity since the early 1990s after their discovery. Despite intensive research, there are no examples of Y1-selective antagonists in clinical testing. The existing Y1 antagonists either lack tractable pharmaceutical properties and pharmacokinetic profiles, and/or are plagued by cardiovascular liabilities [28]. The efficacy of Y5 antagonism has also become controversial. Despite the considerable diversity of small molecule Y5 antagonists available, only two have reached clinical testing. Banyu/Merck have published their phase III results, showing that NPY5R blockade led to statistically significant weight loss for up to 1 year. However, the magnitude of the effect was small and below that deemed clinically meaningful [29]. Shionogi is the only company remaining with a Y5 antagonist in active development ((S-234462; phase I;/Velneperit; phase II) (Table 12.1)). One emerging hypothesis that may help to elucidate the roles of Y1 and Y5 receptor in feeding regulation is that Y1 and Y5 receptors may form hetero-dimers, resulting in altered pharmacology of antagonist interaction [30]. It has therefore been proposed to screen Y1 and Y5 hetero-dimer-selective antagonists for anti-obesity treatment, although the formation of this heterodimer *in vivo* remains to be confirmed. Additionally, a combined treatment using a Y5 antagonist and PYY 3-36 has also demonstrated additive obesity efficacy in rodents, suggesting Y5 may remain a tractable obesity target for combination therapy.

12.1.5
Neuromedin U (NMU) and Neuromedin S (NMS)

The term, NMU, reflects the initial isolation of this peptide from porcine spinal cord and its effects on uterine smooth muscle contraction. Human NMU is a 25-mer (NMU-25). The last 5 amino acids of the highly conserved C-terminal are essential for function. NMU is mainly expressed in the gastrointestinal tract, spinal cord, pituitary, and arcuate nucleus of the hypothalamus. NMU bind to the two NMU receptors (NMUR1 and NMUR2) with equally high affinity [31].

NMU may play an important role in energy homeostasis, since central injection of the peptide resulted in reduced food intake and body weight, along with increased energy expenditure, locomotor activity, grooming, and body temperature. Recently, the functionally inactive mutant R165W co-segregated with childhood-onset obesity. NMU is also involved in other biological functions, including local blood flow control, stress response, circadian rhythm, nociception, smooth muscle contraction, ion transport in the gut, bone health, and reproduction [32].

NMS is another neuropeptide which binds to NMUR1 and NMUR2. NMS, with 36-amino acids, shares a C-term pentapeptide with NMU, but is encoded by a different chromosome. NMS is expressed in the suprachiasmatic nucleus (SCN), testis, and spleen. NMS shows similar *in vitro* potency and biological function to NMU. Its anorexigenic effect is more potent and persistent than NMU, perhaps due to its better metabolic stability [33].

NMUR1 is mainly expressed in peripheral tissues, whereas NMUR2 is more abundant in the brain, especially in the hypothalamus, including the paraventricular nucleus, arcuate nucleus, SCN, and ventromedial nucleus. NMUR1 shares 45–50% amino acid homology to NMUR2. Both receptors belong to GPCR class A, coupled to $G_{q/11}$ and $G_{i/o}$. The genetically modified NMU mice support NMU's critical role in metabolism. NMU transgenic mice that ubiquitously overexpressed mouse proNMU developed and reproduced normally. They showed no behavioral disturbances, hyperthermia, nor hyperactivity. They were, however, hypophagic and lighter, with less somatic and liver fat. They also showed improved insulin sensitivity. In contrast, NMU knockout mice became obese on a normal chow diet. They showed hyperphagia with decreased energy expenditure, hypoactivity and hypometabolism, hyperinsulinemia, late-onset hyperglycemia, hyperleptinemia, and hyperlipidemia. The NMU receptor is clearly an attractive target to treat obesity. Several small molecule NMUR agonists and antagonists of low potency have been reported in the literature; however, there are no NMUR agonists in clinical trials at this time. The therapeutic potential of NMUR agonists for use in the treatment of obesity will be dependent upon whether potential cardiovascular liabilities can be dissociated from efficacy [31].

12.1.6
Opioids

Three families of endogenous opioid peptides have been identified, including β-endorphin, met and leu-enkephalin, dynorphins, and neo-endorphins. These families are derived from either proopiomelanocortin (POMC), proenkephalin (PENK), or prodynorphin (PDYN), respectively [34]. Opioid receptors are part of the class A family of GPCRs, and primarily couple with the G_i/G_o alpha subunits. Activation of opioid receptors leads to inhibition of cAMP production and voltage gated Ca^{++} channels, as well as the stimulation of inwardly rectifying K^+ channels and activation of the mitogen-activated protein (MAP) kinase pathway. The endogenous opioid ligands exhibit different affinities for each opioid receptor. The μ-opioid receptors are located in many areas of the central nervous system that regulate feeding, including the hypothalamus, nucleus accumbens, amygdala, ventral tegmental area, and the nucleus of the tractus solitarius.

Endogenous opioid peptides have long been known to influence eating behavior [35]. The opioid receptor antagonist naloxone was found to cause a significant reduction in short-term food intake in rats. In contrast, activation of μ-opioid receptors with the specific agonist [D-Ala$_2$, N-MePhe$_4$, Gly-ol]-enkephalin] (DAMGO) results in hyperphagia and increased preference for a high fat diet in rats. Furthermore, μ-opioid receptor-deficient mice exhibit diminished food-anticipatory activity, increased body weight in adulthood, and were more resistant to high-fat diet-induced obesity than wild-type mice. Observations that palatable food increased β-endorphin release in the hypothalamus, and evidence that naloxone had a greater effect on the consumption of a sucrose-rich diet compared to a cornstarch-rich diet, led to the hypothesis that endogenous opioids may play a role in the perception of food palatability. The μ-opioid receptor may also play a role in the regulation of glucose and insulin homeostasis, since activation of μ-opioid receptors improves insulin sensitivity in obese rats and genetic deficiency of μ-opioid receptors promotes insulin resistance in mice.

Compared to animal studies, the effects of naltrexone on eating behavior and body weight of human obese subjects has been less consistent [36]. Although naltrexone reduced food intake and induced weight loss in a few studies, it failed to achieve significant efficacy in several other clinical studies. Based on all the clinical data so far, naltrexone monotherapy for obesity is associated with minimal or no weight loss. Most recently, Orexigen® Therapeutics reported their positive results of a large scale phase III study of a combined treatment with sustained-release naltrexone and bupropion (Contrave) [37] (Table 12.1). Subjects taking Contrave lost 5–6.1% of body weight compared to a 1.3% weight loss in the placebo group. Patients taking Contrave also showed a significant reduction in insulin resistance, triglycerides levels, along with improved appetite control. One hypothesis for these effects is that naltrexone may attenuate the negative feedback of β-endorphin on bupropion-stimulated POMC neuron activation. Recent interactions with the United States Food and Drug Administration (FDA), however, resulted in a request for extensive cardiovascular safety studies. As a result, development of Contrave is now on hold.

12.1.7
QRFP

QRFP is a member of the RFamide related peptides, which are a family of peptides that have the motif arginine-phenylanine-amide at their C-terminus. The designation, QRFP, reflects the presence of an N-terminal pyroglutamic acid. There are two forms, QRFP43 and its N-terminal truncated form QRFP26, that may be generated from the precursor peptide for QRFP in human. Both forms of QRFP are endogenous high-affinity ligands for GPR103, which is a Class A GPCR, coupled to G_q and $G_{i/o}$. In human, both QRFP and GPR103 are highly expressed in brain, particularly in the hypothalamus. Interestingly, GPR103 has a single form in human, chimp, rhesus monkey, and dog, whereas two forms, GPR103A and GPR103B, are found in mouse, rat and cow. GPR103A and GPR103B share 80% homology, and their mRNA distributions are virtually without overlap within rodent brain. Central injection of QRFP43 increases food intake, body weight, and fat mass in mice, as well as blood pressure and heart rate [38, 39]. QRFP transcripts are up-regulated under fasted conditions, and in *ob/ob* and *db/db* mice. It is believed that QRFP may act at GPR103 in the arcuate nucleus and stimulate the release of NPY, resulting in inhibition of POMC neurons [40]. The therapeutic potential of GPR103 antagonism for use in the treatment of obesity is promising. No GPR103 antagonists have been reported to date.

12.2
Peripherally Secreted Neuropeptides

12.2.1
Amylin

Amylin, also known as islet amyloid polypeptide (IAPP) and diabetes-associated peptide (DAP), is a 37 amino acid peptide, co-secreted with insulin by the pancreatic β-cells in response to nutrient stimuli after a meal [41]. Circulating amylin, which has a plasma half-life of 15–30 min, rises after a meal and is reduced under fasting conditions. Amylin specifically binds to amylin receptor (AMY) which belongs to the class B family of GPCRs. Activation of amylin receptors by amylin leads to a robust cAMP production in cells. Amylin receptors are formed by the association of calcitonin receptor (CT) and receptor activity modifying protein (RAMP) on the cell surface [42]. Distinct subtypes of human amylin receptor may exist with different combinations of two CT splicing isoforms (CTa and CTb, and three subtypes of RAMPs (I, II, and III). Amylin receptors are predominantly expressed in several regions of the brain, including the nucleus accumbens, area postrema, nucleus of the solitary tract, amygdaloid body, dorsal raphe, and hypothalamus. The localization of each amylin receptor subtype remains a technical challenge to characterize.

The anorexigenic effect of Amylin has been well established in several animal models and appears to be primarily mediated by its receptors in the brain, especially the area postrema (AP) [43]. Peripheral and central administration of amylin reduces food intake and body weight in rodents without inducing taste aversion. Amylin has been shown to reduce meal size without significantly affecting the latency, duration, or intermeal interval. Chronic administration of amylin results in reduced body mass, where the primary mechanism appears to be appetite suppression. Concurrent peripheral administration of amylin and metreleptin has been shown to elicit synergistic weight loss in DIO mice and in obese human subjects [44]. Additionally, amylin has been shown to delay gastric emptying, inhibit gastric acid and glucagon secretion. As a result, the appearance of ingested nutrients (including glucose) in serum is delayed, improving post-prandial glucose homeostasis [45].

The effects of amylin on glucose homeostasis and food intake led to the investigation of amylin agonists as treatments for diabetes mellitus and obesity. Pramlintide, a non-aggregating analog of human amylin, developed by Amylin Pharmaceuticals Inc., has already been launched for a treatment of Type 1 and Type 2 diabetes as an adjunct to insulin therapy. Additionally, administration of pramlintide has been shown to provide a modest reduction in body weight (6–8%) in clinical studies [46]. A late-stage clinical study of a pramlintide/metreleptin combination is currently under investigation (Table 12.1).

12.2.2
Bombesin-Like Peptides (Bombesin and Gastrin-Releasing Peptide)

The natural ligand for bombesin receptor subtype 3 (BRS-3) remains unknown. In the CNS, the highest levels of BRS-3 expression were detected in the rat hypothalamus. BRS-3 knockout mice develop a mild late-onset obesity, associated with metabolic defects, implicating BRS-3 is involved in the regulation of feeding and metabolism. BRS-3 is closely related to two other bombesin receptors, BRS-1 and BRS-2, which mediate the action of natural ligands including bombesin-related peptides, gastrin-releasing peptide, and neuromedin. The BRS-3 receptor, however, does not interact with high affinity with any of these ligands [47, 48].

Merck has recently developed an antagonist for BRS-3 and demonstrated a stimulating effect on food intake and body weight. In contrast, selective agonists for BRS-3 increased metabolic rate and reduced food intake and body weight. In addition, BRS-3 knockout mice lost weight upon treatment with either a MC4R agonist or a CB1R inverse agonist, suggesting BRS-3 has a role in energy homeostasis that complements several well-known pathways [49].

BRS-3 agonists may act indirectly by inhibiting orexin neurons through GABAergic input or may directly activate orexin neurons. [50]. BRS-3 may also play a role in glucose homeostasis by acting at pancreatic islets directly. BRS-3 knockout mice showed a reduced islet size. Further, BRS-3 siRNA or a BRS-3 antagonist reduced glucose-stimulated insulin secretion (GSIS) in rat INS-1 cells. In contrast, a BRS-3 agonist has been shown to enhance GSIS in isolated islets. The development of a BRS-3 agonist to treat metabolic disease remains in the early stages of preclinical discovery at this time, and it is encouraging that there are several small molecule tools available [49].

12.2.3
Cholecystokinin (CCK)

CCK is produced by the enteroendocrine I cells in the intestine in response to the ingestion of a meal. Several molecular forms of CCK exist in plasma as a result of enzymatic cleavage, with CCK-8, CCK-33, and CCK-39 being the most abundant. It is critically involved in many biological functions, including stimulating gall-bladder contraction, pancreatic exocrine secretion, gastrointestinal motility, and satiety. Administration of CCK prior to a meal induced an inhibition of food intake by reducing meal size and duration. This physiological effect has been observed in animals and humans [51].

The CCK peptide interacts with two G-protein coupled receptor subtypes: the CCK1 receptor (CCK1R, also known as CCK-AR) and the CCK2 receptor (CCK2R, also known as CCK-BR). These two receptors both belong to the class A GPCR subfamily, sharing approximately 67% homology. CCK2R is also the gastrin receptor and is located primarily in the stomach and brain, regulating gastric acid secretion and many CNS-related functions. CCK1R is found in the gallbladder, pancreas, pyloric smooth muscle, and the enteric vagal afferent nerves. It is widely accepted that CCK-mediated satiation is largely mediated through the activation of CCK1R on the vagus nerve. CCK1 is also expressed in the brainstem and hypothalamus, which may be involved in relaying satiety signals to the brain. A spontaneous mutation at CCK1R has been identified in the Otsuka Long-Evans Tokushima Fatty rat, which is characterized by hyperphagia-induced obesity [52].

Although CCK was the first hormone identified to reduce food intake, the development of CCK-based therapy has been challenging. It has been shown that after repeated administration of CCK, animals may compensate for reduced meal size by increasing meal frequency [53]. Further, development of tolerance was observed after a continuous CCK infusion [54]. Several series of small molecule CCK1R agonists have been disclosed in the literature. A phase IIB study has revealed that 1,5-benzodiazepine GI181771X alone did not cause weight loss in overweight or obese patients after 24 weeks (Table 12.1). The lack of efficacy may be the result of dose-limiting gastrointestinal adverse effects including vomiting and diarrhea [55]. However, the design of the trial was criticized because it was con-ducted with a hypocaloric diet (600 kcal/day), instead of an *ad libitum* diet, which was employed during an earlier phase IIA trial where efficacy was demonstrated [56]. Currently, there are no other CCKR1 agonists in clinical trials. The future of a small molecule may rely on the development of allosteric modulator, biased agonist, or partial agonist that may selectively agonize the satiety pathways without poten-tiating the pathways associated with side effects such as amylase secretion [51].

CCKR1 agonists may still hold promise as components of a combination therapy. It has been shown, for example, that co-treatment of CCK with leptin may result in a synergistic effect on weight loss [57].

12.2.4
Ghrelin

Ghrelin is a 29 amino acid peptide which is primarily secreted from the X/A-like enteroendocrine cells of the stomach [58]. Circulating ghrelin levels rise and fall before and after meals, respectively. There are 2 major forms of ghrelin in circulation, acyl ghrelin which has an n-octanoyl at the serine in position 3, and a des-acyl ghrelin. The des-acyl ghrelin is the predominate isoform in the circulation. Recently, the enzyme that catalyzed ghrelin octanoylation has been identified as ghrelin O-acyltransferase (GOAT) [59]. Ghrelin was identified as the endogenous ligand of the growth hormone secretagogue receptor type-1a (GHS-R1a) [60]. GHS-R1a is a GPCR which preferentially couples to the G_q alpha subunit which, upon binding to ghrelin, leads to the release of calcium from intracellular stores. The acylation of ghrelin is required for the activation of the type-1 GHS receptor. GHS-R1a is highly expressed in the pituitary, hypothalamus, brainstem, but also in the gastrointestinal tract, adipose tissue, and other peripheral tissues.

Ghrelin has been considered a short-term regulator of food intake, primarily impacting hunger and meal initiation [61]. At present ghrelin is the only known gastrointestinal hormone that increases food intake. In rats, acute and chronic administrations of ghrelin stimulate feeding and body weight gain. There are some reports demonstrating that antagonism of the ghrelin receptor reduces food intake and body weight gain in mice. The orexigenic effects of peripheral ghrelin are primarily mediated via the activation of neurons in the hypothalamic arcuate and paraventricular nuclei, although the brainstem and vagus nerve may also be important in mediating these effects of ghrelin on food intake. GHS-R1a receptor knockout mice eat less food and accumulate less body weight than control mice on a high fat diet (HFD). Some evidence suggests that ghrelin may also play a role in the regulation of glucose and insulin levels. For example, acute administration of ghrelin reduced insulin secretion and caused hyperglycaemia. Further, there is a report showing that GHS-R1a antagonists improved glucose homeostasis in a glucose tolerance test in rats.

In humans, ghrelin levels in plasma are increased in response to fasting and suppressed by food intake. Intravenous administration of ghrelin significantly increases food intake in human subjects [62]. Individuals suffering from Prader–Willi syndrome, a genetic disorder characterized by obesity with a chronic feeling of hunger, have higher plasma ghrelin levels than control subjects. The association of ghrelin with changes in glucose and insulin in humans, however, has been inconsistent.

Pharmacological manipulation of ghrelin has become an attractive target for the treatment of obesity and diabetes [63]. Several antagonists and inverse agonists of GHS-R1a receptor have been discovered. However, there is no report of such compounds in large scale clinical trial yet. Additionally, several other approaches have been explored, including (i) RNA Spiegelmers which bind specifically to GHS-R1a, (ii) a ghrelin-specific neutralizing antibody, and (iii) ghrelin immuno-conjugates to cause an immune response against endogenous ghrelin. The recent discovery of GOAT may provide a unique approach to mediation of ghrelin signals. Several ghrelin agonists are currently in clinical trials for potential anti-cachectic benefits in patients with cancer, HIV, cardiac cachexia, anorexia nervosa, and postoperative patients who usually lose appetite and weight.

12.2.5
Glucagon-like Peptide-1

Glucagon-like peptide-1 (GLP-1) is a 30 amino acid peptide, released by the entero-endocrine L-cells of the small intestine and colon, and the α^c-Cells of the pancreas in response to nutrients from a meal [64]. GLP-1 is a product of its precursor pre-proglucagon which is processed by prohormone convertase 1 and 2 (PC1, PC2). PC1 and PC2 also catalyze the cleavage of pre-proglucagon to oxyntomodulin (OXM), glucagon, and glucagon-like peptide-2. Circulating GLP-1 is elevated after a meal and reduced under fasting conditions. Plasma GLP-1 has a half-life of 5 min due to renal clearance and inactivation by the plasma enzyme dipeptidyl peptidase-IV (DPP-IV). The GLP-1 receptor (GLP-1R) belongs to the class B family of G-protein-coupled receptors. Activation of the GLP-1R leads to an increase in intracellular cAMP accumulation and calcium mobilization. Ligand binding to the GLP-1R can also activate the phospatidylinositol-3 kinase (PI-3K), and MAPK signal transduction pathways. The GLP-1 receptor is expressed in a wide range of tissues, including pancreatic islets, lung, heart, kidney, stomach, intestine, pituitary, skin, vagus nerve, and several regions of the CNS including the hypothalamic ARC, PVN, supraoptic nucleus (SON), and the NTS of the brainstem, which regions have been identified as critical in the mediation of food intake.

Peripheral and central injection of GLP-1 reduces food intake in rats [65]. Further, intracerebroventricular (icv) administration of the GLP-1 receptor antag-onist exendin (9–39) increases food intake and body weight in rats. However, central GLP-1 administration has been shown to elicit conditioned taste aversion in rats [66]. Thus, it is possible that some of the observed reduction in food intake might have been caused by GLP-1-induced malaise in the experimental animals. The GLP-1 anorectic action, as well as the effect on gastric emptying, is partially mediated by the vagal afferents. Additionally, GLP-1 has a well-known incretin effect in that it augments glucose-dependent insulin secretion [64]. GLP-1 also inhibits glucagon release and delays gastric emptying. Mice with a deficiency of the GLP-1 receptor gene show mild fasting hyperglycaemia and impaired glucose tolerance associated with defective insulin release. Interestingly, GLP-1 receptor-deficient mice exhibit normal eating behavior and normal body weight.

Peripheral administration of GLP-1 has an anorectic effect and reduces the rate of gastric emptying in humans. It has been observed that obese subjects have reduced circulating GLP-1 and weight loss is associated with a decrease in GLP-1. Exendin-4, a DPP-IV resistant GLP-1 receptor agonist has been developed as Exenatide and marketed as Byetta for treatment of type 2 diabetes mellitus (T2DM). In addition, Exenatide has been shown to reduce body weight in diabetic patients [67]. Liraglu-tide (Victoza) is another long-acting GLP-1 analog developed by Novo Nordisk. The product was approved for the treatment of type 2 diabetes by the European Medicines Agency (EMEA) and by the US Food and Drug Administration (FDA). Currently a phase III trial of Liraglutide for obesity is on-going (Table 12.1). Specific DPP-IV inhibitors have also been developed, including Januvia (sitagliptin) and Onglyza (Saxagliptin), which are now being used clinically in the treatment of T2DM. These drugs increase the postprandial rise of GLP-1 and increase insulin secretion. However, unlike GLP-1 agonists, DPP-IV inhibitors have only minimal or no effect on body weight in human subjects [68].

12.2.6
Leptin

Leptin is a 16 kDa protein which is secreted from adipocytes and circulates in plasma in proportion to adipose mass. Genetic mutation results in severe obesity and endocrinologic disorders in mice and humans, most of which can be reversed by administration of recombinant leptin [69, 70]. Both peripheral and central administration of leptin reduces food intake and body weight, although efficacy is inversely proportional to the degree of adiposity in the subject (except in the case of the ob mutation) [69]. This, along with data showing that leptin is proportional to adiposity, has led to the conclusion that obesity is a leptin-resistant state. Leptin resistance could be a function of receptor dysfunction. Indeed, the severely obese and diabetic db/db mouse has a truncated form of the leptin receptor and the obese and hyperglycemic fa/fa rat has a mutated form of the leptin receptor which attenuates leptin receptor signaling. However, genetic forms of leptin receptor dysfunction do not appear to be associated with most types of obesity [69].

The leptin receptor is a member of the type 1 cytokine receptor family and is expressed in many brain areas, including the POMC neurons of the ARC. Leptin receptor activation promotes the secretion of anorexigenic peptides, such as POMC and inhibits the secretion of orexigenic peptides such as AGRP and NPY [69, 71]. Leptin binding initiates a signaling cascade beginning with the autopho-sphorylation of Janus-kinase 2 (Jak2), involving the extracellular signal regulated kinase (ERK) cascade and ultimately leading to the phosphorylation of the tran-scription factor, signal transducer and activator of transcription-3 (STAT3) which mediates the regulation of gene expression. Leptin signaling is negatively regulated by the suppressor of cytokine signaling-3 (SOCS-3) [71].

Leptin and the leptin receptor have been intensely pursued as targets for anti-obesity therapeutics since the cloning and characterization of leptin in 1994 [72]. Unfortunately, recombinant human leptin failed to produce significant weight loss in phase II clinical trials, although it has been suggested that leptin could be effective in obese subpopulations with reduced leptin levels [69]. Recently, Amylin Pharmaceuticals has shown that pre-treatment with the hormone amylin followed by combination with leptin produces synergistic levels of efficacy in phase II trials

[69]. This, along with preclinical data, suggests that amylin may be able to restore leptin signal transduction in the brain [44].

12.2.7
Oxyntomodulin (OXM)

OXM is another cleavage product of preproglucagon which is released primarily from L-cells of the intestine, as well as from the central nervous system (CNS) to a lesser degree [73]. It is secreted following ingestion of a meal. OXM is now well established as a gut peptide, which promotes satiety in both rodents and humans [74]. Peripheral (intraperitoneal) administration of OXM to rodents inhibits fasting-induced food intake. Central administration of OXM to rats reduces food intake as well. A specific OXM receptor has not been identified so far and it has been postulated that OXM may signal through the GLP-1 receptor. The anorectic effect of peripheral OXM is blocked by the GLP-1 receptor antagonist exendin (9–39) and is absent in GLP-1 receptor knockout mice. OXM has also been shown to increase insulin release and improve glucose homeostasis in rodents. However, there is no strong evidence indicating an incretin effect of OXM in humans.

OXM has also been shown to reduce food intake and body weight in human volunteers [73]. In one study, the intravenous administration of OXM to human subjects reduced food intake by 19.3% at a buffet meal. In a second study, the preprandial subcutaneous administration of OXM to overweight and obese humans over 4 weeks led to a significant reduction in body weight of 2.3 kg compared with 0.5 kg in the control group. Although oxyntomodulin peptide had been under early clinical development, it is not listed as being under clinical development at this time.

12.2.8
PYY3-36 and PP

PYY is produced by the intestinal endocrine L-cells, and is rapidly converted by DPP-IV to the Y2-selective peptide PYY3-36 in the circulation. PP is mainly produced in endocrine cells located at the head of the pancreas. Both PYY3-36 and PP are satiety factors which are secreted in response to meal ingestion and are reduced upon fasting, although with different kinetics. It has been shown that patients with morbid obesity have reduced basal and meal-stimulated PYY3-36 and PP levels. In the case of PP, its expression is also blunted in ob/ob mice and in patients with Prader–Willi syndrome (a genetic form of obesity characterized by extreme hyperphagia). In contrast, patients with anorexia, or weight loss after bypass surgery, have higher plasma PYY3-36 and PP. Importantly, peripheral injection of either PYY3-36 or PP has been shown to reduce food intake, body weight, and rate of gastric emptying in various species including humans [75, 76].

The anorectic effect of PYY3-36 is primarily mediated via the Y2 receptor which is located in vagal afferents and in the hypothalamus. Circulating PYY3-36 may stimulate afferent vagal discharges, as well as act at presynaptic Y2 receptors in the arcuate nucleus to inhibit NPY neurons and disinhibit POMC neurons. Based on a brain fMRI study, PYY3-36 may also affect the orbitofrontal cortex, a region implicated in reward processing, suggesting PYY3-36 may affect energy intake by modulating feeding behavior [77]. PYY knockout mice displayed hyperphagia and increased adiposity [78, 79]. In contrast, PYY transgenic mice are protected against diet-induced and genetic obesity [80]. These phenotypes are consistent with PYY agonism reducing food intake and body weight.

PP selectively binds to the Y4 receptor, which is expressed mainly in the periphery, particularly in the gastrointestinal tract. Y4 expression in the brain is limited to regions such as the area postrema and nucleus tractus solitarus. It is believed that Y4 in the area postrema, which is a circumventricular organ, may be the primary target of circulating PP. The Y4 activation in this brain region may modulate vagal input, resulting in feeding inhibition [81]. Consistently, PP transgenic mice are leaner, with lower food intake and fat mass, validating the role of Y4 agonism in inducing satiety [82].

The half-life of both PYY3-36 and PP in plasma is extremely short, less than 10 min, rendering neither one in its native form suitable as a therapeutic agent. Currently, no small molecule Y2 or Y4 agonists have been reported. Several PYY or PP peptidic homologues are in clinical trials (Table 12.1). An attempt to use intranasally-delivered PYY3-36 has failed to demonstrate significant weight loss efficacy at a phase II clinical trial, due to dose-limiting adverse effects including vomiting and nausea [83]. It should be noted that the intranasally-delivered PYY3-36 may be exposed to the centrally expressed orexigenic Y1 and Y5 receptors, which also have significant affinity to PYY3-36, thus canceling out the efficacy. A more selective Y2 agonist may have better efficacy. Finally, Obineptide (7TM Pharma), which is a Y2/Y4 dual acting peptide, is currently in phase I/II clinical trials.

12.3
Summary

The neural network which regulates food intake is composed of a diverse array of neuropeptide modulators, which can act as nutrient sensors or as components of a complex information integration system. These neuropeptides and their cognate receptors should provide a rich source of potential therapeutic targets for the treatment of obesity. Indeed, selective modulators of some neuropeptide targets are now in clinical testing and will hopefully provide a new avenue for the future in metabolic disease drug discovery.

References

1 Bray, G.A. and Greenway, F.L. (2007) Pharmacological treatment of the overweight patient. *Pharmacol. Rev.*, **59**, 151–184.

2 US Department of Health and Human Services, Food and Drug Administration, Center for Drug Evaluation and Research (Revision 1)

(2007) Guidance for industry developing products for weight management, 3.

3 Field, A.E., Coakley, E.H., Must, A., Spadano, J.L., Laird, N., Dietz, W.H., Rimm, E., and Colditz, G.A. (2001) Impact of overweight on the risk of developing common chronic disease during a 10-year period. *Arch. Intern. Med.*, **161**, 1581–1586.

4 Rogers, R.P., Bemelmans, W.J.E., Hoogenveen, R.T., Boshuizen, H.C., Woodward, M., Knekt, P., van Dam, R.M., Hu, F.B., Visscher, T.L.S., Menotti, A., Thorpe, R.J., Jamrozik, K., Calling, S., Strand, B.H., and Shipley, M.J. (2007) Association of overweight with increased risk of coronary heart disease partly independent of blood pressure and cholesterol levels. *Arch. Intern. Med.*, **167** (16), 1720–1728.

5 Valentino, M.A., Lin, J.E., and Waldman, S.A. (2010) Central and peripheral molecular targets for antiobesity pharmacotherapy. *Clin. Pharmacol. Therapeut.*, **87**, 652–662.

6 Powell, L.M., Han, E., and Chaloupka, F.J. (2010) Economic contextual factors, food consumption and obesity among US adolescents. *J. Nutr.*, **140**, 1175–1180.

7 Donnelly, J.E., Smith, B., Jacobsen, D.J., Kirk, E., DuBose, K., Bailey, B., and Washburn, R. (2004) The role of exercise for weight loss and maintenance. *Best Practice and Research Clinical Gastroenterology*, **18**, 1009–1029.

8 Arora, S.A (2006) Role of neuropeptides in appetite regulation and obesity – a review. *Neuropeptides*, **40**, 375–401.

9 Badman, M.K. and Flier, J.S. (2005) The gut and energy balance: visceral allies in the obesity wars. *Science*, **307**, 1909–1914.

10 Cooke, D. and Bloom, S. (2006) The obesity pipeline: current strategies in the development of anti-obesity drugs. *Nat. Rev, Drug Discov.*, **5**, 919–931.

11 Berthoud, H.R. and Morrison, C. (2008) The brain, appetite and obesity. *Annu. Rev. Psychol.*, **59**, 55–92.

12 Schwartz, J.H. (2000) Neurotransmitters, in *Principles of Neural Science*, 4th edn (eds E.R. Kandel, J.H. Schwartz, and T.M. Jessell), McGraw-Hill Co., pp. 286–290.

13 Vale, W., Spiess, J., Rivier, C., and Rivier, J. (1981) Characterization of a 41-residue ovine hypothalamic peptides that stimulates secretion of corticotropin and beta-endorphin. *Science*, **213**, 1394–1397.

14 Richard, D., Lin, Q., and Timofeeva, E. (2002) The corticotropin-releasing factor family of peptides and CRF receptors: their roles in the regulation of energy balance. *Eur. J. Pharmacol.*, **440**, 189–197.

15 Vaughan, J., Donaldson, C., Bittencort, J., Perrin, M.H., Lewis, K., Sutton, S., Chan, R., Turnbull, A.V., Lovejoy, D., Rivier, C., Rivier, J., Sawchenko, P.E., and Vale, W. (1995) Urocortin, a mammalian neuropeptide related to fish urotensin I and to corticotropin-releasing factor. *Nature*, **378**, 287–292.

16 Reyes, T.M., Lewis, K., Perrin, M.H., Kunitake, K.S., Vaughan, J., Arias, C.A., Hogenexch, J.B., Gulyas, J., Rivier, J., Vale, W.W., and Sawchenko, P.E. (2001) Urocortin II: a member of the corticotropin releasing factor (CRF) neuropeptide family that is selectively bound by type 2 CRF receptors. *Proc. Natl. Acad. Sci. U.S.A.*, **98**, 2843–2848.

17 Lewis, K., Li, C., Perrin, M.H., Blount, A., Kunitake, K., Donaldson, C., Vauthan, J., Reyes, T.M., Gulyas, J., Fischer, W., Bilezikjian, L., Rivier, J., Sawchenko, P.E., and Vale, W.W. (2001) Identification of urocortin III, an additional family member of the corticotropin releasing factor (CRF) family with high affinity for the CRF2 receptor. *Proc. Natl. Acad. Sci. U.S.A.*, **98**, 7570–7575.

18 Pissios, P. and Maratos-Flier, E. (2003) Melanin-concentrating hormone: from fish to skinny mammals. *Trends in Endocrinol. Metab.*, **14** (5), 243–248.

19 Luthin, D.R. (2007) Anti-obesity effects of small molecule melanin-concentrating hormone receptor 1 (MCHR1) antagonists. *Life Sci.*, **81**, 423–440.

20 Zimanyi, I.A. and Pelleymounter, M.A. (2003) The role of melanocortin peptides and receptors in regulation of energy balance. *Curr. Pharm. Des.*, **9**, 1–14.

21 Ellacott, K.L.J. and Cone, R.D. (2004) The central melanocortin system and the integration of short and long-term regulators of energy homeostasis. *Recent Prog. Horm. Res.*, **59**, 395–408.

22 Cone, R.D. (2006) Studies on the physiological functions of the melanocortin system. *Endocrine Rev.*, **27**, 736–749.

23 Wikberg, J.E.S. and Mutulis, F. (2008) Targeting melanocortin receptors: an approach to treat weight disorders and sexual dysfunction. *Nat. Rev. Drug Discov.*, **7**, 307–323.

24 Krishna, R., Gumbiner, B., Stevens, C., Musser, B., Mallick, M., Suryawanshi, S., Maganti, L., Zhu, H., Han, T.H., Scherer, L., Simpson, B., Cosgrove, D., Gottesdiener, K., Amatruda, J., Rolls, B.J., Blundell, J., Bray, G.A., Fujioka, K., Heymsfield, S.B., Wagner, J.A., and Herman, G.A. (2009) *Clin. Pharmacol. Ther.*, **86**, 659–666.

25 MacNeil, D.J. (2007) NPY Y1 and Y5 receptor selective antagonists as anti-obesity drugs. *Curr. Top. Med. Chem.*, **7** (17), 1721–1733.

26 Herzog, H. (2003) Neuropeptide Y and energy homeostasis: insights from Y receptor knockout models. *Eur. J. Pharmacol.*, **480** (1–3), 21–29.

27 Pesonen, U. (2008) NPY L7P polymorphism and metabolic diseases. *Regul. Pept.*, **149** (1–3), 51–55.

28 Sato, N., Ogino, Y., Mashiko, S., and Ando, M. (2009) Modulation of neuropeptide Y receptors for the treatment of obesity. *Expert Opin. Ther. Pat.*, **19** (10), 1401–1415.

29 Erondu, N., Gantz, I., Musser, B., Suryawanshi, S., Mallick, M., Addy, C., Cote, J., Bray, G., Fujioka, K., Bays, H., Hollander, P., Sanabria-Bohorquez, S.M., Eng, W., Langstrom, B., Hargreaves, R.J., Burns, H.D., Kanatani, A.T. Fukami, T., MacNeil, D.J., Gottesdiener, K.M., Amatruda, J.M., Kaufman, K.D., and Heymsfield, S.B. (2006) Neuropeptide Y5 receptor antagonism does not induce clinically meaningful weight loss in overweight and obese adults. *Cell. Metab.*, **4** (4), 275–282.

30 Gehlert, D.R., Schober, D.A., Morin, M., and Berglund, M.M. (2007) Co-expression of neuropeptide Y Y1 and Y5 receptors results in heterodimerization and altered functional properties. *Biochem. Pharmacol.*, **74** (11), 1652–1664.

31 Budhiraja, S. and Chugh, A. (2009) Neuromedin U: physiology, pharmacology and therapeutic potential. *Fundam. Clin. Pharmacol.*, **23** (2), 149–157.

32 Mitchell, J.D., Maguire, J.J., and Davenport, A.P. (2009) Emerging pharmacology and physiology of neuromedin U and the structurally related peptide neuromedin S. *Br. J. Pharmacol.*, **158** (1), 87–103.

33 Mori, K., Miyazato, M., and Kangawa, K. (2008) Neuromedin S: discovery and functions. *Results Probl. Cell Differ.*, **46**, 201–212.

34 Waldhoer, M., Bartlett, S.E., and Whistler, J.L. (2004) Opioid receptors. *Annu. Rev. Biochem.*, **73**, 953–990.

35 Bodnar, R.J. (2004) Endogenous opioids and feeding behavior: a 30-year historical perspective. *Peptides*, **25**, 697–725.

36 Lee, M.W. and Fujioka, K. (2009) Naltrexone for the treatment of obesity: review and update. *Expert Opin. Pharmacother.*, **10**, 1841–1845.

37 Greenway, F.L., Fujioka, K., Plodkowski, R.A., Mudaliar, S., Guttadauria, M., Erickson, J., Kim, D.D., and Dunayevich, E. (2010) Effect of naltrexone plus bupropion on weight loss in overweight and obese adults (COR-I): a multicentre, randomised, double-blind, placebo-controlled, phase 3 trial. *The Lancet*, **376**, 595–605.

38 Moriya, R., Sano, H., Umeda, T., Ito, M., Takahashi, Y., Matsuda, M., Ishihara, A., Kanatani, A., and Iwaasa, H. (2006) RFamide peptide QRFP43 causes obesity with hyperphagia and reduced thermogenesis in mice. *Endocrinology*, **147** (6), 2916–2922.

39 Takayasu, S., Sakurai, T., Iwasaki, S., Teranishi, H., Yamanaka, A., Williams, S.C., Iguchi, H., Kawasawa, Y.I., Ikeda, Y., Sakakibara, I., Ohno, K., Ioka, R.X., Murakami, S., Dohmae, N., Xie, J.,

Suda, T., Motoike, T., Ohuchi, T., Yanagisawa, M., and Sakai, J. (2006) A neuropeptide ligand of the G protein-coupled receptor GPR103 regulates feeding, behavioral arousal, and blood pressure in mice. *Proc. Natl. Acad. Sci. U. S. A.*, **103** (19), 7438–7443.

40 Lectez, B., Jeandel, L., El-Yamani, F.Z., Arthaud, S., Alexandre, D., Mardargent, A., Jegou, S., Mounien, L.,Bizet, P., Magoul, R., Anouar, Y., and Chartrel, N. (2009) The orexgenic activity of the hypothalamic neuropeptide 26RFa is mediated by the neuropeptide Y and proopiomelanocortin neurons of the arcuate nucleus. *Endocrinology*, **150** (5), 2342–2350.

41 Cooper, G.J.S., Day, A.J., Willis, A.C., Roberts, A.N., Reid, K., and Leighton, B. (1989) Amylin and the amylin gene: structure, function and relationship to islet amyloid and to diabetes mellitus. *Biochim. Biophys. Acta*, **1014**, 247–258.

42 Poyner, D.R., Sexton, P.M., Marshall, I., Smith, D.M., Quirion, R., Born, W., Muff, R., Fischer, J.A., and Foord, S.M. (2002) International Union of Pharmacology. XXXII. The mammalian calcitonin gene-related peptides, adrenomedullin, amylin, and calcitonin receptors. *Pharmacol. Rev.*, **54**, 233–246.

43 Lutz, T.A. (2006) Amylinergic control of food intake. *Physiol. Behav.*, **89**, 465–471.

44 Roth, J.D., Roland, B.L., Cole, R.L. *et al.* (2008) Leptin responsivenss restored by amylin agonism in diet-induced obesity: evidence from clinical and non-clinical studies. *Proc. Natl. Acad. Sci. U.S.A.*, **105**, 7257–7262.

45 Schmitz, O., Brock, B., and Rungby, J. (2004) Amylin agonists: a novel approach in the treatment of diabetes. *Diabetes*, **53**, S233–S238.

46 Ravussin, E., Smith, S.R., Mitchell, J.A., Shringarpure, R., Shan, K., Maier, H., Koda, J.E., and Weyer, C. (2009) Enhanced weight loss with pramlintide/ metreleptin: an integrated neurohormonal approach to obesity pharmacotherapy. *Obesity (Silver Spring, Md.)*, **17**, 1736–1743.

47 Jensen, R.T., Battey, J.F., Spindel, E.R., and Benya, R.V. (2008) International

Union of Pharmacology. LXVIII. Mammalian bombesin receptors: nomenclature, distribution, pharmacology, signaling, and functions in normal and disease states. *Pharmacol. Rev.*, **60** (1), 1–42.

48 Gonzalez, N., Moody, T.W., Igarashi, H., Ito, T., and Jensen, R.T. (2008) Bombesin-related peptides and their receptors: recent advances in their role in physiology and disease states. *Curr. Opin. Endocrinol. Diabetes Obes.*, **15** (1), 58–64.

49 Guan, X.M., Chen, H., Dobbelaar, P.H., Dong, Y., Fong, T.M., Gagen, K., Gorski, J., He, S., Howard, A.D., Jian, T., Jiang, M., Kan, Y., Kelly, T.M., Kosinski, J., Lin, L.S., Liu, J., Marsh, D.J., Metzger, J.M., Miller, R., Nargund, R.P., Palyha, O., Shearman, L., Shen, Z., Stearns, R., Strack, A.M., Stribling, S., Tang, Y.S., Wang, S.P., White, A., Yu, H., and Reitman, M.L. (2010) Regulation of energy homeostasis by bombesin receptor subtype-3: selective receptor agonists for the treatment of obesity. *Cell Metab.*, **11** (2), 101–112.

50 Furutani, N., Hondo, M., Tsujino, N., and Sakurai, T. (2010) Activation of bombesin receptor subtype-3 influences activity of orexin neurons by both direct and indirect pathways. *J. Mol. Neurosci.*, **42** (1), 106–111.

51 Cawston, E.E. and Miller, L.J. (2010) Therapeutic potential for novel drugs targeting the type 1 cholecystokinin receptor. *Br. J. Pharmacol.*, **159** (5), 1009–1021.

52 Moran, T.H. (2008) Unraveling the obesity of OLETF rats. *Physiol. Behav.*, **94** (1), 71–78.

53 West, D.B., Fey, D., and Woods, S.C. (1984) Cholecystokinin persistently suppresses meal size but not food intake in free-feeding rats. *Am. J. Physiol.*, **246** (5 Pt 2), R776–R787.

54 Crawley, J.N. and Beinfeld, M.C. (1983) Rapid development of tolerance to the behavioural actions of cholecystokinin. *Nature*, **302** (5910), 703–706.

55 Jordan, J., Greenway, F.L., Leiter, L.A., Li, Z., Jacobson, P., Murphy, K., Hill, J., Kler, L., and Aftring, R.P. (2008)

Stimulation of cholecystokinin-A receptors with GI181771X does not cause weight loss in overweight or obese patients. *Clin. Pharmacol. Ther.*, **83** (2), 281–287.

56 Roses, A.D. (2009) Stimulation of cholecystokinin-A receptors with GI181771X: a failed clinical trial that did not test the pharmacogenetic hypothesis for reduction of food intake. *Clin. Pharmacol. Ther.*, **85** (4), 362–365.

57 Matson, C.A., Reid, D.F., and Ritter, R. C. (2002) Daily CCK injection enhances reduction of body weight by chronic intracerebroventricular leptin infusion. *Am. J. Physiol. Regul. Integr. Comp. Physiol.*, **282** (5), R1368–R1373.

58 Date, Y., Kojima, M., Hosoda, H., Sawaguchi, A., Mondal, M.S., Suganuma, T., Matsukura, S., Kangawa, K., and Nakazato, M. (2000) Ghrelin, a novel growth hormone-releasing acylated peptide, is synthesized in a distinct endocrine cell type in the gastrointestinal tracts of rats and humans. *Endocrinology*, **141**, 4255–4261.

59 Yang, J., Brown, M.S., Liang, G., Grishin, N.V., and Goldstein, J.L. (2008) Identification of the acyltransferase that octanoylates ghrelin, an appetite-stimulating peptide hormone. *Cell*, **132**, 387–396.

60 Kojima, M., Hosoda, H., Matsuo, H., and Kangawa, K. (2001) Ghrelin: discovery of the natural endogenous ligand for the growth hormone secretagogue receptor. *Trends Endocrin. Metab.*, **12**, 118–122.

61 Castaneda, T.R., Tong, J., Datta, R., Culler, M., and Tschöp, M.H. (2010) Ghrelin in the regulation of body weight and metabolism. *Frontiers Neuroendocrinol.*, **31**, 44–60.

62 Dostálová, I. and Haluzík, M. (2009) The role of ghrelin in the regulation of food intake in patients with obesity and anorexia nervosa. *Physiol. Res.*, **58**, 159–170.

63 Moulin, A., Ryan, J., Martinez, J., and Fehrentz, J.A. (2007) Recent developments in ghrelin receptor ligands. *ChemMedChem*, **2**, 1242–1259.

64 Baggio, L.L. and Drucker, D.J. (2007) Biology of incretins: GLP-1 and GIP. *Gastroenterology*, **132**, 2131–2157.

65 Hayes, M.R., De Jonghe, B.C., and Kanoski, S.E. (2010) Role of the glucagon-like-peptide-1 receptor in the control of energy balance. *Physiol. Behav.*, **100**, 503–510.

66 Thiele, T.E., Van Dijk, G., Campfield, L. A., Smith, F.J., Burn, P., Woods, S.C., Bernstein, I.L., and Seeley, R.J. (1997) Central infusion of GLP-1, but not leptin, produces conditioned taste aversions in rats. *Am. J. Physiol.*, **272** (2Pt 2), R726–R730.

67 Bradley, D.P., Kulstad, R., and Schoeller, D.A. (2010) Exenatide and weight loss. *Nutrition*, **26**, 243–249.

68 Neumiller, J.J. (2009) Differential chemistry (structure), mechanism of action, and pharmacology of GLP-1 receptor agonists and DPP-4 inhibitors. *J. Am. Pharm. Assoc.*, **49**, 16–29.

69 Friedman, J.M. (2009) Leptin at 14 y of age: an ongoing story. *Am. J. Clin. Nutr.*, **89** (Supp.), 973S–979S.

70 Farooqi, I.S. and O'Rahilly, S. (2009) Leptin: a pivotal regulator of human energy homeostasis. *Am. J. Clin. Nutr.*, **89** (Supp.), 980S–984S.

71 Villanueva, E.C. and Myers, M.G. Jr (2008) Leptin receptor signaling and the regulation of mammalian physiology. *Int. J. Obes. (Lond.)*, **32** (Supp. 7), S8–S12.

72 Zhang, Y., Proenca, P., Maffei, M., Barone, M., Leopold, L., and Friedman, J.M. (1994) Positional cloning of the mouse obese gene and its human homologue. *Nature*, **372**, 425–432.

73 Wynne, K., Park, A.J., Small, C.J., Patterson, M., Ellis, S.M., Murphy, K.G., Wren, A.M., Frost, G.S., Meeran, K., and Ghatei, M.A. (2005) Subcutaneous oxyntomodulin reduces body weight in overweight and obese subjects. *Diabetes*, **54**, 2390–2395.

74 Druce, M.R. and Bloom, S.R. (2006) Oxyntomodulin: a novel potential treatment for obesity. *Treat. Endocrinol.*, **5**, 265–272.

75 Batterham, R.L. and Bloom, S.R. (2003a) The gut hormone peptide YY regulates

appetite. *Ann. N. Y. Acad. Sci.*, **994**, 162–168.

76 Batterham, R.L., Le Roux, C.W., Cohen, M.A., Park, A.J., Ellis, S.M., Patterson, M., Frost, G.S., Ghatei, M.A., and Bloom, S.R. (2003b) Pancreatic polypeptide reduces appetite and food intake in humans. *J. Clin. Endocrinol. Metab.*, **88** (8), 3989–3992.

77 Batterham, R.L., ffytche, D.H., Rosenthal, J.M., Zelaya, F.O., Barker, G. J., Withers, D.J., and Williams, S.C. (2007) PYY modulation of cortical and hypothalamic brain areas predicts feeding behaviour in humans. *Nature*, **450** (7166), 106–109.

78 Boey, D., Lin, S., Karl, T., Baldock, P., Lee, N., Enriquez, R., Couzens, M., Slack, K., Dallmann, R., Sainsbury, A., and Herzog, H. (2006) Peptide YY ablation in mice leads to the development of hyperinsulinaemia and obesity. *Diabetologia*, **49** (6), 1360–1370.

79 Batterham, R., Heffron, L.H., Kapoor, S., Chivers, J.E., Chandarana, K., Herzog, H., Le Roux, C.W., Thomas, E.L., Bell, J.D., and Withers, D.J. (2006) Critical role for peptide YY in protein-mediated satiation and body-weight regulation. *Cell Metab.*, **4** (3), 223–233.

80 Boey, D., Lin, S., Enriquez, R.F., Lee, N. J., Slack, K., Couzens, M., Baldock, P.A., Herzog, H., and Sainsbury, A. (2008) PYY transgenic mice are protected against diet-induced and genetic obesity. *Neuropeptides*, **42** (1), 19–30.

81 Kojima, S., Ueno, N., Asakawa, A., Sagiyama, K., Naruo, T., Mizuno, S., and Inui, A. (2007) A role for pancreatic polypeptide in feeding and body weight regulation. *Peptides*, **28** (2), 459–463.

82 Ueno, N., Inui, A., Iwamoto, M., Kaga, T., Asakawa, A., Okita, M., Fujimiya, M., Nakajima, Y., Ohmoto, Y., Ohnaka, M., Nakaya, Y., Miyazaki, J.I., and Kasuga, M. (1999) Decreased food intake and body weight in pancreatic polypeptide-overexpressing mice. *Gastroenterology*, **117** (6), 1427–1432.

83 Gantz, I., Erondu, N., Mallick, M., Musser, B., Krishna, R., Tanaka, W.K., Snyder, K., Stevens, C., Stroh, M.A., Zhu, H., Wagner, J.A., Macneil, D.J., Heymsfield, S.B., and Amatruda, J.M. (2007) Efficacy and safety of intranasal peptide YY3–36 for weight reduction in obese adults. *J. Clin. Endocrinol. Metab.*, **92** (5), 1754–1757.

13
Translation of Motilin and Ghrelin Receptor Agonists into Drugs for Gastrointestinal Disorders

Gareth J. Sanger, John Broad, and David H. Alpers

13.1
Introduction

13.1.1
Similarities and Differences Between Motilin and Ghrelin

Both hormones activate G protein-coupled receptors (the motilin receptor was previously known as GPR38 and the ghrelin receptor as the growth hormone secretagogue receptor), and share such a high sequence homology that ghrelin was originally named as the motilin-related peptide [1, 2]. However, the receptors have poor affinity for the natural ligand of the other [3, 4]. The motilin receptor is found in multiple mammalian species (including humans, dogs, ferrets, cats, rabbits), but may exist only as a pseudogene in mice [5] rats and guinea-pigs [6]. By contrast, a functional ghrelin system has been detected in all mammalian species studied so far, including rodents. The reasons for the deletion of motilin function in rodents are unknown but may be related to the peculiar inability of these animals to vomit [7].

Ghrelin mRNA is most abundant in the gastric mucosa, but is also found in nearly all human tissues [8]. In contrast to ghrelin, motilin is found almost exclusively in the gut, with very limited detection of mRNA reported elsewhere [1]. Both hormones are located in large amounts in endocrine cells of the gastro-duodenal mucosa [9–11] and both are released during fasting. The release of motilin is believed to play a part in the cyclic pattern of gastrointestinal (GI) motility which occurs during fasting, known as the migrating motor complex (MMC). MMCs consist of a prolonged period of near-quiescence (phase I) followed by irregular, non-propulsive contractions (phase II) and then a short burst of high amplitude propulsive contractions (phase III). In humans and dogs, the release of motilin occurs in association with the phase III contractions which begin in the stomach [9], but not with those which begin in the small intestine [12].

Peptide Drug Discovery and Development: Translational Research in Academia and Industry, First Edition.
Edited by Miguel Castanho and Nuno C. Santos.
© 2011 WILEY-VCH Verlag GmbH & Co. KGaA, Weinheim.
Published 2011 by WILEY-VCH Verlag GmbH & Co. KGaA

The released motilin is thought to at least partly mediate the gastric phase III activity, as a motilin antibody inhibits this activity [13]. These propulsive movements help clear undigested material and prevent bacterial overgrowth in the upper gut [14, 15]. Gastric MMCs may also correlate with feelings of hunger [16, 17], perhaps by motilin releasing ghrelin to enhance appetite [18], and/or directly activating the vagus nerve [19, 20] to transmit information about the empty stomach to the brain.

Blood plasma concentrations of ghrelin peak just before a meal, supporting a role in stimulation of appetite [21], metabolism [22], and, perhaps, inhibition of emesis [23]. It has been suggested that this release of ghrelin is unable to significantly increase gastric emptying [24] but when higher plasma concentrations are achieved by administration of exogenous ghrelin, gastric emptying can be increased and phase III MMC-like activity induced [24, 25]. Away from the gut, smaller amounts of ghrelin are widely distributed in different regions and organs of the mammalian body [26, 22]. Whereas only one form of motilin is known, there are at least two forms of ghrelin – an acylated form created by post-translational modification of the peptide and active at the ghrelin receptor, and a non-acylated form (des-acylated ghrelin). The latter has been measured in blood plasma in amounts exceeding that of acylated ghrelin [22] and may act via a receptor that is distinct from the ghrelin receptor [27, 28], sometimes opposing the actions of acylated ghrelin (e.g., inhibition, not stimulation of rat gastric motility [29]).

13.1.2
Clinical Potential of Motilin and Ghrelin Receptor Agonists

The discovery that the antibiotic drug erythromycin could also activate the motilin receptor [30] provided a valuable tool to investigate the functions of motilin. Studies provided evidence that, in addition to stimulating phase III-like activity during fasting, motilin receptor activation can increase gastric emptying of meals. As such, erythromycin is used in patients requiring rapid intubation or endoscopy or the removal of gastric contents prior to endoscopy or surgery. The drug is also used to facilitate enteral feeding, help control blood glucose levels in diabetic patients and treat symptoms in patients with diabetic- or non-diabetic gastroparesis [7]. Erythromycin is generally without prokinetic activity in the colon [31]. In the upper gut, the prokinetic effects of high doses of erythromycin (250–400 mg, 4 × daily) are tolerated with repeat dosing [32], whereas the effects of lower doses appear well maintained (e.g., 50–100 mg 3 × daily and at bedtime [33]). Similarly, DiBiase and Quigley [34] titrated the dose of intravenous erythromycin in individual patients to achieve tolerance and efficacy during repeat administration. Nevertheless, erythromycin is an antibiotic drug and there are concerns over its use for GI disorders when antibiotic resistance continues to rise [35]. An ability of erythromycin to inhibit the cytochrome P450 enzyme CYP3A4 [36] also suggests an urgent need for a selective motilin receptor agonist.

Much has been written about ghrelin as a drug target, especially as a potential treatment of cachexia and inflammation [37, 38]. In addition, the upper GI prokinetic properties of ghrelin, together with its ability to promote appetite, suggest possible roles in the treatment of several different conditions, as exemplified by experiments on animal models of post-operative gastric ileus [39], septic ileus [40], dyspepsia [41], vomiting [23], and diabetic gastroparesis [42], and also by early clinical data with the ghrelin receptor agonist TZP-101 in patients with post-operative ileus [43] and gastroparesis [44]. At present, the use is for patients requiring relatively short-term treatments, until the widespread increase in endocrine functions caused by ghrelin is more fully understood. The need for caution is exemplified by a fall in insulin sensitivity caused by constant intravenous infusion of ghrelin [45].

An ability of ghrelin to increase colonic motility has not been observed in humans [46] although small molecule, brain-penetrant ghrelin receptor agonists may stimulate colonic motility, at least in rats [47].

13.2
Motilin and Ghrelin Receptor Agonists Under Development

Table 13.1 summarizes the compounds in development for GI disorders; older motilin receptor agonists no longer in development are described elsewhere, along with the reasons for their withdrawal [7, 48]. These older compounds were derivatives of erythromycin (known as "macrolides"; a term derived from a large macrocyclic lactone ring to which deoxy sugars are attached) and are often referred to as "motilides". The obvious difficulty in determining structure–activity relationships is now giving way to small molecule chemistry, in which more precise drug design can be achieved.

13.3
Translational Value of Preclinical Assays

With all receptor agonists it is essential to know that the potency, intrinsic activity, and desensitization liability of the molecule at the recombinant receptor (where most compounds are initially screened) correctly translates to the native receptor in therapeutically-relevant tissues. Thus, the coupling of a recombinant receptor to an effector mechanism in a host cell may not reflect that which exists in the native tissue.

13.3.1
Motilin

13.3.1.1 Assays Relevant to the Therapeutic Mechanism of Action
There is a large body of literature on the recombinant receptor (transfected into host cells) which looks at the ability of motilin receptor agonists to cause tachyphylaxis [65]. However, anomalies in correlating results from these studies with

Table 13.1 Motilin and ghrelin receptor agonists in development for GI disorders.

Approach	Compound	Significant activity
Motilin receptor agonist	Mitemcinal (GM-611)	• Macrolide, originally characterized as a molecule which mimicked the ability of motilin to cause short-lived contraction of rabbit isolated duodenal muscle, then profiled *in vivo* using a large number of different animal models [49]
		• Increased gastric emptying [50] and symptomatic relief has been obtained over a three-month period in a subset of patients with diabetic gastroparesis, a body mass index of <35 kg/m^2 and good glycemic control [51]
	GSK962040	• Non-macrolide small molecule, characterized using the recombinant receptor where translation to native tissues was confirmed by studies with rabbit and human isolated stomach [52]
		• Long-lasting facilitation of motor nerve activity demonstrated in human isolated stomach [53]
		• Increased gastric emptying in healthy volunteers [54] an effect maintained during 14 days of repeat dosing; adverse events were mild and comparable to placebo [55]
	RQ-00201894	• Non-macrolide small molecule active at the human recombinant receptor
		• Increased gastric emptying in dogs [56]
Ghrelin receptor agonist	TZP-101 (ulimorelin)	• Macrocyclic peptidomimetic. Affinity and efficacy determined by using the recombinant ghrelin receptor expressed in a host cell. May increase rat gastric emptying at doses which do not increase growth hormone secretion [57]
		• Dose-ranging phase II trial improved GI recovery in patients with post-operative ileus after abdominal surgery [58]. In another dose-ranging trial, 4 days of 30 min intravenous infusions improved symptoms of vomiting in patients with diabetic gastroparesis [59]
		• Dose-ranging phase II trial selected optimal dose (80 µg/kg IV infusion) which improved symptoms (loss of appetite, vomiting, postprandial fullness) 4 days after treatment in patients with diabetic gastroparesis [44]

Approach	Compound	Significant activity
	TZP-102	• Details not published for critical review but said to be orally-available and to have gastric prokinetic properties [60]
	Ipamorelin	• Pentapeptide, identified as a growth hormone secretagogue and shown to increase growth hormone release from rat primary pituitary cells, anesthetized rats and conscious pigs [61] • Intravenous infusions effective in rat model of post-operative ileus [62]
	ST-1141	• Said to be orally active, for the treatment of opioid-induced bowel dysfunction, but details not published for critical review [63]
	EX-1314	• Evaluated only by using the recombinant receptor expressed in a host cell, prior to *in vivo* studies; selectivity similarly determined against responses to the recombinant motilin receptor. GI prokinetic activity and ability to stimulate food intake studied in rodents [64]

the results of clinical trials have questioned how the recombinant systems should be used.

Lamian *et al.* [66] showed marked ligand-dependent differences in the kinetics of motilin receptor internalization in recombinant cells. ABT-229, a motilin receptor agonist without symptomatic benefit in patients with functional dyspepsia or diabetes [67, 68], displayed far greater tachyphylaxis than motilin or erythromycin. This was demonstrated by repeated application of the ligands in CHO cells (calcium mobilization response) and also in duodenal longitudinal muscle preparations (where motilin acts directly to cause muscle contraction) [65]. Further studies indicated that motilin, erythromycin, and ABT-229 encourage trafficking through G-protein receptor kinases and β-arrestin. ABT-229 was also phosphorylated by protein kinase C which has been implicated in longer desensitization times for a number of receptors; in CHO cells the time taken for the motilin receptor to recover from desensitization was 3 h and 1 h for motilin and erythromycin, respectively, but 26 h for ABT-229 [69]. Thus, one of several reasons generated to explain the clinical failure of ABT-229 is the strong tachyphylaxis found in these assays.

The concept that *in vitro* studies could predict the desensitization liability of a compound was subsequently confused by studies on the motilin receptor agonist mitemcinal. In rabbit duodenal muscle this compound caused a greater degree of tachyphylaxis that ABT-229 itself [70], yet in CHO cells expressing the human receptor, the desensitizing effect was less than that for ABT-229 [49]. In the clinic, repeat dosing with mitemcinal is an effective gastric prokinetic agent and may provide symptomatic relief over a 3-month period in a subset of patients with diabetic gastroparesis [49]. Similarly, repeated administration of low doses of erythromycin provides a maintained increase in gastric emptying [3, 34], further confusing the translational value of the *in vitro* assays described above.

Dass *et al.* [3] and Jarvie *et al.* [71] developed an alternative model, which looked at the ability of motilin receptor agonists to facilitate cholinergically-mediated contractions of rabbit isolated gastric antrum, caused by electrical stimulation of the intrinsic nerves. The approach was based on the observation that low doses of erythromycin stimulate gastric motility by increasing cholinergic activity [72], so an assay measuring the ability of motilin to enhance cholinergic activity must be a more physiologically-relevant system. Using this model, it was discovered that low concentrations of erythromycin facilitated cholinergic activity in a long-lasting manner, whereas a similar ability of $[Nle^{13}]$-motilin (a more stable analogue of the peptide) to excite cholinergic activity was relatively short; the difference was unaffected by peptidase inhibitors. Interestingly, higher concentrations of both compounds acted directly on the muscle to cause contractions which were in both cases were short-lived. Thus, these observations suggest that, for the native receptor, the kinetics of responses to motilin receptor agonists vary according to the ligand or to the cell-type in which the receptor is expressed (muscle or nerve). The reasons for these variations are unknown, but speculation has focused on the suggestion that motilin and erythromycin share a common binding site on the motilin receptor [73], whereas motilin, but not erythromycin, may occupy a second binding site on the receptor [74]. Perhaps the different binding sites promote ligand- and cell-dependent differences in how the receptor is desensitized and internalized downstream.

Similar observations have now been made using human isolated gastric antrum (Figure 13.1), in which both motilin and the motilin receptor agonist GSK962040 facilitated cholinergically-mediated contractions evoked by electrical stimulation. Again, the facilitation caused by motilin was significantly shorter than that caused by GSK962040 (times for the responses to fade by 50% were 21 min for motilin and >45 min for GSK962040 [53]). Importantly, the ability of GSK962040 to increase gastric emptying in healthy volunteers [54] was found to be sustained during repeated dosing [55]. Although preliminary, these data suggest that assays which measure enhancement of cholinergic activity *in vitro* are likely to provide meaningful assessments of both activity and desensitization liability *in vivo*.

An alternative to rabbits is provided by the house musk shrew of the order Insectivora, *Suncus murinus*. This small animal is capable of vomiting [75], a reflex absent in rodents or rabbits, and is, therefore, closer to the physiology of humans. The animals also express functional motilin receptors [55] and motilin receptor agonists produce a small enhancement of cholinergically-mediated contractions of the gastric antrum (unpublished observations). To date, insufficient studies have been carried out using these animals to determine how well the effects observed with different motilin receptor agonists translate in terms of *in vivo* efficacy.

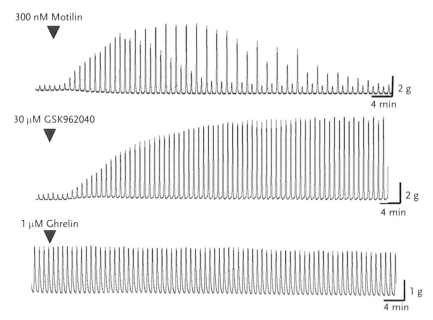

300 nM Motilin

30 μM GSK962040

1 μM Ghrelin

Figure 13.1 Facilitation of cholinergic activity in human isolated stomach by motilin and by the motilin receptor agonist GSK962040, but not by ghrelin. (Preparations were from the gastric antrum, cut in the direction of the circular muscle. Cholinergically-mediated contractions (prevented by atropine or by tetrodotoxin) were evoked by electrical field stimulation [53]. Ligands were added at maximal concentrations. Application of motilin facilitated the contractions but the facilitation becomes irregular and fades rapidly. GSK962040 facilitates electrically evoked contractions with no apparent fade in activity. Ghrelin has no effect on evoked contractions).

13.3.1.2 Assays Relevant to Possible Non-GI Activity

Most investigators have been unable to locate a functional motilin system in rodents, so reports describing actions of motilin in the brain of rats and mice must be treated with caution [6]. Elsewhere, some reports describe an action of motilin within the cardiovascular system. One abstract describes an ability of motilin to cause small contraction (maximum $\sim 19.8\%$ of that evoked by KCl) of human coronary arteries from six patients receiving a transplant because of cardiac or lung disease, but no effect of motilin in arteries from three other transplant patients, or a tiny maximum response ($<5\%$ KCl) in three others [76]. The possibility that these data might translate to a general cardiovascular effect is not supported by a study with critically ill patients, in which erythromycin (200 mg IV) increased gastric emptying but did not change systemic blood pressure or heart rate [77]. In another study erythromycin 300 mg oral was reported to cause a small reduction in systolic blood pressure [78]. In dogs, transient hypotensive activity could be evoked by [Leu^{13}]-motilin *in vivo* and *in vitro*, but in contrast to the ability of the peptide to stimulate gastric motility, this action was not prevented by appropriate concentrations of the motilin receptor antagonist GM-109 [79].

Similarly, motilin has been reported to relax precontracted porcine coronary artery muscle strips in an endothelium-dependent manner [80], but only at concentrations considerably higher (>3 μM) than those which activate the motilin receptor in other species.

13.3.2
Ghrelin

13.3.2.1 Assays Relevant to the Therapeutic Mechanism of Action

"Growth hormone secretagogues" were characterized in native tissues by studying their ability to stimulate growth hormone release, usually from rat isolated pituitary cells [37]. However, for compounds identified for GI use (Table 13.1), characterizations using recombinant receptors have been followed by studies *in vivo* rather than on isolated GI tissues. This reflects the difficulty of modeling the GI effects of ghrelin *in vitro*. For example, ghrelin facilitates cholinergic (and tachykinergic) activity in rat isolated stomach (in a manner qualitatively similar to that described above for motilin in rabbit stomach) but the effect is small [81] and insufficiently robust to survive the rigors of a full drug discovery screening cascade. Similar effects of ghrelin have been observed in mouse isolated stomach [82]. In human gastric antrum, ghrelin 10^{-6}M enhanced neuronally-mediated contractions evoked by electrical field stimulation, [46] but in our laboratory we have been unable to replicate this activity using a method which detects the prokinetic-like actions of motilin receptor agonists (Figure 13.1), again illustrating the lack of robustness of this type of response to ghrelin. Small differences in protocol, such as the presence or absence of mucosa, and the orientation of the muscle strips, may account for this variation. Excitatory activity was not detected in rabbit stomach (where the prokinetic-like effects of motilin are clearly apparent) [3] or in guinea-pigs (where ghrelin facilitated a nitrergic pathway instead), an animal in which ghrelin did increase gastric emptying *in vivo*, via a mechanism prevented by capsaicin pretreatment [83]. Others have shown that increased gastric emptying caused by ghrelin in rodents may be prevented by vagotomy [6]. Together, these studies suggest that the prokinetic activity of ghrelin is more dependent on vagal [84] than on enteric nerve activity.

Ghrelin receptor agonists progressed for GI use have been profiled by measuring their ability to increase gastric emptying and/or stimulate feeding, usually in rats or mice. For example, following determination of affinity and intrinsic activity at the recombinant human receptor only, the ghrelin receptor agonists EX-1314 and EX-1315 were shown to increase rat gastric emptying, and mouse small intestinal transit, feeding, and fecal output [64]. The route for progression of TZP-101 is not clear, but from presentations on the Trazyme website, it may be assumed that gastric emptying and feeding by rodents were key assays used to characterize the compound before further development.

13.3.2.2 Assays Relevant to Non-GI Activity

Ghrelin receptor agonists may have a variety of beneficial cardiovascular activities, including cardioprotection and a potential use as an adjunct therapy in end-stage heart failure [85, 86]. However, for GI uses of a ghrelin receptor agonist, a concern must be the fall in blood pressure caused by reduced peripheral artery resistance, observed during intravenous infusion of ghrelin at a plasma concentration approximately eight times higher than peak levels measured in normal fasted individuals [87]. Nevertheless, in healthy volunteers, a range of different intravenously-infused doses of the ghrelin receptor agonist TZP-101 increased the release of growth hormone and were well tolerated (except at the highest dose tested where transient bradycardia was observed, arguably because of increased parasympathetic drive) [88]. In patients with diabetic gastroparesis, the safety profiles associated with all doses of TZP-101 (including measurements of orthostatic hypotension and electrocardiograms) were similar to placebo [44].

13.4
Clinical Translation: Selecting the "Right" Patient Population

The critical questions to ask regarding any drug's possible efficacy are (i) what is the mechanism of action and (ii) what clinical symptoms or disease will be benefited by altering that particular action? There are good data regarding the effects on motility of exogenous motilin and ghrelin, derived from studies in humans (Table 13.2). Although it is clear that these prokinetic agents can alter motility patterns in expected ways, many studies do not show a close correlation between symptoms produced in healthy volunteers and motility effects [89].

The problem of finding the correct link between mode of action and clinical symptoms for motilin or ghrelin receptor agonists is complicated by the incomplete relationship between delayed gastric emptying and symptom pathogenesis. Nausea, vomiting, and fullness/distension are symptoms that empirically appear to correlate best with a delay in gastric emptying [90]. A more systematic attempt to correlate symptoms with mechanisms of action is reflected in the Gastroparesis Cardinal Symptom Index [91]. This index was based on patient reported assessment

Table 13.2 Physiological functions in humans resulting from motilin and ghrelin agonists.

Function	Motilin	Ghrelin
Improved gastric emptying	Y	Y
Increased LES pressure	Y	?
Induction of MMC phase III	Y (non-vagal)	Y (vagal)
Increased gallbladder emptying	Y	?
Increased colonic motility	?	?
Improved appetite	N	Y
Increased growth hormone release	N	Y

Yes (Y) or No (N).From [6, 24].

of symptoms, divided into three subscales with items related to post-prandial fullness, nausea or vomiting and bloating. Only the first two symptom sets were related to gastric emptying in a prospective series of 226 patients, and there was overlap between those with and without delayed gastric emptying [92].

The second cause of uncertainty between delayed gastric emptying and symptom generation is the heterogeneity of many of the disorders presenting with nausea, vomiting, or fullness. These symptoms might be related to gastro-intestinal, abdominal, or central nervous system abnormalities. Thus, it is not unexpected that symptom assignment to patients with delayed gastric emptying is not precise. The initial step in narrowing the clinical focus should be to select a disorder in which a high percentage of patients have delayed gastric emptying or other related physiological abnormality, such as low lower esophageal sphincter (LES) pressure or anorexia. Table 13.3 lists many of these conditions, classified by the associated abnormal function.

Depending on the stage of the disease, there may be differences in the prevalence of the abnormality. Some disorders appear to have progressively increased abnormality (e.g., type I diabetes mellitus, Parkinson's disease), while in others, the abnormality may be independent of disease stage (e.g., gastro-esophageal reflux disease (GERD), functional dyspepsia). The next section will discuss in more detail the considerations that might lead to selecting the "right" patient population for each clinical condition.

Table 13.3 Clinical disorders resulting from alterations in gastric emptying, upper GI motility or appetite.

Physiological function	Clinical disorder	Mechanism-related endpoints	Potential for motilin (M) or ghrelin (G) receptor agonists
Delayed gastric emptying, normal stomach	Critically ill patients	calorie provision, aspiration	M, G
	Major surgery	calorie provision	
	Migraine	nausea	
Delayed gastric emptying, abnormal stomach (gastroparesis)	Parkinson's disease	drug absorption	M,G
	Diabetes mellitus	symptoms: nausea, vomiting, bloating	
	Cyclic nausea & vomiting	symptoms	
	Post-viral	calorie provision	
	Functional dyspepsia	symptoms	
Low Lower Esophageal Sphincter pressure	GERD	reflux events	M,G
Decreased appetite	Cancer	calorie provision	G
	Anorexia nervosa	calorie provision	
	Post-prandial anorexia in elderly	calorie provision	

13.4.1
Critically Ill Patients with Delayed Gastric Emptying

Critically ill patients are subject to many alterations in GI function, among which is delayed gastric emptying (Table 13.4). This abnormality is clinically relevant, as it affects the ability to deliver an optimal enteral regimen of calories during the critical illness. Gastric emptying is frequently impaired (50–80%) in critically ill patients [93, 94]. One quarter of such patients have abnormal to absent MMC patterns [95]. The delayed gastric emptying seen in critically ill patients should be completely reversible with gastric prokinetics, because the pre-illness stomach of such patients should be normal. Consistent with this concept, prokinetic drugs (metoclopramide or erythromycin) are capable of restoring abnormal emptying rates to normal [96]. Some evidence suggests that intolerance to feeding may be related to hyperglycemia from inadequate blood glucose control [97]. However, it is difficult to stratify optimal nutritional management separate from intensive insulin therapy, so the two risk factors are not really independent. Moreover, intensive insulin therapy has led to decreased caloric provision in some trials, so the benefit in terms of altered gastric emptying and improved caloric provision cannot be properly assessed [98]. Thus, hyperglycemia is not included in Table 13.3.

Early enteral nutrition, within 36 h, leads to better intestinal immunity and decreased end-organ complications [100, 101]. Intolerance to nasogastric feeding due to slow gastric emptying occurs in up to half of critically ill patients, so that slow gastric emptying prevents early delivery of enteral nutrition [102]. Although the critically ill patients form a heterogenous group, patients selected for delayed gastric emptying should be reasonably similar in terms of gastric physiology, provided that confounders such as medication and hypotension are accounted for.

13.4.2
Patients with Gastroparesis

Gastroparesis is a term that refers to any condition in which delayed gastric emptying is observed in the absence of mechanical obstruction [103]. Thus, it is comparable to a symptom, not a disease. However, the diagnosis of gastroparesis often implies a relationship with other, specific gastrointestinal symptoms (see below) [104]. Causes of gastroparesis include post-surgical conditions, infections, CNS disorders (strokes, seizures, multiple sclerosis, dysautonomias), connective tissues diseases, and neuromuscular diseases (chronic intestinal pseudo-obstruction, myotonic dystrophy, amyloidosis). In most of these conditions the component of the presenting disease due to gastroparesis is relatively small. Some of the conditions listed above do indeed present with the symptoms felt to be related to delayed gastric emptying (i.e., nausea, vomiting, early satiety). These include chronic intestinal pseudoobstruction and post-infectious gastroparesis [105]. However, some patients with these conditions do not respond to currently available gastric prokinetic agents, perhaps because the underlying neuromuscular

Table 13.4 Mechanisms of abnormal GI motility in critically ill patients.

Organ	Abnormality	Mechanism	Evaluative test
Esophagus	• ineffective peristalsis • reduced LES pressure	• low blood pressure, sepsis • medication	manometry, tracheal reflux luminal impedence
Stomach	• increased gastric emptying	• increased pyloric tone • reduced antral motility • reduced fundic tone, drugs hyperglycemia, reduced vagal tone, increased retrograde duodenal waves	scintigraphy, CO_2 breath test acetaminophen absorption gastric residual volume
Small bowel	• increased phase III pattern • retrograde peristalsis • MMC from duodenum • reduced fat absorption, bacterial overgrowth	• opioids, other medications • post-operative neural changes • endotoxemia, increased PYY and cholecystokinin	manometry
Colon	• dilation • delayed transit time	• same as small bowel	imaging hydrogen breath test

From [94, 99].

physiology is so abnormal that no major improvement in gastric emptying is possible [33, 103] and/or because these drugs have poor efficacy as prokinetic agents. Erythromycin appears to be effective in improving symptoms in patients with gastroparesis, although the studies included in the meta-analysis were small, of short duration, and with inadequate symptom assessment [106].

There are diseases included in the differential diagnosis of gastroparesis in which a subgroup presents with gastroparesis-related symptoms that are dominant, and in which the underlying stomach still appears to be responsive to prokinetic agents. These syndromes may be better clinical targets for drug development of gastric prokinetics and are discussed below.

13.4.2.1 Diabetic Gastroparesis

This condition is often over diagnosed, and should be made only when symptoms are associated with delayed gastric emptying [104]. This definition of diabetic gastroparesis is not so easy to make in practice, as there is not a good correlation between gastric emptying abnormalities, blood sugar concentration, and symptoms [107]. Many studies in diabetic patients used a full pattern of upper GI symptoms (including abdominal pain and dyspepsia), rather than only nausea, vomiting, and early satiety, felt to reflect delayed gastric emptying [108, 109].

Delayed gastric emptying improves following oral erythromycin in diabetics [110], and the drug has even been reported to improve glycemic control, presumably by creating a more normal pattern of food delivery into the duodenum [111]. Ghrelin also improved gastric emptying in insulin-requiring diabetic patients [112]. Another motilin agonist, mitemcinal, accelerated gastric emptying, and improved symptomatic response in a subgroup of patients without obesity and with moderate glycemic control [50]. As with other studies in patients with gastroparesis, although the most common symptoms were nausea, early satiety, and bloating, over half the patients had abdominal pain. Thus, the evidence suggests that motilin agonists improve gastric emptying and symptoms in diabetic patients, but the proper patient subgroup has not yet been identified for pivotal drug development studies.

13.4.2.2 Parkinson's Disease

Delayed gastric emptying occurred in about 40% of a series of consecutive cases [113, 114], and is especially likely in patients with muscular rigor and tremor [113]. Delayed gastric emptying also occurs in the Parkinson-like syndrome of multiple system atrophy (MSA) diagnosed by similar clinical picture but with a different brain pattern on magnetic resonance imaging [115]. MSA has an estimated prevalence of 2–5/100 000, but not all MSA cases present with Parkinsonian features. It is unclear whether delayed gastric emptying is the cause of symptoms in patients with Parkinson's disease, but it does change the pharmacokinetics of levodopa absorption [116, 117]. Vomiting and postprandial abdominal fullness have not been associated with a delay in gastric emptying in Parkinson's patients, but this may be related to the nausea and vomiting that occur as adverse events from dopaminergic agents [113]. Longitudinal data relating neurological and gastrointestinal symptoms are needed to explore this relationship further.

13.4.2.3 Cyclic Nausea and Vomiting

Cyclic vomiting syndrome (CVS) is a disorder characterized by recurrent episodes of intractable nausea and vomiting with symptom-free intervals [118]. It is more often seen in children but can occur at all ages. Co-morbid migraine is found in 40 –60% of patients, and some experts consider this a variant of the migraine spectrum [119]. Assessing gastric emptying during episodes of nausea and vomiting has been difficult during acute attacks, but delayed emptying has been found when the test could be performed [120]. Between attacks rapid emptying has been found in some patients, but in others motility abnormalities were found, but without rapid emptying [121]. Electrogastrography has shown tachygastria and blunted wave amplitude following meals [120, 121]. One explanation for these discordant results is the finding of impaired antral contraction postprandially during, but not between, episodes [122]. Consistent with this observation is the response to erythromycin of children with cyclic vomiting who did not respond to metoclopramide [123]. These studies suggest that this group of patients develop their symptoms in response to inadequate gastric motility and decreased postprandial gastric emptying.

13.4.2.4 Migraine

Migraine is accompanied by symptoms suggesting abnormal autonomic function, including nausea and vomiting. Nausea has been reported in 46–56% of migraine patients, and vomiting in 18–24% of such patients [124]. Delayed gastric emptying has been reported both during and between migraine attacks [125], and in visually-induced migraine as well as in spontaneous episodes [126]. Metoclopramide has been reported to work as well as triptans in acute migraine, when it was combined with analgesic medication [127]. These data suggest that a subset of patients with migraine may have symptoms that are related to a delay in gastric emptying, and that the gastric dysfunction may persist even during interictal periods.

13.4.2.5 Functional Dyspepsia (FD)

This condition is a symptom complex that includes some of the symptoms felt to reflect delayed gastric emptying (nausea, vomiting, early satiety), but also epigastric pain, bloating, epigastric burning, and belching [128]. About one-third of patients show altered gastric emptying, although the correlation with specific symptoms has been poor [129]. FD has been reported to occur with an incidence of 15–30%, but this frequency is based on self-reported questionnaires of infrequent symptoms. Moreover, more than half of the patients with FD have irritable bowel syndrome, raising the possibility that these two conditions are different manifestations of the same disorder [129]. Because of the prevalence of the disorder, and the presence of delayed gastric emptying in a subgroup of patients, FD seems an attractive target for drug development.

Many attempts have been made to identify appropriate subgroups for use in studies with gastric prokinetics. FD is a syndrome that requires abdominal pain for its definition, and the patients with most pain correlated less well with delayed gastric emptying, although there was much overlap between the groups [130]. Factor analysis of symptom patterns of FD patients with weight loss showed that nausea, vomiting, early satiety, postprandial fullness, and bloating were most associated with visceral hypersensitivity and delayed gastric emptying [131]. Pain and epigastric burning were associated with severity of symptoms, but not so much with gastric emptying abnormalities. These studies do not clearly identify a subgroup that might respond to prokinetics, but suggest that pain is not a symptom that should respond reliably to such intervention. Consistent with this conclusion is the finding that erythromycin improves gastric emptying in FD patients, but without an effect on meal-related symptom severity [132]. Azithromycin, another macrolide antibiotic, has a similar effect on gastric emptying, but the effect on symptoms was not reported [133]. Patients with IBS have high interdigestive and postprandial motilin levels, suggesting that increasing motilin effect might not be useful in IBS, and, by implication, in FD [134]. Currently there is no agreement on a subgroup of FD that would provide an appropriate target for either motilin or ghrelin agonists.

13.4.2.6 Gastroesophageal Reflux Disease (GERD)

The process of gastric emptying is maximized by increased lower esophageal pressure, preventing the reflux of gastric contents during periods of increased intragastric pressure. These pressure differentials are responsible for part of the propulsive effects of gastric contractions, but the degree of this contribution is not known. It seems clear that symptoms of reflux that persist during acid suppressive therapy are related to non-acid reflux components [135]. Thus, prokinetics have seemed a logical addition to the management of GERD. Initial studies with prokinetics (especially cisapride) showed symptom improvement over placebo, but with the discovery of H_2 receptor antagonists (H_2RAs) and proton pump inhibitors (PPIs), and the much greater efficacy of these drugs by decreasing the acid refluxate, prokinetics are no longer licensed for this indication [136]. Addition of the prokinetic, mosapride, to lansoprazole in patients with GERD showed some added effect in those patients with the most symptoms [137]. Additional support for an additive effect of preventing reflux comes from the finding that reflux symptoms in patients with gastroparesis are improved by radioablation treatment of the cardia and esophageal junction [138]. In fact, the gastroparesis improved in these patients, suggesting an abnormality in vagal tone to explain the gastroparesis.

In children with reflux, symptoms are improved by Gaviscon and by H_2RAs, but the evidence is less good for the prokinetics domperidone and metoclopramide [139]. However, erythromycin appears to be effective, along with acid suppression, in treating GERD in preterm infants [140]. These data would support the use of gastric prokinetics in patients with GERD who continue to have reflux and reflux-induced symptoms while taking optimal doses of PPIs. Other potential study groups include prevention of pulmonary aspiration due to reflux in lung transplant and other critically ill patients [141].

13.4.2.7 **Anorexia and Decreased Appetite (Ghrelin Agonists Only)**

Anorexia and decreased appetite are usually symptoms of complex diseases, and have proved relatively resistant to any intervention. Cancer anorexia has been the most studied, but even in that condition the causes are poorly understood. They include abnormal neurohormonal signaling in regulating appetite and satiety, and in overproduction of pro-inflammatory cytokines [142]. Pharmacological options have included corticosteroids and progestational agents, most commonly meges-trol acetate [143]. These agents demonstrate modest efficacy, but the effects are relatively short lived. Megestrol is most commonly used, but its efficacy seems related to the portion of weight loss that is due to pain [144]. Ghrelin has been suggested as potentially useful in tumors such as head-neck cancer, in which the inability to eat is more related to radiation therapy rather than widespread tumor invasion [145]. Patients in whom the anorexia is not related to the underlying tumor, but to adverse effects of radiation or chemotherapy, may provide the best groups to first test the utility of ghrelin agonists on appetite, but the effect on cancer anorexia will require a highly selected group with advanced cancer and perhaps a more complex study design to provide a period of clinical stability.

13.5
Clinical Development of Motilin and Ghrelin Receptor Agonists

The most advanced motilin receptor agonist currently in clinical development, is the motilide mitemcinal [146]. This compound was assessed in a phase II study in patients with idiopathic and diabetic gastroparesis who showed delayed gastric emptying, and was then re-evaluated in diabetic patients with symptomatic gas-troparesis and normal or delayed gastric emptying. The first study confirmed the ability of mitemcinal to increase gastric emptying over a month of repeated dosing, but the overall symptomatic benefit was unimpressive; increased gastric emptying not, therefore, always lead to symptomatic relief in these patients [50]. In the latter study [51], a *post hoc* analysis showed that the compound provided symptomatic relief over three months in a subset of patients with diabetic gastroparesis, a body mass index of $<35\,\mathrm{kg/m^2}$ and good glycemic control; a high placebo response was argued to explain the modest response. Overall, these data suggest that at least some benefit may be obtained by motilin receptor activation, but that care needs to be taken to select the correct patient population.

The small molecule motilin receptor agonist GSK962040 has shown an ability to increase gastric emptying ($[^{13}C]$-octanoic acid breath method) in healthy volunteers when the compound was administered as a single dose [54], an effect maintained during a 14 day repeat dose phase I trial in which mild adverse events were distributed evenly between the drug-treated and placebo-treated groups [55].

The most advanced ghrelin receptor agonist in development for GI disorders is TZP-101 (ulimorelin). This is an intravenously-administered compound, well tolerated in healthy volunteers and shown to increase growth hormone release [88]. In patients with diabetes and symptomatic gastroparesis, gastric emptying was increased by a single infusion of TZP-101 [147]. In a dose-ranging phase II trial, TZP-101 was given daily for up to 7 days and improved GI recovery in patients with post-operative ileus after abdominal surgery [58]. A further trial showed that daily 30 min intravenous infusions of TZP-101 over 4 days reduced the severity of vomiting in hospitalized patients with diabetic gastroparesis; a range of doses was apparently studied but the doses were not stated in the abstract [59].

13.6
Conclusions

There is a great unmet clinical need for a new and effective gastric prokinetic agent, suitable for use in a number of different disorders associated with delayed gastric emptying; selective motilin and ghrelin receptor agonists are being developed for this purpose.

Until recently, motilin receptor agonists were complex macrolide structures, hampering structure–activity studies and drug design. There was also a misconception that motilin receptor activation caused rapid desensitization of its own response, limiting enthusiasm for the target [6]. However, these difficulties are beginning to be overcome by studies with mitemcinal and by the discovery of small molecule motilin receptor agonists. Successful development of this class of agent will now depend on their evaluation in an uncomplicated, non-symptomatic model of a disease in which an increased gastric emptying is likely to be of benefit.

The complex biology of ghrelin receptor agonists makes these agents interesting in terms of the type of patient population which may be treated, but also more risky because of the danger of unwanted endocrine-mediated adverse events. Perhaps this complexity explains why the preclinical characterization of ghrelin receptor agonists has not been as rigorous as those for motilin. For example, the difficulty of designing therapeutically-meaningful isolated tissue assays for ghrelin has meant that the intrinsic activities of new molecules have often only been evaluated using the recombinant receptor before testing *in vivo*. Nevertheless, encouraging preliminary data have been obtained with one compound under evaluation for GI disorders, and others are following.

For each type of molecule, progress in the clinic must now be followed with great interest.

References

1 McKee, K.K., Tan, C.P., Palyha, O.C., Liu, J., Feighner, S.D., Hreniuk, D.L., Smith, R.G., Howard, A.D., and Van der Ploeg, L.H.T. (2007) Cloning and characterization of two human G protein-coupled receptor genes (GPR38 and GPR39) related to the growth hormone secretagogue and neurotensin receptors. *Genomics*, **46**, 426–434

2 Folwaczny, C., Chang, J.K., and Tschöp, M. (2001) Ghrelin and motilin: two sides of one coin?. *Eur. J. Endocrinol.*, **144**, R1–R3.

3 Dass, N.B., Hill, J., Muir, A., Testa, T., Wise, A., and Sanger, G.J. (2003) The rabbit motilin receptor: molecular characterisation and pharmacology. *Br. J. Pharmacol.*, **140**, 948–954.

4 Peeters, T.L. (2003) Central and peripheral mechanisms by which ghrelin regulates gut motility. *J. Physiol. Pharmacol.*, **54** (Suppl. 4), 95–103.

5 He, J., Irwin, D.M., Chen, R., and Zhang, Y. (2010) Stepwise loss of motilin and its specific receptor genes in rodents. *J. Mol. Endocrinol.*, **44**, 37–44.

6 Sanger, G.J. (2008) Motilin, ghrelin and related neuropeptides as targets for the treatment of GI diseases. *Drug Discov. Today*, **13**, 234–239.

7 Sanger, G.J., Holbrook, J.D., and Andrews, P.L. (2011) The translational value of rodent gastrointestinal functions: a cautionary tale. *Trends Pharmacol Sci*, **32** (7), 402–409.

8 Gnanapavan, S., Bustin, B., Morris, D. G., McGee, P., Fairclough, P., Bhattacharya, S., Carpenter, R., Grossman, A.B., and Korbonits, M. (2002) The tissue distribution of the mRNA of ghrelin and subtypes of its receptor, GHS-R in humans. *J. Clin. Endocrinol. Metab.*, **87**, 2988–2991.

9 Itoh, Z. (1997) Motilin and clinical application. *Peptides*, **18**, 593–608.

10 Kojima, M., Hosoda, H., Date, Y., Nakazato, M., Matsuo, H., and Kangawa, K. (1999) Ghrelin is a growth-hormone-releasing acylated peptide from stomach. *Nature*, **402**, 656–660.

11 Wierup, N., Björkqvist, M., Westrom, B., Pierzynowski, S., Sundler, F., and Sjölund, K. (2007) Ghrelin and motilin are cosecreted from a prominent endocrine cell population in the small intestine. *J. Clin. Endocrinol. Metab.*, **92**, 3573–3581.

12 Nakajima, H., Mochiki, E., Zietlow, A., Ludwig, K., and Takahashi, T. (2010) Mechanism of interdigestive migrating motor complex in conscious dogs. *J. Gastroenterol.*, **45**, 506–514.

13 Lee, K.Y., Chang, T.M., and Chey, W.Y. (1983) Effect of rabbit antimotilin serum on myoelectric activity and plasma motilin concentration in fasting dog. *Am. J. Physiol.*, **245**, G547–G553.

14 Vantrappen, G., Janssens, J., Peeters, T.L., Bloom, S.R., Christofides, N.D., and Hellmans, J. (1979) Motilin and the interdigestive migrating motor complex in man. *Dig. Dis. Sci.*, **24**, 497–500.

15 Husebye, E. (1999) The patterns of small bowel motility: physiology and implications in organic disease and functional disorders. *Neurogastroenterol. Motil.*, **11**, 141–161.

16 Ang, D.C., Nicolai, H., Vos, R., Berghe, P.V., Sifrim, D., Depoortere, I., Peeters, T.L., Janssens, J., and Tack, J.F. (2008) Hunger scores correlate with the occurrence of pharmacologically induced gastric phase 3 in man. *Gastroenterology*, **134** (4, S1), A–285.

17 Ang, D.C., Nicolai, H., Vos, R., Berghe, P.V., Sifrim, D., Depoortere, I., Peeters, T.L., Janssens, J., and Tack, J.F. (2008) Gastric phase 3 is a hunger signal in the interdigestive state in man. *Gastroenterology*, **134** (4, S1), A–314.

18 Zeitlow, A.M., Ludwig, K.A., and Takahashi, T. (2010) Association between plasma ghrelin and motilin levels during interdigestive MMC cycle in conscious dogs. *Gastroenterology*, **138** (5, S1), S–737.

19 Mochiki, E., Inui, A., Satoh, M., Mizumoto, A., and Itoh, Z. (1997) Motilin is a biosignal controlling cyclic release of pancreatic polypeptide via the vagus in fasted dogs. *Am. J. Physiol.*, **272**, G224–G232.

20 Suzuki, H., Mochiki, E., Haga, N., Satoh, M., Mizumoto, A., and Itoh, Z. (1998) Motilin controls cyclic release of insulin through vagal cholinergic muscarinic pathways in fasted dogs. *Am. J. Physiol.*, **274**, G87–G95.

21 Cummings, D.E., Purnell, J.Q., Frayo, R.S., Schmidova, K., Wisse, B.E., and Weigle, D.S. (2001) A preprandial rise in plasma ghrelin levels suggests a role in meal initiation in humans. *Diabetes*, **50**, 1714–1719.

22 Chen, C.-Y., Asakawa, A., Fujimya, M., Lee, S.-D., and Inui, A. (2009) Ghrelin

gene products and the regulation of food intake and gut motility. *Pharmacol. Rev.*, **61**, 430–481.

23 Rudd, J.A., Ngan, M., Wai, M.K., King, A.G., Witherington, J., Andrews, P.L.R., and Sanger, G.J. (2006) Anti-emetic activity of ghrelin in ferrets exposed to the cytotoxic anti-cancer agent cisplatin. *Neurosci. Lett.*, **392**, 79–83

24 Camilleri, M., Papathanasopoulos, A., and Odunsi, S.T. (2009) Action and therapeutic pathways of ghrelin for gastrointestinal disorders. *Nature Rev. Gastroenterol. Hepatol.*, **6**, 343–352.

25 Tack, J., Depoortere, I., Bisschops, R., Delporte, C., Coulie, B., Meulemans, A., Janssens, J., and Peeters, T. (2006) Influence of ghrelin on interdigestive gastrointestinal motility in humans. *Gut*, **55**, 327–333.

26 Ghelardoni, S., Carnicelli, V., Frascarelli, S., Ronca-Testoni, S., and Zucchi, R. (2006) Ghrelin tissue distribution: comparison between gene and protein expression. *J. Endocrinol. Invest.*, **29**, 115–121.

27 Toshinai, K., Yamaguchi, H., Sun, Y., Smith, R.G., Yamanaka, A., Sakurai, T., Date, Y., Mondal, M.S., Shimbara, T., Kawagoe, T., Murakami, N., Miyazato, M., Kangawa, K., and Nakazato, M. (2006) Des-acyl ghrelin induces food intake by a mechanism independent of the growth hormone secretagogue receptor. *Endocrinology*, **147**, 2306–2314.

28 Lear, P.V., Iglesias, M.J., Feijóo-Bandin, S., Rodriguez-Penas, D., Mosquera-Leal, A., Garcia-Rua, V., Gualilo, O., Ghè, C., Arnoletti, E., Muccioli, G., Diéguez, C., González-Juanatey, J.R., and Lago, F. (2010) Des-acyl ghrelin has specific binding sites and different metabolic effects from ghrelin cardiomyocytes. *Endocrinology*, **151**, 3286–3298

29 Fujimiya, M., Asakawa, A., Ataka, K., and Inui, A. (2008) Different effects of ghrelin, des-acyl ghrelin and obestatin on gastroduodenal motility in conscious rats. *World J. Gastroenterol.*, **14**, 6318–6326.

30 Peeters, T., Matthijs, G., Depoortere, I., Cachet, T., Hoogmartens, J., and Vantrappen, G. (1989) Erythromycin is a motilin receptor agonist. *Am. J. Physiol.*, **257**, G470–G474.

31 Venkatasubramani, N., Rudolph, C.D., and Sood, M.R. (2008) Erythromycin lacks colon prokinetic effect in children with functional gastrointestinal disorders: a retrospective study. *BMC Gastroenterol.*, **8**, 38 (http://www.biomedcentral.com/1471-230X/8/38).

32 Richards, R.D., Davenport, K., and McCallum, R.W. (1993) The treatment of idiopathic and diabetic gastroparesis with acute intravenous and chronic oral erythromycin. *Am. J. Gastroenterol.*, **88**, 203–207.

33 Dhir, R. and Richter, J.E. (2004) Erythromycin in the short- and long-term control of dyspepsia symptoms in patients with gastroparesis. *J. Clin. Gastroenterol.*, **38**, 237–242.

34 Dibaise, J.K. and Quigley, E.M. (1999) Efficacy of prolonged administration of intravenous erythromycin in an ambulatory setting as treatment of severe gastroparesis: one centre's experience. *J. Clin. Gastroenterol.*, **28**, 131–134.

35 Hawkyard, C.V. and Koerner, R.J. (2007) The use of erythromycin as a gastrointestinal prokinetic agent in adult critical care: benefits versus risks. *J. Antimicrob. Chemother.*, **59**, 347–358.

36 Zhou, S., Chan, E., Lim, L.Y., Boelsterli, U.A., Li, S.C., Wang, J., Zhang, Q., Huang, M., and Xu, A. (2004) Therapeutic drugs that behave as mechanism-based inhibitors of cytochrome P450 3AA. *Curr. Drug Metab.*, **5**, 415–442.

37 Moulin, A., Ryan, J., Martinez, J., and Fehrentz, J.-A. (2007) Recent developments in ghrelin receptor ligands. *ChemMedChem*, **2**, 1242–1259.

38 Ashitani, J.-I., Matsumoto, N., and Nakazato, M. (2009) Ghrelin and its therapeutic potential for cachectic patients. *Peptides*, **30**, 1951–1956.

39 Trudel, L., Bouin, M., Tomasetto, C., Eberling, P., St-Pierre, S., Bannon, P., L'Heureux, M.C., and Poitras, P. (2003)

Two new peptides to improve post-operative gastric ileus in dog. *Peptides*, **24**, 531–534.

40 De Winter, B.Y., De Man, J.G., Seerden, T.C., Depoortere, I., Herman, A.G., Peeters, T.L., and Pelckmans, P. A. (2004) Effect of ghrelin and growth hormone-releasing peptide 6 on septic ileus in mice. *Neurogastroenterol. Motil.*, **16**, 439–446.

41 Liu, Y.-L., Malik, N.M., Sanger, G.J., and Andrews, P.L. (2006) Ghrelin alleviates cancer chemotherapy-associated dyspepsia in mice. *Cancer Chemother. Pharmacol.*, **58**, 326–333.

42 Qiu, W.C., Wang, Z.G., Wang, W.G., Yan, J., and Zheng, Q. (2008) Gastric motor effects of ghrelin and growth hormone releasing peptide 6 in diabetic mice with gastroparesis. *World J. Gastroenterol.*, **14**, 1419–1424.

43 Popescu, I., Fleshner, P., Pezzullo, J., Charlon, P., Kosutic, G., and Senagore, A. (2010) The ghrelin agonist TZP-101 for management of postoperative ileus after partial colectomy: a randomized, dose-ranging, placebo-controlled clinical trial. *Dis. Colon Rectum*, **53**, 126–134.

44 Ejsjaer, N., Dimcevski, G., Wo, J., Hellström, P.M., Gormsen, L.C., Sarosiek, I., Softeland, E., Nowak, T., Pezzullo, J.C., Shaugnessy, L., Kosutic, G., and McCallum, R. (2010) Safety and efficacy of ghrelin agonist TZP-101 in relieving symptoms in patients with diabetic gastroparesis: a randomized, placebo-controlled study. *Neurogastroenterol. Motil.*, doi 10.1111sj.1365–2982.2010.01519.x.

45 Vestergaard, E.T., Hansen, T.K., Gormsen, L.C., Jakobsen, P., Moller, N., Christiansen, J.S., and Jorgensen, J. O.L. (2007) Constant intravenous ghrelin infusion in healthy young men: clinical pharmacokinetics and metabolic effects. *Am. J. Physiol.*, **292**, E1829–E1836.

46 Falkén, Y., Hellström, P.M., Sanger, G. J., Dewit, O., Dukes, G., Grybäck, P., Holst, J.J., and Näslund, E. (2010) Actions of prolonged ghrelin infusion on gastrointestinal transit and glucose

homeostasis in humans. *Neurogastroenterol. Motil.*, **22**, e192–200.

47 Shafton, A.D., Sanger, G.J., Witherington, J., Brown, J.D., Muir, A., Butler, S., Abberley, L., Shimizu, Y., and Furness, J.B. (2009). Oral administration of a centrally-acting ghrelin receptor agonist to conscious rats triggers defecation. *Neurogastroenterol. Motil.*, **21**, 71–77.

48 Westaway, S.M. and Sanger, G.J. (2009) The identification and rationale for drugs which act at the motilin receptor. *Prog. Med. Chem.*, **48**, 31–80 (ed. G. Lawton and D. Witty).

49 Takanashi, H. and Cynshi, O. (2009) Motilides: a long and winding road: lessons from mitemcinal (GM-611) on diabetic gastroparesis. *Reg. Pept.*, **155**, 18–23.

50 McCallum, R.W., Cynshi, O., and Investigator team. (2007) Effects of a motilin agonist (mitemcinal) on gastric emptying in patients with gastroparesis: a randomized, multi-center, placebo-controlled trial. *Aliment Pharmacol. Ther.*, **26**, 1121–1130.

51 McCallum, R.W., Cynshi, O., and Investigator team. (2007) Efficacy of mitemcinal, a motilin receptor agonist, on gastrointestinal symptoms in patients with symptoms suggesting diabetic gastropathy: a randomized, multi-centere, placebo-controlled trial. *Aliment. Pharmacol. Ther.*, **26**, 107–116.

52 Sanger, G.J., Westaway, S.M., Barnes, A.A., MacPherson, D.T., Muir, A.I., Jarvie, E.M., Bolton, V., Cellek, S., Näslund, E., Hellström, P.M., Borman, R.A., Unsworth, W.P., Matthews, K.L., and Lee, K. (2009) GSK962040: a small molecule, selective motilin receptor agonist, effective as a stimulant of human and rabbit gastrointestinal motility. *Neurogastroenterol. Motil.*, **21**, 657–666.

53 Broad, J., Mukherjee, S., Boundouki, G., Dukes, G.E., and Sanger, G.J. (2010) Different abilities of [Nle[13]]-motilin and the motilin receptor agonist GSK962040 to facilitate cholinergic and nitrergic activity in human isolated stomach. *Neurogastroenterol. Motil.*, **22** (S1), 84.

54 Dukes, G.E., Barton, M., Dewit, O., Hicks, K., Vasist, L., Van Hecken, A., De Hoon, J., Verbeke, K., Young, M., Williams, P., and Alpers, D. (2009) Pharmacokinetics, safety/tolerability, and effect on gastric emptying of the oral motilin receptor agonist, GSK962040, in healthy male and female volunteers. *Neurogastroenterol. Motil.*, **21** (S1), 84.

55 Dukes, G.E., Barton, M., Dewit, O., Stephens, K., Vasist, L., Young, M., Richards, D., Alpers, D., and Williams, P. (2010) Safety/tolerability, pharmacokinetics (PK), and effect on gastric emptying(GE) with 14-days repeat oral dosing of the motilin receptor agonist, GSK962040, in healthy male and female volunteers. *Neurogastroenterol. Motil.*, **22** (S1), 14–15.

56 Takahashi, N., Koba, N., Yamamoto, T., and Sudo, M. (2010) Characterization of a novel, potent, and selective small molecule motilin receptor agonist, RQ-00201894. *Gastroenterology*, **138** (5, S1), S–713.

57 Fraser, G.L., Hoveyda, H.R., and Tannenbaum, G.S. (2005) Pharmacological demarcation of the growth hormone, gut motility and feeding effects of ghrelin using a novel ghrelin receptor agonist. *Endocrinology*, **149**, 6280–6288.

58 Popescu, I., Fleshner, P.R., Pezzullo, J.C., Charlton, P.A., Kosutic, G., and Senagore, A.J. (2010). The ghrelin agonist TZP-101 for management of postoperative ileus after partial colectomy: a randomized, dose-ranging, placebo-controlled clinical trial. *Dis. Colon Rectum*, **53**, 126–134.

59 Wo, J., Malik, R., Nowak, T., Snape, W., Hellström, P.M., Shaughnessy, L., Kosutic, G., and McCallum, R. (2010) TZP-101 (ghrelin agonist) effects on daily vomiting due to diabetic gastroparesis (GP): phase 2 subset analysis. *Neurogastroenterol. Motil.*, **22** (S1), 13–14.

60 http://www.tranzyme.com/pipeline.html

61 Raun, K., Hansen, B.S., Johansen, N.L., Thogersen, H., Madsen, K., Ankersen, M., and Andersen, P.H. (1998) Ipamorelin, the first selective growth hormone secretagogue. *Eur. J. Endocrinol.*, **139**, 552–561

62 Venkova, K., Mann, W., Nelson, R., and Greenwood-Van Meerveld, B. (2009) Efficacy of ipamorelin, a novel ghrelin mimetic, in a rodent model of postoperative ileus. *J. Pharmacol. Exp. Ther.*, **329**, 1110–1116.

63 http://www.helsinn.com/

64 Charoenthongtrakul, S., Giuliana, D., Longo, K.A., Govek, E.K., Nolan, A., Gangne, S., Morgan, K., Hixon, J., Flynn, N., Murphy, B.J., Hernández, A.S., Li, J., Tino, J.A., Gordon, D.A., DiStefano, P.S., and Geddes, B.J. (2009) Enhanced gastrointestinal motility with orally active ghrelin receptor agonists. *J. Pharmacol. Exp. Ther.*, **329**, 1178–1188.

65 Thielemans, L., Depoortere, I., Perret, J., Robberecht, P., Liu, Y., Thijs, T., Carreras, C., Burgeon, E., and Peeters, T.L. (2005) Desensitization of the human motilin receptor by motilides. *J. Pharmacol. Exp. Ther.*, **313**, 1397–1405.

66 Lamian, V., Rich, A., Ma, Z., Li, J., Seethala, R., Gordon, D., and Dubaquie, Y. (2006) Characterization of agonist-induced motilin receptor trafficking and its implications for tachyphylaxis. *Mol. Pharmacol.*, **69**, 109–118.

67 Talley, N.J., Verlinden, M., Snape, W., Beker, J.A., Ducrotte, P., Dettmer, A., Brinkhoff, H., Eaker, E., Ohning, G., Miner, P.B., Mathias, J.R., Fumagalli, I., Staessen, D., and Mack, R.J. (2000) Failure of a motilin receptor agonist (ABT-229) to relieve the symptoms of functional dyspepsia in patients with and without delayed gastric emptying: a randomized double-blind placebo-controlled trial. *Aliment. Pharmacol. Ther.*, **14**, 1653–1661.

68 Talley, N.J., Verlinden, M., Geenen, D., Hogan, R., Riff, D., McCallum, R., and Mack, R. (2001) Effects of a motilin receptor agonist (ABT-229) on upper gastrointestinal symptoms in type 1 diabetes mellitus: a randomised, double blind, placebo controlled trial. *Gut*, **49**, 395–401.

69 Mitselos, A., Vanden Berghe, P., Peeters, T.L., and Depoortere, I. (2008) Differences in motilin receptor desensitization after stimulation with motilin or motilides are due to alternative receptor trafficking. *Biochem. Pharmacol.*, **75**, 1115–1128.

70 Carreras, C.W., Claypool, M., Santi, D. V., Schuurkes, J.A.J., Peeters, T.L., and Johnson, R.G. (2004) Tachyphylaxis assays for motilin agonist drug development, *Gastroenterology*, **126** (4 Suppl. 2), A–276.

71 Jarvie, E.M., North Laidler, V., Corcoran, S., Bassil, A., and Sanger, G. J. (2007) Differences between the abilities of tegaserod and motilin receptor agonists to stimulate gastric motility *in vitro. Br. J. Pharmacol.*, **150**, 455–462.

72 Coulie, B., Tack, J., Peeters, T., and Janssens, J. (1998) Involvement of two different pathways in the motor effects of erythromycin on the gastric antrum in humans. *Gut*, **43**, 395–400.

73 Xu, L., Depoortere, I., Vertongen, P., Waelbroeck, M., Robberecht, P., and Peeters, T.L. (2005) Motilin and erythromycin-A share a common binding site in the third transmembrane segment of the motilin receptor. *Biochem. Pharmacol.*, **70**, 879–887.

74 Matsuura, B., Dong, M., Naik, S., Miller, L.J., and Onji, M. (2006) Differential contributions of motilin receptor extracellular domains for peptide and non-peptidyl agonist binding and activity. *J. Biol. Chem.*, **281**, 12390–12396.

75 Ueno, S., Matsuki, N., and Saito, H. (1987) Suncus murinus: a new experimental model in emesis research. *Life Sci.*, **41**, 513–518.

76 Maguire, J.J., Kuc, R.E., and Davenport, A.P. (2004) Motilin mediates vasoconstriction in human coronary artery *in vitro. Proc. Br. Pharmacol. Soc.*, at http://www.pa2online.org/ Vol2Issue2abst116P.hyml

77 Nguyen, N.Q., Mangoni, A.A., Fraser, R.J., Chapman, M., Brtyant, L., Burgstad, C., and Holloway, R.H. (2006) Prokinetic therapy with erythromycin has no significant impact on blood pressure and heart rate in critically ill patients. *Br. J. Clin. Pharmacol.*, **63**, 498–500.

78 Mangoni, A.A., Close, J.C., Rodriguez, S., Sherwood, R.A., Bryant, C.A., Swift, C.G., and Jackson, S.H. (2004) Acute hypotensive effects of oral cisapride and erythromycin in healthy subjects. *Br. J. Clin. Pharmacol.*, **58**, 223–224.

79 Iwai, T., Nakamura, H., Takanashi, H., Yogo, K., Ozaki, K., Ishizuka, N., and Asano, T. (1998) Hypothensive mechanism of [Leu13]motilin in dogs *in vivo* and *in vitro. Can. J. Physiol. Pharmacol.*, **76**, 1103–1109.

80 Higuchi, Y., Nishimura, J., and Kanaide, H. (1994) Motilin induces the endothelium-dependent relaxation of smooth muscle and the elevation of cytosolic calcium in endothelial cells *in situ. Biochem. Biophys. Res. Commun.*, **202**, 346–353.

81 Bassil, A., Dass, N.M., and Sanger, G.J. (2006) The gastric prokinetic-like activity of ghrelin in rat isolated stomach is mediated via cholinergic and tachykininergic motor neurones. *Eur. J. Pharmacol.*, **544**, 146–152.

82 Kitazawa, T., De Smet, B., Verbeke, K., Depoortere, I., and Peeters, T.L. (2005) Gastric motor effects of peptide and non-peptide ghrelin agonists in mice *in vivo* and *in vitro. Gut*, **54**, 1078–1084.

83 Nakamura, T., Onaga, T., and Kitazawa, T. (2010) Ghrelin stimulates gastric motility of the guinea-pig through activation of a capsaicin-sensitive neural pathway: *in vivo* and *in vitro* functional studies. *Neurogastroenterol. Motil.*, **22**, 446–452.

84 Page, A.J., Slattery, J.A., Milte, C., Laker, R., O'Donnell, T., Dorian, C., Brierley, S.M., and Blackshaw, L.A. (2007) Ghrelin selectively reduces mechanosensitivity of upper gastrointestinal vagal afferents. *Am. J. Physiol.*, **292**, G1376–G1384.

85 Garcia, E.A. and Korbonitis, M. (2005) Ghrelin and cardiovascular health. *Curr. Opin. Pharmacol.*, **6**, 142–147.

86 Tesauro, M., Schinzari, F., Caramanti, M., Lauro, R., and Cardillo, C. (2010) Metabolic and cardiovascular effects of ghrelin. *Int. J. Pept.*, Article ID 864342. doi 10.1155/2010/864342.

87 Nagaya, N., Kojima, M., Uematsu, M., Yamagishi, M., Hosoda, H., Oya, H., Hayashi, Y., and Kangawa, K. (2001) Hemodynamic and hormonal effects of human ghrelin in healthy volunteers. *Am. J. Physiol.*, **280**, R1483–R1487.

88 Lasseter, K.C., Shaughnessy, L., Cummings, D., Pezzullo, J.C., Wargin, W., Gagnon, R., Oliva, J., and Kosutic, G. (2008) Ghrelin agonist (TZP-101): Safety, pharmacokinetics and pharmacodynamic evaluation in healthy volunteers: a phase I, first-in-human study. *J. Clin. Pharmacol.*, **48**, 193–202.

89 Korimilli, A. and Parkman, H.P. (2009) Effect of atilmotin, a motilin receptor agonist, on esophageal, lower esophageal sphincter, and gastric pressures. *Dig. Dis. Sci.*, **55**, 300–306.

90 Quigley, E.M. (2004) Review article: gastric emptying in functional gastrointestinal disorders. *Aliment. Pharmacol. Ther.*, **20** (Suppl. 7), s56–s60.

91 Revicki, D.A., Reutz, A.M., Dubois, D., Kahrilas, P., Stanghellini, V., Talley, N.J., and Tack, J. (2004) Gastroparesis Cardinal Symptom Index (GCSI): development and validation of a patient-reported assessment of severity of gastroparesis symptoms. *Qual. Life Res.*, **13**, 833.

92 Cassilly, D.W., Wang, Y.R., Friedenberg, F.K., Nelson, D.B., Maurer, A.H., and Parkman, H.P. (2008) Symptoms of gastroparesis: use of the gastroparesis cardinal symptom index in symptomatic patients referred for gastric emptying scintigraphy. *Digestion*, **78**, 144–171.

93 Booth, C.M., Heyland, D.K., and Paterson, W.G. (2002) Gastrointestinal promotility drugs in the critical care

setting: a systematic review of the evidence. *Crit. Care Med.*, **30**, 1429–1435.

94 Ritz, M.A., Fraser, R., Tam, W., and Dent, J. (2000) Impacts and patterns of disturbed gastrointestinal function in critically ill patients. *Am. J. Gastroenterol.*, **95**, 3044–3052.

95 Dive, A., Miesse, C., Jamart, J., Evrard, P., Gonzalez, M., and Installe, E. (1994) Duodenal motor response to continuous enteral feeding is impaired in mechanically ventilated critically ill patients. *Clin. Nutr.*, **13**, 302–306.

96 Landzinski, J., Kiser, T.H., Fish, D.N., Wischmeyer, P.E., and MacLaren, R. (2008) Gastric motility function in critically ill patients tolerant vs intolerant to gastric nutrition. *J. Parenter. Enteral. Nutr.*, **32**, 45–50.

97 Nguyen, N.Q., Chapman, M.J., Fraser, R.J., Bryant, L.K., and Holloway, R.H. (2007) Erythromycin is more effective than metoclopramide in the treatment of feed intolerance in critical illness. *Crit. Care Med.*, **35**, 483–489.

98 Berger, M.M. and Mechanick, J.I. (2010) Continuing controversy in the intensive care unit: why tight glycemic control, nutrition support, and nutritional pharmacology are each necessary therapeutic considerations. *Curr. Opin. Clin. Nutr. Metab. Care*, **13**, 167–169.

99 Ukleja, A. (2010) Altered GI motility in critically ill patients: current understanding of pathophysiology, clinical impact, and diagnostic approach. *Nutr. Clin. Pract.*, **25**, 16–25.

100 Dhaliwal, R. and Heyland, D.K. (2005) Nutrition and infection in the intensive care unit: what does the evidence show?. *Curr. Opin. Crit. Care*, **11**, 461–467.

101 Marik, P.E. and Zaloga, G.P. (2001) Early enteral nutrition in acutely ill patients: a systematic review. *Crit. Care Med.*, **29**, 2264–2270.

102 Mentec, H., Dupont, H., Bocchetti, M., Cani, P., Ponche, F., and Bleichner, G. (2001) Upper digestive intolerance during enteral nutrition in critically ill patients: frequency, risk factors, and complications. *Crit. Care Med.*, **29**, 1955 –1961.

103 Waseem, S., Moshiree, B., and Draganov, P.V. (2009) Gastroparesis: current diagnostic challenges and management considerations. *World J. Gastroenterol.*, **15**, 25–37.

104 Samsom, M., Bharucha, A., Gerich, J. E., Herrmann, K., Limmer, J., Linke, R., Maggs, D., Schirra, J., Vella, A., Worle, H.J., and Goke, B. (2009) Diabetes mellitus and gastric emptying: questions and issues in clinical practice. *Diabetes Metab. Res. Rev.*, **25**, 502–514.

105 Naftali, T., Yishai, R., Zanghen, T., and Levine, A. (2007) Post-infectious gastroparesis: clinical and electrogastrographic aspects. *J. Gastroenterol. Hepatol.*, **22**, 1422–1426.

106 Maganti, K., Onyemere, K., and Jones, M.P. (2003) Oral erythromycin and symptomatic relief of gastroparesis: a systematic review. *Am. J. Gastroenterol.*, **98**, 259–263.

107 Ma, J., Rayner, C.K., Jones, K.L., and Horowitz, M. (2009) Diabetic gastroparesis: diagnosis and management. *Drugs*, **69**, 971–986.

108 Quan, C., Talley, N.J., Jones, M.P., Howell, S., and Horowitz, M. (2008) Gastrointestinal symptoms and glycemic control in diabetes mellitus: a longitudinal population study. *Eur. J. Gastroenterol. Hepatol.*, **20**, 888–897.

109 Punkkinen, J., Farkkila, M., Mätzke, S., Korppi-Tommola, T., Sane, T., Piirilä, P., and Koskenpato, J. (2008) Upper abdominal symptoms in patients with type I diabetes: unrelated to impairment in gastric emptying caused by autonomic neuropathy. *Diabetic Med.*, **25**, 570–577.

110 Desautels, S.G., Hutson, W.R., Christian, P.E., Moore, J.G., and Datz, F.L. (1995) Gastric emptying response to variable oral erythromycin dosing in diabetic gastroparesis. *Dig. Dis. Sci.*, **40**, 141–146.

111 Ueno, N., Inui, A., Asakawa, A., Takao, F., Tani, S., Komatsu, Y., Itoh, Z., and Kasuga, M. (2000) Erythromycin improves glycaemic control in patients with type II diabetes mellitus. *Diabetologia*, **43**, 411–415.

112 Murray, C.D.R., Martin, N.M., Patterson, M., Taylor, S.A., Ghatei, M. A., Kamm, M.A., Johnston, C., Bloom, S.R., and Emmanuel, A.V. (2005) Gherlin enhances gastric emptying in diabetic gastroparesis: a double blind, placebo controlled, crossover study. *Gut*, **54**, 1693–1698.

113 Goetze, O., Wieczorek, J., Mueller, T., Przuntek, H., Schmidt, W.E., and Woitalla, D. (2005) Impaired gastric emptying of a solid test meal in patients with Parkinson's disease using 13C-sodium octanoate breath test. *Neurosci. Lett.*, **375**, 170–173.

114 Hardoff, R., Sula, M., Tamir, A., Soil, A., Front, A., Badarna, S., Honigman, S., and Giladi, N. (2001) Gastric emptying time and gastric motility in patients with Parkinson's disease. *Movement Disorders*, **16**, 1041–1047.

115 Thomaides, T., Karapanayiotides, T., Zoukos, Y., Haeropoulos, C., Kerezoudi, E., Demacopoulos, N., Floodas, G., Papageorgiou, E., Armakola, F., Thomopoulos, Y., and Zaloni, I. (2005) Gastric emptying after semi-solid food in multiple system atrophy and Parkinson disease. *J. Neurol.*, **252**, 1055–1059.

116 Muller, T., Erdmann, C., Bremen, D., Schmidt, W.E., Muhlack, S., Woitalla, D., and Goetze, O. (2006) Impact of gastric emptying on levodopa pharmacokinetics in Parkinson disease patients. *Clin. Neuropharmacol.*, **29**, 61–67.

117 Nyholm, D. and Lennernas, H. (2008) Irregular gastrointestinal drug absorption in Parkinson's disease. *Exp. Opin. Drug Metab. Toxicol.*, **4**, 193–203.

118 Abell, T.L., Adams, K.A., Boles, R.G., Bousvaros, A., Chong, S.K., Fleisher, D.R., Hasler, W.L., Hyman, P.E., Issenman, R.M., Li, B.U., Linder, S.L., Mayer, E.A., McCallum, R.W., Olden, K., Parkman, H.P., Rudolph, C.D., Taché, Y., Tarbell, S., and Vakil, N. (2008) Cyclic vomiting syndrome in adults. *Neurogastroenterol. Motil.*, **20**, 269–284.

119 Pareek, N., Fleisher, D.R., and Abell, T. (2007) Cyclic vomiting syndrome: what a gastroenterologist needs to know. *Am. J. Gastroenterol.*, **102**, 2832–2840.

120 Namin, F., Patel, J., Lin, Z., Sarosiek, I., Foran, P., Esmaeili, P., and McCallum, R. (2007) Clinical, psychiatric and manometric profile of cyclic vomiting syndrome in adults and response to tricyclic therapy. *Neurogastroenterol. Motil.*, **19**, 196–202.

121 Abell, T.L., Kim, C.H., and Malagelada, J.R. (1988) Idiopathic cyclic nausea and vomiting-a disorder of gastrointestinal motility?. *Mayo Clin. Proc.*, **63**, 1169–1173.

122 Kerlin, P. (1989) Postprandial antral hypomotility in patients with idiopathic nausea and vomiting. *Gut*, **30**, 54–59.

123 Vanderhoof, J.A., Young, R., Kaufman, S.S. and Ernst, L. (1993) Treatment of cyclic vomiting in childhood with erythromycin. *J. Pediatr. Gastroenterol. Nutr.*, **17**, 387–391.

124 Kelman, L. (2006) Migraine changes with age: IMPACT on migraine classification. *Headache*, **46**, 1161–1171.

125 Aurora, S.K., Kori, S.H., Borrodale, P., McDonald, S.A., and Haseley, D. (2006) Gastric stasis in migraine: more than just a paroxysmal abnormality during a migraine attack. *Headache*, **46**, 57–63.

126 Aurora, S., Kori, S., Barrodale, P., Nelsen, A., and McDonald, S. (2007) Gastric stasis occurs in spontaneous, visually induced, and interictal migraine. *Headache*, **47**, 1443–1446.

127 Azzopardi, T.D. and Brooks, N.A. (2008) Oral metoclopramide as an adjunct to analgesics for the outpatient treatment of acute migraine. *Ann. Pharmacother.*, **42**, 397–402.

128 Tack, J., Bisschops, R., and Sarnelli, G. (2004) Pathophysiology and treatment of functional dyspepsia. *Gastroenterol.*, **127**, 1239–1255.

129 Reidl, A., Schmitdmann, M., Stengel, A., Goebel, M., Wisser, A.S., Klapp, B. F., and Monnikes, H. (2008) Somatic comorbidities of irritable bowel syndrome: a systematic analysis. *J. Psychosom. Res.*, **64**, 573–82.

130 Karamanolis, G., Caenepeel, P., Arts, J., and Tack, J. (2006) Association of the predominant symptom with clinical characteristics and pathophysiological mechanisms in functional dyspepsia. *Gastroenterol.*, **30**, 276–303.

131 Tack, J., Jones, M.P., Karamanolis, G., Coulie, B., and Dubois, D. (2010) Symptom pattern and pathophysiological correlates of weight loss in tertiary-referred functional dyspepsia. *Neurogastrointest. Motil.*, **22**, 29–34.

132 Arts, J., Caenepeel, P., Verbeke, K., and Tack, J. (2005) Influence of erythromycin on gastric emptying and meal related symptoms in functional dyspepsia with delayed gastric emptying. *Gut*, **54**, 455–60.

133 Moshiree, B., McDonald, R., Hou, W., and Toskes, P.P. (2010) Comparison of the effect of azithromycin versus erythromycin on antroduodenal pressure profiles of patients with chronic functional gastrointestinal pain and gastroparesis. *Dig. Dis. Sci.*, **55**, 675–583.

134 Simren, M., Bjornsson, E.S., and Abrahamsson, H. (2005) High interdigestive and postprandial motilin levels in patients with the irritable bowel syndrome. *Neurogastroenterol. Motil.*, **17**, 51–57.

135 Tack, J. (2006) Review article: the role of bile and pepsin in the pathophysiology and treatment of gastro-oesophageal reflux disease. *Aliment. Pharmacol. Ther.*, **24** (Suppl 2), 10–16.

136 Donnellan, C., Sharma, N., Preston, C., and Moayyedi, P. (2005) Medical treatments for the maintenance therapy of reflux oesophagitis and endoscopic negative reflux disease. *Cochrane Database Syst. Rev.*, **2**, CD003245.

137 Hsu, Y.C., Yang, T.H., Hsu, W.L., Wu, H.T., Cheng, Y.C., Chiang, M.F., Wang, C.S., and Lin, H.J. (2010) Mosapride as an adjunct to lansoprazole for symptom relief of

reflux oesophagitis. *Br. J. Clin. Pharmacol.*, **70**, 171–179.

138 Noar, M.D. and Noar, E. (2008) Gastroparesis associated with gastroesophageal reflux disease and corresponding reflux symptoms may be corrected by radiofrequency ablation of the cardia and esophageal junction. *Surg. Endoscopy*, **22**, 240–244.

139 Tighe, M.P., Afzal, N.A., Bevan, A., and Beattie, RM. (2009) Current pharmacological management of gastro-esophageal reflux in children: an evidence-based systematic review. *Paediatr. Drugs*, **11**, 185–202.

140 Chicella, M.F., Batres, L.A., Heesters, M.S., and Dice, J.E. (2005) Prokinetic drug therapy in children: a review of current options. *Ann. Pharmacother.*, **39**, 706–711.

141 Martens, V., Blondeau, K., Pauwels, A., Farre, R., Vanaudenaerde, B., Vos, R., Verleden, G., Van Raemdonck, D.E., Dupont, L.J., and Sifrim, D. (2009) Azithromycin reduces gastroesophageal reflux and aspiration in lung transplant patients. *Dig. Dis. Sci.*, **54**, 972–979.

142 Schragge, J.E., Wismer, W.V., Olson, K.L., and Baracos, V.E. (2006) The management of anorexia by patients with advanced cancer: a critical review of the literature. *Palliative Medicine*, **20**, 623–629.

143 Behl, D. and Jatoi, A. (2007) Pharmacological options for advanced cancer patients with loss of appetite and weight. *Expert Opin. Pharmacother.*, **8**, 1085–1090.

144 Lesniak, W., Bala, M., Jaeschke, R., and Krzakowski, M. (2008) Effects of megestrol acetate in patients with cancer anorexia-cachexia syndrome – a systematic review and meta-analysis. *Polskie Archiwum Medycyny Wewnetrznej*, **118**, 1–10.

145 Guney, Y., Turkcu, U.O., Hicsonmez, A., Andrieu, M.N., and Kurtman, C. (2007) Ghrelin may reduce radiation-induced mucositis and anorexia in head-neck cancer. *Medical Hypotheses*, **68**, 538–540.

146 Takanashi, H. and Cynshi, O. (2009) Motilides: a long and winding road. Lessons from mitemcinal (GM-611) on diabetic gastroparesis. *Reg. Pept.*, **155**, 18–23.

147 Ejsjaer, N., Vestergaard, E.T., Hellström, P.M., Gormsen, L.C., Madsbad, S., Madsen, J.L., Jensens, T. A., Pezzullo, J.C., Christianseen, J.S., Shaugnessy, L., and Kosutic, G. (2009) Ghrelin receptor agonist (TZP-101) accelerates gastric emptying in adults with diabetes and symptomatic gastroparesis. *Aliment. Pharmacol. Ther.*, **29**, 1179–1187.

148 Tsutsui, C., Kajihara, K., Yanaka, T., Sakata, I., Itoh, Z., and Oda S-i, S.T. (2009) House musk shrew (*Suncus murinus*, Order: Insectivora) as a new animal model for motilin study. *Peptides*, **30**, 318–329.

14
Of Mice and Men: Translational Research on Amylin Agonism

Jonathan D. Roth, Christine M. Mack, James L. Trevaskis, and David G. Parkes

14.1
Overview of Amylin Physiology

In response to nutrient intake and energy balance, the β-cell hormone insulin is a critical hormone acting directly upon peripheral tissues for glucose disposal and centrally, via the hypothalamus, as a long-term signal of adiposity. Conversely, insulin's co-localized and co-secreted β-cell partner hormone amylin acts as a short-term signal for meal termination, primarily through amylin receptors residing within the area postrema (AP) in the hindbrain. The physiological actions of amylin complement those of insulin in regulating the appearance of glucose in the circulation through at least three mechanisms that include reducing food intake, decreasing the rate of gastric emptying, and suppressing post-meal glucagon secretion (Figure 14.1).

Whereas these physiological features serve to maintain optimal glucose control and weight regulation in healthy individuals, it is instructive to consider their consequences in disease states such as diabetes mellitus. In type 1 diabetes there is an absence of secretion of β-cell hormones whereas β-cell dysregulation in type 2 diabetes (depending on its severity) can range from mild to severe. Since insulin's discovery in 1922, treatment of type 1 and late stage type 2 diabetes has consisted of exogenous insulin dosing in response to glucose measurements. While insulin monotherapy has been a life-saving strategy, even optimally controlled patients exhibit glycemic hyper-variability in response to relatively modest perturbations in fuel balance. It is becoming more widely appreciated that adjunctive therapies that enable reductions in exogenous insulin are quite desirable. For example, in a percentage of patients (~ 12–40%) [1], long-term insulin monotherapy is associated with development of metabolic syndrome. This is felt to be mediated by inducing a persistent state of hyperinsulinemia wherein exogenous insulin is circulating in blood at higher concentrations than is needed at target tissues. In turn, individuals that develop metabolic syndrome are at an increased risk of developing clinical micro- and macro-vascular complications and mortality. One rational candidate for adjunctive therapy with insulin would be its partner hormone amylin, which is also deficient in type 1 diabetes.

Peptide Drug Discovery and Development: Translational Research in Academia and Industry, First Edition.
Edited by Miguel Castanho and Nuno C. Santos.
© 2011 WILEY-VCH Verlag GmbH & Co. KGaA, Weinheim.
Published 2011 by WILEY-VCH Verlag GmbH & Co. KGaA

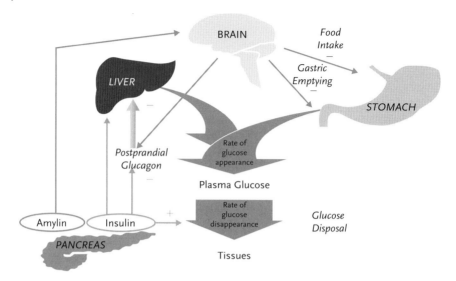

Figure 14.1 Complementary roles of amylin and insulin to regulate plasma glucose (see text for details).

Table 14.1 Amino acid sequence and homology of rat amylin, human amylin and pramlintide

	1		20		30	
rat amylin	KCNTATCATQRLANFLVR	SSNNLGPVLPPTNVGSNTY				37
human amylin	KCNTATCATQRLANFLVH	SSNNFGAILSSTNVGSNTY				37
pramlintide	KCNTATCATQRLANFLVH	SSNNFGPILPPTNVGSNTY				37

C-2:C-7 disulfide bond; shading indicates homology

14.2
Pramlintide: An Amylin Agonist

Pramlintide is a synthetic and equipotent analogue of human amylin and is used as an adjunctive therapy to patients treated with insulin. It differs from the natural peptide by three amino acids; prolines were substituted at positions 25, 28, and 29 (Table 14.1). These substitutions were necessary to overcome several physico-chemical properties which make human amylin unsuitable for pharmacologic delivery, including poor stability in solution and a propensity to aggregate and adhere to surfaces. Hence, amylin's biology and therapeutic potential in humans is almost exclusively assessed using pramlintide. By contrast, reports on the actions of amylin in rodents have been assessed using either rat amylin (which also possesses favorable pharmaceutical properties) or pramlintide.

14.3
Amylin Agonism: Translational Research in Insulin-Dependent Diabetes

In this section, we briefly highlight selected pre-clinical and clinical findings that bridge the endogenous biology and physiology of amylin with the utility of pramlintide as an adjunctive therapy to insulin to improve glycemic control in insulin-dependent diabetes, a state of combined amylin/insulin deficiency. Two translational aspects detailed here are the effects of amylin agonism on gastric emptying and post-prandial hyperglucagonemia. Although food intake is also an important component in regulating glucose, the anorexigenic properties of amylin agonists are discussed in more detail as they relate to obesity (below). For a comprehensive review of all aspects of amylin physiology and pharmacology we refer the reader to [2].

14.3.1
Post-Prandial Hyperglucagonemia and Diabetes

As noted above, the optimal treatment of diabetes requires more than insulin replacement because of the involvement of multiple hormonal systems involved in maintaining tight glycemic control. Juxtaposed to insulin/amylin-containing pancreatic β-cells are α-cells which release glucagon in order to maintain blood glucose levels at the appropriate concentration. In non-diabetic individuals glucagon prevents hypoglycemia by causing the liver to convert stored glycogen into glucose, which is released into the bloodstream. As part of an elegant feedback system, glucagon also stimulates the release of insulin, which enables glucose to be taken up and used by insulin-dependent tissues, and then insulin, in turn, also acts directly upon α-cells to suppress glucagon release. However, in patients with diabetes, α-cells are deprived of insulin signaling, leading to abnormally high glucagon concentrations, especially notable during the post-prandial period, in turn, further contributing to hyperglycemia. Although exogenous insulin replacement ultimately stimulates the α-cells to suppress glucagon, the concentrations of insulin required also stimulate the liver and muscle, resulting in a blockade in hepatic glucose production and increasing peripheral glucose disposal. Collectively, this hormonal milieu is felt to contribute to suboptimal glycemic control.

14.3.2
Amylin Agonism and Glucagon: Preclinical and Clinical Studies

Glucagonostatic effects of amylin were first demonstrated in anesthetized rats through the use of an arginine tolerance test (as amino acids are a stimulus for glucagon release). These studies revealed that amylin's effects to suppress glucagon were quite potent (achieved at an EC_{50} of 18 pM, which is in the physiological range for endogenously secreted amylin in rats) [3]. Subsequent rodent studies confirmed a similar profile for pramlintide. Interestingly, amylin antagonism with the selective amylin receptor antagonist AC187 increased glucagon levels ~2-fold, implying that amylinergic pathways may exert a tonic suppression upon glucagon secretion. Amylin's glucagonostatic properties do not appear to be modulated via direct effects of amylin upon α-cells as they are not evident *ex vivo* (e.g., isolated perfused pancreas) or *in vitro* (e.g., isolated pancreatic islets) [4]. Rather, these effects are most likely mediated via amylin activation of hindbrain receptors and vagally mediated, although this remains to be demonstrated experimentally. Finally, amylin's glucagonostatic effects are not evident in the face of insulin-induced hypoglycemia [3]. This phenemona is referred to as a "hypoglycemic override mechanism" and is a desirable feature from a therapeutic perspective.

In patients with type 1 diabetes, postprandial secretion of glucagon is elevated and was inhibited by the administration of pramlintide [5–6]. Pramlintide also prevented the abnormal meal-related rise in glucagonemia in insulin-treated patients with type 1 diabetes [7]. However, while evident during normoglycemia, the glucagonostatic effects of pramlintide were not evident during insulin-induced hypoglycemia [5]. Insulin-treated type 2 diabetes also presents with impaired suppression of glucagon secretion and hepatic glucose production which contribute to unsatisfactory glycemic control. In this patient group pramlintide infusions were also demonstrated to reduce post-prandial hyperglucagonemia [8]. Hence, the effects of amylin on glucagon secretion identified in rodents appear to translate into the clinic to address an important metabolic derangement in diabetes.

14.3.3
Gastric Emptying and Diabetes

A second contributor to the regulation of post-prandial glucose levels is the rate of gastric emptying. *Vice versa*, gastric emptying has also been reported to be regulated by glycemic status; it is slowed by hyperglycemia and accelerated by hypoglycemia. As such, one potential contributing factor to increased postprandial glucose excursions in diabetes could be accelerated gastric emptying. Indeed, gastric emptying has been shown to be accelerated in some rodent models of type 1 diabetes (e.g., BioBreeding rats [9] and streptozotocin-treated rats [10–11]) and type 2 diabetes (e.g., Fatty Zucker rats, [11]). Hypermotility has also been noted in clinical studies of type 1 diabetic individuals [12] and to a greater extent type 2 diabetics, especially during its 'early' stages [13]. However, impaired motility has not been uniformly observed across clinical studies (reviewed in [14]). Nevertheless, from a therapeutic perspective slowing gastric emptying represents one viable strategy for reducing the rate of post-meal glucose excursions.

14.3.4
Amylin Agonism and Gastric Emptying: Preclinical and Clinical Studies

In preclinical studies gastric emptying has been assessed by quantifying the rate of appearance following oral delivery of a variety of markers (e.g., phenol red, acetaminophen, radio-labeled nutrients). These techniques consistently suggest that amylin agonism dose-dependently slows the rate of gastric emptying. The effects of rat amylin are quite potent (ED_{50} estimated at $0.42+/-0.07$ nmol/kg $+/-$ SE of log) even in comparison to other peptidic regulators of nutrient uptake (e.g., GLP-1 and CCK have estimated ED_{50}s of 6.1 $+/-$ 0.12 and 8.5 $+/-$ 0.20 nmol/kg $+/-$ SE of log, respectively; [15]). Similar ED_{50} values in rodents have been obtained with pramlintide. At high doses rat amylin can fully inhibit gastric emptying in both normal and diabetic rats [16]. Amylin inhibition of gastric emptying is thought to be primarily centrally mediated. First, aspiration of the AP abolishes amylin's effects on gastric emptying [17]. More recently, amylin inhibition of gastric emptying was demonstrated in rats with a sub-diaphragmatic vagal deafferentiation (e.g., in which vagal afferent fibers are destroyed but efferent fibers remain intact) supporting the hypothesis that amylin acts via hormonal mechanisms to stimulate the AP and transmits signals to the gut via efferent vagal fibers [18].

The effects of pramlintide on gastric emptying have also been assessed in a number of clinical studies. Infusion of pramlintide delayed solid and liquid gastric emptying in patients with type 1 diabetes [19], and these effects were subsequently shown to be dose-dependent and no longer evident after 4 h [20]. When the gastric emptying effects of pramlintide were compared in individuals with type 1 or type 2 diabetes, they were determined to be equally effective. Likewise, in non-diabetic volunteers pramlintide delayed gastric emptying without affecting small bowel or colonic transit [21]. Hence, the effects of amylin agonism on gastric emptying have been recapitulated in the clinic and are evident irrespective of disease state.

14.4
Amylin Agonism: Translational Research in Obesity

To date, clinical studies have evaluated the use of pramlintide alone as well as in combination with other agents (e.g., metreleptin, sibutramine or phentermine) for its anti-obesity potential. Selected pre-clinical and clinical observations are reviewed below.

14.4.1
Food Intake and Body Weight: Role of Endogenous Amylin

In rodents, endogenous amylin fulfills the main criteria for a peripheral satiety signal [22]. Namely, amylin's anorexigenic effects are evident at near-physiological concentrations and plasma amylin concentrations increase proportionally with meal size. At low doses peripherally administered amylin reduces meal size (satiation) and increases the post-meal interval/meal size ratio (an index of satiety) [23] [24]. Endogenous amylin may also contribute to the physiological control of food intake and body weight. Acute amylin receptor antagonism with AC187 stimulates feeding and, with continuous intracerebroventricular infusion, increased adiposity by $\sim 30\%$ although body weight was unchanged [25–26]. Nevertheless, amylin gene deletion against two background strains of mice resulted in only modest and transient defects with respect to energy balance [27, 28] suggesting that amylin's endogenous role is not as critical as other signals such as leptin whose deletion results in morbid obesity/metabolic disease.

14.4.2
Food Intake and Body Weight: Pre-clinical Studies

The pharmacological inhibition of food intake by amylin has been described in numerous species and has been well described in the literature (confirmed in more than 100 publications, reviewed in [29]). An example of decreased food intake in overnight fasted rats is shown in Figure 14.2a. [23]. Amylin's ability to decrease food intake in rodents does not appear to be due to malaise or the induction of competing behavior/s such as conditioned taste aversion or avoidance [30, 31]. Agents that reduce food intake via induction of nauseau/emesis or general malaise may also elicit pica behavior, the ingestion of non-nutritive substances such as the synthetic white clay kaolin. Doses of amylin that decrease food intake do not elicit pica behavior nor do they introduce competing locomotor activities or suppress general locomotor activities [23].

As with gastric emptying, amylin's anorexigenic effects are centrally mediated via the hindbrain AP. Direct application of amylin to the AP decreases food intake, whereas application of the amylin antagonist AC187 to the AP increases food intake (and blocks the anorexigenic effects of peripherally administered amylin [32]). Moreover, lesioning the AP abolishes the anorexigenic effect of amylin [33], as well as amylin-induced c-fos expression throughout the neuro-axis [34]. An intact vagus is not required for the expression of amylin's anorexigenic effects [35], but under normal physiological conditions, vagal transmission, and gastric emptying can certainly serve to enhance amylin's central effects. For example, amylin suppression of "sham" feeding (e.g., a technique where liquid food drains from the stomach so that gastric food stimuli related to the accumulation of food in the stomach, intestinal food stimuli, and post-absorptive food stimuli are absent or greatly reduced) requires higher doses compared to those required to decrease "real" feeding [36].

Diet-induced obese prone (DIO) rats exhibit many characteristics of human obesity (increased fat mass, obesity-related disturbances, e.g., dyslipidemia, hyperinsulinemia), and lack genetic disruption of key feeding-related central signaling pathways [37]. Importantly, the anorexigenic effects of peripheral amylin, which were largely demonstrated in acute tests in lean animals, translated into meaningful weight loss in these models [23, 38]. In DIO rats, peripherally-administered rat amylin (3–300 µg/kg/d) for 4 weeks reduced food intake and decreased body weight by 10–14% at the highest doses tested (Figure 14.3a). Pair-feeding studies revealed some important differences between amylin-induced weight loss and that induced by caloric restriction alone [38]. While food intake reduction was the predominant mode of action for overall weight loss, the composition of weight loss was notably different across treatment groups. In amylin-treated rats,

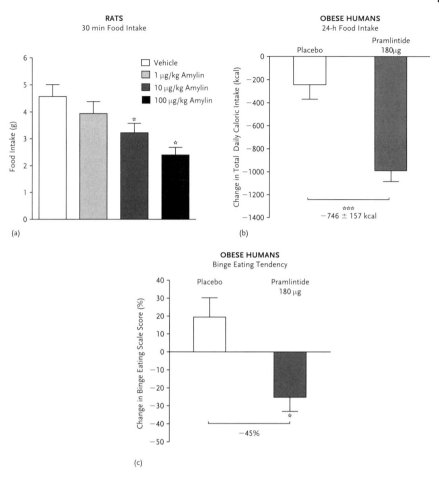

Figure 14.2 Effect of amylin (1, 10, or 100 μg/kg, IP) on 30 min food intake in fasted rats (*N* = 5–7/group) (a). Effect of pramlintide on food intake and binge-eating in obese subjects (b, c) (Evaluable *N* = 84). Subjects were treated with pramlintide (180 μg TID) or placebo for 6 weeks; change in 24 h total caloric intake placebo lead-in (Day 1) to Day 3 at three *ad libitum* buffets (b) and change in Binge Eating Scale score from baseline to Day 42 (c). Mean ± SE. $*P < 0.05$, $**P < 0.01$, $***P < 0.001$ versus vehicle/placebo. Adapted from [23, 43].

weight loss was entirely attributable to reductions in fat mass, with relative preservation of lean mass. In contrast, pair-fed control animals experienced reductions in both fat and lean body mass. Amylin-induced weight loss was also demonstrated not to be associated with counter-regulatory decreases in energy expenditure typically associated with a reduced weight state. When amylin's weight- and fat-reducing properties were evaluated across a variety of nutritive states, they were determined to still be evident following a diet "lead-in" regimen [39–40]. Finally, amylin monotherapy seems to be similarly effective in reducing body weight, irrespective of starting body weight; in other words, there does not

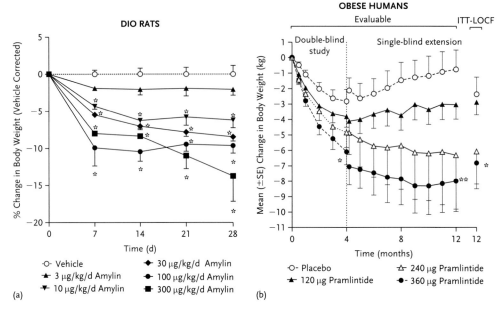

Figure 14.3 Effect of amylin on body weight in diet-induced obese rats (a). Change in body weight (percent vehicle corrected) of rats receiving amylin (3–300 μg/kg/d) for 4 weeks via SC implanted osmotic minipumps. Effect of pramlintide on body weight in obese subjects (b). Changes in body weight from baseline (month 0) for placebo ($n=17$), 120 μg pramlintide ($n=24$) 240 μg pramlintide ($n=17$) or 360 μg pramlintide ($n=21$) twice daily (Evaluable population). Mean ± SE. *$P<0.05$, **$P<0.01$, versus vehicle/placebo. Adapted from [23] (a) and [45] (b).

appear to be "amylin resistance" to the weight-lowering actions of amylin with increasing obesity (reviewed in [41]).

14.4.3
Food Intake and Body Weight: Clinical Studies

The food intake lowering effects of pramlintide have been confirmed in several clinical studies. Obese subjects receiving a single injection of pramlintide 1 h prior to a buffet meal decreased their food intake by 16% compared to placebo [42]. Pramlintide also elicited a 58% increase in the satiety quotient, indicating that consuming less food was required to promote meal-related satiation. In other studies, pramlintide durably reduced total daily food intake (by 15–20%) in obese subjects when measured both early during the study and after 6 weeks of administration (Figure 14.2b) [43]. Pramlintide was also shown to be associated with acute and sustained reductions in the intake of highly palatable high-fat, high-sugar foods at a "fast-food challenge" and to improve perceived control of eating, as demonstrated by a 45% placebo-corrected reduction in binge eating scores (Figure 14.2c). These findings suggest that the nuances of changes in feeding behavior (e.g., decreased meal size while concomitantly increasing satiety, reduced intake and preference for palatable foods) observed in preclinical models with amylin may also be recapitulated in the clinic with pramlintide.

Weight lowering effects of pramlintide have also been established in a variety of clinical studies. In patients with type 1 and 2 diabetes pramlintide generally led to weight loss, whereas insulin treatment tended to promote weight gain [44]. In a phase 2b dose ranging study pramlintide was evaluated in conjunction with life-style intervention [45]. The design also included a single-blind placebo controlled extension to examine the weight lowering effects of pramlintide for up to 12 months. During the first 4 months of this study, weight loss from baseline was 3.8–6.1 kg in the pramlintide-treated subjects versus 2.8 kg in the life-style intervention alone group. After 12 months, those subjects that continued to the extension protocol experienced a mean weight loss of up to 6.8 and 8.0 kg from baseline compared with 0.7 kg in the placebo group. In these obesity studies, the most commonly reported adverse event was nausea associated with pramlintide compared with placebo treatment, which was typically mild to moderate in intensity and decreased over time. Collectively, these studies suggest that obese subjects treated with pramlintide alone, or as an adjunct to life-style intervention can achieve weight loss and enhanced long-term maintenance of weight loss. Translational findings of amylin agonism on food intake and body weight are depicted in Figures 14.2 and 14.3 and summarized in Table 14.2.

Table 14.2 Comparison of the effects of amylin (in rodents) and the amylin analog pramlintide (in humans) on food intake and body weight.

	Rodent	Human
Food Intake		
Meal Size	↓ during dark-cycle feeding	↓ after buffet meal
Intermeal interval	no increase in meal frequency	no change in intermeal interval
Satiation	↔ satiating efficiency	↔ satiety quotient
Control of Eating	↓ stress-induced eating	↓ binge eating score
Malaise	No malaise at doses that ↓ food intake	Food intake dissociated from nausea
Food Intake (Chronic)	↓ daily food intake for 8 weeks	↓ daily food intake for 6 weeks
Body Weight-Monotherapy		
Weight loss	↓ (durable up to 12 weeks)	↓ (progressive up to 16 weeks)
Fat Mass	↓ (weight loss is fat specific)	tbd
Lean Mass	↔ (weight loss is lean sparing)	tbd
Body Weight-Combination Therapy		
Amylin + Sibutramine	↓ (additive)	↓ (additive)
Amylin + Leptin	↓ (synergistic)	↓ (synergistic)

14.4.4
Combination Studies

As with other chronic diseases such as hypertension, cancer and diabetes, combinatorial approaches have gained significant traction for the potential treatment of obesity. While individual agents may be initially effective at reducing body weight, the overall percentage of weight loss is typically modest, in the single digit range, if at all, and typically body weight plateaus, and even rebounds to pretreatment levels. Analogous to diabetes, monotherapy-based approaches for obesity target only a single aspect of a multi-hormonal disease state. As such, a single agent is either unable to break through the multiple systems to elicit meaningful weight loss and/or fails to overcome, or counter, the subsequent metabolic adaptations for weight loss to be maintained. These adaptations are complex and include psychological, autonomic and neuroendocrine changes that are deeply rooted in evolution (for a review of these mechanisms we refer the reader to [46, 47]). A series of translational research studies have demonstrated the potential utility of combined amylin agonism with small molecule anorexigenic agents (e.g., phentermine or sibutramine) or with an analog of the long-term adiposity signal leptin (e.g., metreleptin) that may be useful in overcoming these adaptations to promote double-digit body weight loss.

14.4.5
Amylin Agonism and Small Molecule Agents

Preclinical studies demonstrated additive food intake, weight- and fat-lowering effects when amylin was combined with either phentermine hydrochloride (a catacholaminergic agent) or sibutramine hydrochloride (a serotonin/norepinephrine reuptake inhibitor; Figure 14.4a). Detailed analyses of feeding patterns with amylin and phentermine suggest that these effects may be achieved by a $\sim$2-fold increase in the satiety ratio compared to either agent alone [48]. In terms of off-target behavioral effects, amylin neither enhanced nor reduced the known actions of phentermine (which is an amphetamine derivate) to stimulate activity [49].

In a clinical study that enrolled obese or overweight, non-diabetic subjects, the effects of pramlintide, pramlintide combined with sibutramine, or pramlintide combined with phentermine were compared relative to a pramlintide placebo control group. Mean weight loss ($\pm$SEM) achieved at week 24 with either combination treatment ($11.1\pm1.1\%$ with pramlintide combined with sibutramine, $11.3\pm0.9\%$ with pramlintide combined with phentermine) was significantly greater than treatment with either pramlintide alone ($3.7\pm0.7\%$) or placebo ($2.2\pm0.7\%$; Figure 14.4b). No novel safety or tolerability issues were observed with pramlintide or either of the combinations. The off-target effects of the small molecules to modestly increase heart rate and blood pressure were neither enhanced nor reduced in the presence of pramlintide [50].

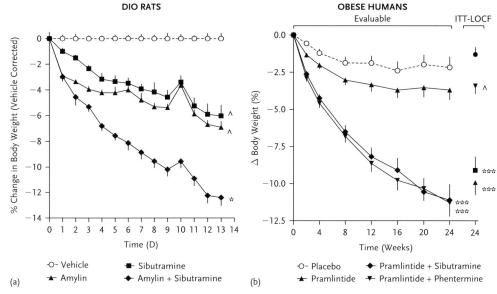

Figure 14.4 Effect of amylin, sibutramine, or amylin + sibutramine on body weight in diet-induced obese rats (a). Change in body weight (percent vehicle corrected) of rats receiving vehicle, 100 µg/kg/d amylin, 3 mg/kg/d sibutramine, or 100 µg/kg/d amylin + 3 mg/kg/d sibutramine ($ns = 5$ /group) for 4 weeks via SC implanted osmotic minipumps. Effect of pramlintide, pramlintide + sibutramine, or pramlintide + phentermine on body weight in obese subjects (b). Changes in body weight from baseline (week 0) to week 24 for placebo ($n = 32$), 120 µg pramlintide three times daily ($n = 44$), 120 µg pramlintide 3 times daily + 10 mg oral sibutramine once daily ($n = 41$), or 120 µg pramlintide 3 times daily + 37.5 mg oral phentermine once daily ($n = 45$) (Evaluable population). Mean ± SE. $^{\wedge}P < 0.05$ compared to vehicle/placebo; $*P < 0.05$ and $***P < 0.001$ compared to monotherapy alone and vehicle/placebo. Adapted from [48] (a) and [50] (b).

14.4.6
Combined Amylin and Leptin Agonism

Although the adipokine leptin is regarded as the prototypical long-term signal of energy balance, obese rodents and humans are largely nonresponsive to exogenous leptin administration. In several preclinical studies, exogenous pharmacological amylin was shown to synergize with leptin to induce marked and sustained fat-specific body weight loss in leptin-resistant DIO rats (Figure 14.5a) [51–53]. Weight loss synergy was specific to amylin treatment, compared with other anorexigenic peptides, and dissociable from amylin's effect on food intake. Mechanistic studies suggest that the presence of amylin "primes" the hypothalamus to respond to leptin by enhancing leptin receptor number and/or signaling capacity (for a recent review of the physiological, neurobiological, and molecular mechanisms mediating these interactions see [41]).

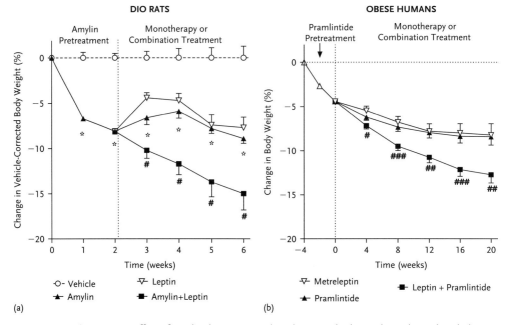

Figure 14.5 Effect of amylin, leptin, or amylin + leptin on body weight in diet-induced obese rats (a). Change in body weight (percent vehicle corrected) of rats pretreated for 14 d with 100 μg/kg/d amylin, and then maintained on 100 μg/kg/d amylin or switched to either 500 μg/kg/d leptin monotherapy or 100 μg/kg/d amylin + 500 μg/kg/d leptin combination therapy ($N = 6$–8/group). Compounds were delivered for 6 weeks via SC implanted osmotic minipumps. Effect of metreleptin, pramlintide, or metreleptin + pramlintide combination on body weight in obese subjects (b). Changes in body weight from enrolment (week 4) for subjects pretreated with pramlintide (titrated from 180 μg to 360 ig) twice and then treated with 360 μg pramlintide twice daily, 5 mg metreleptin twice daily, or pramlintide + metreleptin combination treatment. (93=Evaluable population). Mean ± SE. *$P < 0.05$ compared to vehicle; #$P < 0.05$, ##$P < 0.01$, ###$P < 0.001$ compared to monotherapies. Adapted from [51].

Clinical proof-of-concept for combined amylin/leptin agonism induced weight loss was obtained in a clinical study in subjects with overweight and obesity. Co-administration of metreleptin and pramlintide for 20 weeks (after a 4-week lead-in treatment period with pramlintide alone) elicited significantly more weight loss (approximately 13%) than either treatment alone (Figure 14.5b) [51, 54]. The greater reduction in body weight with the combination was significant as early as week 4, and weight loss continued throughout the study, without evidence of a plateau. The most common adverse events with pramlintide/metreleptin were injection site events and nausea, which were mostly mild to moderate and decreased over time. These results support further development of pramlintide/metreleptin as a novel, integrated neurohormonal approach to obesity pharmacotherapy.

14.4.7
Future Areas for Amylin Agonism-Based Translational Research

With the arsenal of available therapies for metabolic diseases continuing to evolve, it is likely that sub-groups of target populations will exhibit differential responsiveness to any given pharmacological agent. Just as there exist large differences between males and females in the regulation of energy homeostasis, it is not unreasonable to assume that therapeutic modalities will be more, or less, efficacious as concentrations of gonadal hormones fluctuate during development and aging. Sexually dimorphic effects are especially relevant with respect to neurohormone-based therapies for metabolic disease/s as pharmacological and neurobiological studies have convincingly demonstrated a role for estradiol in the central control of energy balance. These studies generally predict that the presence of estradiol enhances the anorexigenic properties of short-term signals of satiation (e.g., cholecystokinin) and long-term signals of adiposity (e.g., leptin), while concomitantly decreasing the potency of orexigenic signals (e.g., melanin concentrating hormone, neuropeptide Y, ghrelin; reviewed in [55–57]). Recently, we explored whether estradiol signaling impacted the weight regulatory and metabolic effects of amylin agonism [58]. Our studies elucidated a surprising, ~2-fold increase in amylin's weight-lowering efficacy in a state of estradiol deficiency (DIO ovariectomized (OVX) rat model; Figure 14.6a) compared to sham operated controls. Detailed metabolic studies revealed that amylin reversed the decline in energy expenditure and fat oxidation linked to an estradiol-deficient state via food intake dependent (reduction in respiratory exchange ratio) and independent (maintenance of metabolic rate) mechanisms. Given that post-menopausal women comprise a large majority of patients for whom weight loss agents are prescribed, the extent to which these preclinical observations translate into the clinical use of the amylin agonist pramlintide warrants further investigation.

A second area that merits further attention involves intriguing observations that amylin agonism may also hold utility in the treatment of neuropsychiatric disease. The neural circuitry modulating energy homeostasis interacts and even overlaps with pathways implicated in cognition, reward, and stress [59]. Thus signals involved in modulating metabolic tone may also possess beneficial effects on emotional behavior and cognitive function. In preclinical studies, amylin administration has been linked to anti-depressive and anxiolytic effects. Coupled with classic resetting of the hypothalamic–pituitary–adrenal axis, animals exposed to chronic stress increase their intake of palatable foods, leading to increased visceral adiposity. In one study rats were given access to standard lab chow and sucrose solutions and were exposed to chronic stressors (e.g., daily restraint stress). Vehicle-treated rats increased their consumption of sucrose and increased visceral adiposity. By contrast, amylin-treated rats decreased their stress-induced sucrose consumption following restraint stress, while maintaining their intake of standard lab chow [60]. Next, given the link between estradiol deficiency and depression, we evaluated whether amylin exhibited anti-depressive effects in our OVX model using the forced swim test [58]. As expected OVX-vehicle treated rats displayed

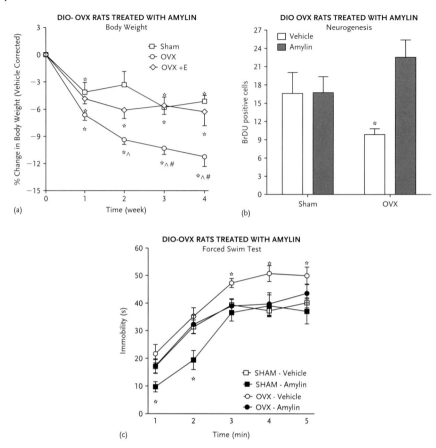

Figure 14.6 Effect of ovariectomy (OVX) or OVX with estrogen replacement (OVX + E) in amylin-treated diet-induced obese (DIO) rats (a). Change in body weight (percent vehicle corrected) of Sham-Vehicle, OVX, or OVX + E rats treated for 4 weeks with amylin (50 μg/kg/d) via SC implanted osmotic pumps ($N = 6$/group). Effect of amylin on neurogenesis on OVX rats (b). Average cell counts of the hippocampus with diaminobenzidine staining of Sham and OVX DIO rats infused 2 weeks with vehicle or amylin (50 μg/kg/d) ($N = 6$/group). BrdU (75 mg/kg, IP) was administered d 6–12, twice daily (b). Effect of amylin in OVX DIO rats in the forced swim test. The time spent immobile in Sham and OVX DIO rats infused for 4 weeks with vehicle or amylin (50 μg/kg/d) ($N = 9$/group) (c). Mean ± SE. *$P < 0.05$ versus Sham-Vehicle, ^$P < 0.05$ versus SHAM-Amylin, #$P < 0.05$ versus OVX + E. Adapted from [58].

increased immobility (a depressed phenotype) as compared to sham operated controls. Amylin-treatment of OVX rats normalized their immobility scores to a similar extent as intact vehicle-treated controls. To gain insight into the central mechanisms mediating these effects we quantified hippocampal neurogenesis, a process known to be diminished in models of depression as well as estrogen deficiency, and restored by the administration of anti-depressants or estrogen replacement. Within the hippocampus, decreased neurogenesis (by ∼40%) was evident in vehicle-treated OVX rats relative to intact vehicle-treated rats based on BrdU incorporation studies. Although amylin infusion had no effect on neurogenesis in intact rats, amylin restored hippocampal neurogenesis in OVX rats (Figure 14.6b and c). Collectively these preclinical findings raise the intriguing possibility that the integrated mechanisms of amylin may improve metabolic and behavioral processes and represent an important area for future clinical research.

References

1 McGill, M. *et al.* (2008) The metabolic syndrome in type 1 diabetes: does it exist and does it matter?. *J. Diabetes Complications*, **22** (1), 18–23.

2 Young, A. (2005) Clinical studies. *Adv. Pharmacol.*, **52**, 289–320.

3 Gedulin, B.R., Rink, T.J., and Young, A. A. (1997) Dose-response for glucagonostatic effect of amylin in rats. *Metabolism*, **46** (1), 67–70.

4 Silvestre, R.A. *et al.* (2001) Selective amylin inhibition of the glucagon response to arginine is extrinsic to the pancreas. *Am. J. Physiol. Endocrinol. Metab.*, **280** (3), E443–E449.

5 Nyholm, B. *et al.* (1996) Acute effects of the human amylin analog AC137 on basal and insulin-stimulated euglycemic and hypoglycemic fuel metabolism in patients with insulin-dependent diabetes mellitus. *J. Clin. Endocrinol. Metab.*, **81** (3), 1083–1089.

6 Levetan, C. *et al.* (2003) Impact of pramlintide on glucose fluctuations and postprandial glucose, glucagon, and triglyceride excursions among patients with type 1 diabetes intensively treated with insulin pumps. *Diabetes Care*, **26** (1), 1–8.

7 Fineman, M.S. *et al.* (2002) The human amylin analog, pramlintide, corrects postprandial hyperglucagonemia in patients with type 1 diabetes. *Metabolism*, **51** (5), 636–641.

8 Fineman, M. *et al.* (2002) The human amylin analog, pramlintide, reduces postprandial hyperglucagonemia in patients with type 2 diabetes mellitus. *Horm. Metab. Res.*, **34** (9), 504–508.

9 Nowak, T.V. *et al.* (1994) Accelerated gastric emptying in diabetic rodents: effect of insulin treatment and pancreas transplantation. *J. Lab. Clin. Med.*, **123** (1), 110–116.

10 Granneman, J.G. and Stricker, E.M. (1984) Food intake and gastric emptying in rats with streptozotocin-induced diabetes. *Am. J. Physiol.*, **247** (6 Pt 2), R1054–R1061.

11 Green, G.M. *et al.* (1997) Accelerated gastric emptying of glucose in Zucker type 2 diabetic rats: role in postprandial hyperglycaemia. *Diabetologia*, **40** (2), 136–142.

12 Nakanome, C. *et al.* (1983) Disturbances of the alimentary tract motility and hypermotilinemia in the patients with diabetes mellitus. *Tohoku J. Exp. Med.*, **139** (2), 205–215.

13 Jones, K.L. *et al.* (1996) Gastric emptying in early noninsulin-dependent diabetes mellitus. *J. Nucl. Med.*, **37** (10), 1643–1648.

14 Ma, J. *et al.* (2009) Insulin secretion in healthy subjects and patients with Type 2 diabetes – role of the gastrointestinal tract. *Best Pract. Res. Clin. Endocrinol. Metab.*, **23** (4), 413–424.

15 Young, A.A., Gedulin, B.R., and Rink, T. J. (1996) Dose-responses for the slowing of gastric emptying in a rodent model by glucagon-like peptide (7–36) NH2, amylin, cholecystokinin, and other possible regulators of nutrient uptake. *Metabolism*, **45** (1), 1–3.

16 Young, A.A. *et al.* (1995) Gastric emptying is accelerated in diabetic BB rats and is slowed by subcutaneous injections of amylin. *Diabetologia*, **38** (6), 642–648.

17 Young, A. (2005) Inhibition of gastric emptying. *Adv. Pharmacol.*, **52**, 99–121.

18 Wickbom, J. *et al.* (2008) Gastric emptying in response to IAPP and CCK

in rats with subdiaphragmatic afferent vagotomy. *Regul. Pept.*, **148** (1–3), 21–25.

19 Kong, M.F. *et al.* (1997) Infusion of pramlintide, a human amylin analogue, delays gastric emptying in men with IDDM. *Diabetologia*, **40** (1), 82–88.

20 Kong, M.F. *et al.* (1998) The effect of single doses of pramlintide on gastric emptying of two meals in men with IDDM. *Diabetologia*, **41** (5), 577–583.

21 Samsom, M. *et al.* (2000) Pramlintide, an amylin analog, selectively delays gastric emptying: potential role of vagal inhibition. *Am. J. Physiol. Gastrointest. Liver Physiol.*, **278** (6), G946–G951.

22 Lutz, T.A. (2005) Pancreatic amylin as a centrally acting satiating hormone. *Curr. Drug Targets*, **6** (2), 181–189.

23 Mack, C. *et al.* (2007) Pharmacological actions of the peptide hormone amylin in the long-term regulation of food intake, food preference, and body weight. *Am. J. Physiol. Regul. Integr. Comp. Physiol.*, **293** (5), R1855–R1863.

24 Lutz, T.A. *et al.* (1995) Amylin decreases meal size in rats. *Physiol. Behav.*, **58** (6), 1197–1202.

25 Rushing, P.A. *et al.* (2001) Inhibition of central amylin signaling increases food intake and body adiposity in rats. *Endocrinology*, **142** (11), 5035.

26 Reidelberger, R.D. *et al.* (2004) Amylin receptor blockade stimulates food intake in rats. *Am. J. Physiol. Regul. Integr. Comp. Physiol.*, **287** (3), R568–R574.

27 Turek, V.F. *et al.* (2010) Mechanisms of amylin/leptin synergy in rodent models. *Endocrinology*, **151** (1), 143–152.

28 Gebre-Medhin, S. *et al.* (1998) Increased insulin secretion and glucose tolerance in mice lacking islet amyloid polypeptide (amylin). *Biochem. Biophys. Res. Commun.*, **250** (2), 271–277.

29 Young, A. (2005) Inhibition of food intake. *Adv. Pharmacol.*, **52**, 79–98.

30 Rushing, P.A. *et al.* (2002) Acute 3rd-ventricular amylin infusion potently reduces food intake but does not produce aversive consequences. *Peptides*, **23** (5), 985–988.

31 Chance, W.T. *et al.* (1992) Tests of adipsia and conditioned taste aversion following the intrahypothalamic injection of amylin. *Peptides*, **13** (5), 961–964.

32 Mollet, A. *et al.* (2004) Infusion of the amylin antagonist AC 187 into the area postrema increases food intake in rats. *Physiol. Behav.*, **81** (1), 149–155.

33 Lutz, T.A. *et al.* (1998) Lesion of the area postrema/nucleus of the solitary tract (AP/NTS) attenuates the anorectic effects of amylin and calcitonin gene-related peptide (CGRP) in rats. *Peptides*, **19** (2), 309–317.

34 Rowland, N.E. and Richmond, R.M. (1999) Area postrema and the anorectic actions of dexfenfluramine and amylin. *Brain Res.*, **820** (1–2), 86–91.

35 Lutz, T.A., Del Prete, E., and Scharrer, E. (1995) Subdiaphragmatic vagotomy does not influence the anorectic effect of amylin. *Peptides*, **16** (3), 457–462.

36 Asarian, L., Eckel, L.A. and Geary, N. (1998) Behaviorally specific inhibition of sham feeding by amylin. *Peptides*, **19** (10), 1711–1718.

37 Levin, B.E. *et al.* (1997) Selective breeding for diet-induced obesity and resistance in Sprague-Dawley rats. *Am. J. Physiol.*, **273** (2 Pt 2), R725–R730.

38 Roth, J.D. *et al.* (2006) Antiobesity effects of the beta-cell hormone amylin in diet-induced obese rats: effects on food intake, body weight, composition, energy expenditure, and gene expression. *Endocrinology*, **147** (12), 5855–5864.

39 Roth, J.D. *et al.* (2007) Effects of prior or concurrent food restriction on amylin-induced changes in body weight and body composition in high-fat fed female rats. *Am. J. Physiol. Endocrinol. Metab.*, **293** (4), E1112–E1117.

40 Wielinga, P.Y. *et al.* (2010) Central amylin acts as an adiposity signal to control body weight and energy expenditure. *Physiol. Behav.*, **101** (1), 45–52.

41 Trevaskis, J.L., Parkes, D.G., and Roth, J.D. (2010) Insights into amylin-leptin synergy. *Trends Endocrinol. Metab.*, **21** (8), 473–479.

42 Chapman, I. *et al.* (2005) Effect of pramlintide on satiety and food intake in obese subjects and subjects with type 2 diabetes. *Diabetologia*, **48** (5), 838–848.

43 Smith, S.R. *et al.* (2007) Pramlintide treatment reduces 24-h caloric intake and meal sizes and improves control of eating in obese subjects: a 6-wk translational research study. *Am. J. Physiol. Endocrinol. Metab.*, **293** (2), E620 –E627.

44 Pullman, J., Darsow, T., and Frias, J.P. (2006) Pramlintide in the management of insulin-using patients with type 2 and type 1 diabetes. *Vasc. Health Risk Manag.*, **2** (3), 203–212.

45 Smith, S.R. *et al.* (2008) Sustained weight loss following 12-month pramlintide treatment as an adjunct to lifestyle intervention in obesity. *Diabetes Care*, **31** (9), 1816–1823.

46 Levin, B.E. (2006) Central regulation of energy homeostasis intelligent design: how to build the perfect survivor. *Obesity (Silver Spring)*, **14** (Suppl. 5), 192S–196S.

47 Rosenbaum, M. *et al.* (2010) Energy intake in weight-reduced humans. *Brain Res.*, **1350**, 95–102.

48 Roth, J.D. *et al.* (2008) Antiobesity effects of the beta-cell hormone amylin in combination with phentermine or sibutramine in diet-induced obese rats. *Int. J. Obes. (Lond.)*, **32** (8), 1201–1210.

49 Roth, J.D. and Rowland, N.E. (1998) Efficacy of administration of dexfenfluramine and phentermine, alone and in combination, on ingestive behavior and body weight in rats. *Psychopharmacology (Berlin)*, **137** (1), 99–106.

50 Aronne, L.J. *et al.* (2010) Enhanced weight loss following coadministration of pramlintide with sibutramine or phentermine in a multicenter trial. *Obesity (Silver Spring)*, **18** (9), 1739–1746.

51 Roth, J.D. *et al.* (2008) Leptin responsiveness restored by amylin agonism in diet-induced obesity: evidence from nonclinical and clinical studies. *Proc Natl Acad Sci U S A*, **105** (20), 7257–7262.

52 Trevaskis, J.L. *et al.* (2008) Amylin-mediated restoration of leptin responsiveness in diet-induced obesity: magnitude and mechanisms. *Endocrinology*, **149** (11), 5679–5687.

53 Trevaskis, J.L. *et al.* (2010) Interaction of leptin and amylin in the long-term maintenance of weight loss in diet-induced obese rats. *Obesity (Silver Spring)*, **18** (1), 21–26.

54 Ravussin, E. *et al.* (2009) Enhanced weight loss with pramlintide/ metreleptin: an integrated neurohormonal approach to obesity pharmacotherapy. *Obesity (Silver Spring)*, **17** (9), 1736–1743.

55 Brown, L.M. *et al.* (2010) Metabolic impact of sex hormones on obesity. *Brain Res.*, **1350**, 77–85.

56 Asarian, L. and Geary, N. (2006) Modulation of appetite by gonadal steroid hormones. *Philos. Trans. R. Soc. Lond. B Biol. Sci.*, **361** (1471), 1251–1263.

57 Butera, P.C. (2010) Estradiol and the control of food intake. *Physiol. Behav.*, **99** (2), 175–180.

58 Trevaskis, J.L. *et al.* (2010) Enhanced amylin-mediated body weight loss in estradiol-deficient diet-induced obese rats. *Endocrinology*, **151** (12): 5657–5668.

59 Berthoud, H.R. (2006) Homeostatic and non-homeostatic pathways involved in the control of food intake and energy balance. *Obesity (Silver Spring)*, **14** (Suppl. 5), 197S–200S.

60 Roth, J.D. *et al.* (2009) Implications of amylin receptor agonism: integrated neurohormonal mechanisms and therapeutic applications. *Arch. Neurol.*, **66** (3), 306–310.

15
Peptides and Polypeptides as Immunomodulators and Their Consequential Therapeutic Effect in Multiple Sclerosis and Other Autoimmune Diseases

Ruth Arnon, Michael Sela, and Rina Aharoni

15.1
Introduction

Peptides and polypeptides, from either natural resources or synthetic, are the predominant agents in the immune system. They play a major role in the induction of immune response, thus providing protection against infection; they may induce immune response to self body components, thus leading to various autoimmune disorders; but they may also suppress the immune response, thus leading to either tolerance or immunomodulation, and, consequently, to an influence on the immune response to various antigens, including autoantigens. When such immunomodulation affects autoimmune responses it results in alleviation of the pathologies involved.

The majority of naturally occurring antigens consist of proteins. However, as early as 1960, studies from our laboratory showed that a completely synthetic protein-like polymer can also be endowed with antigenic properties. Thus, a multichain amino acid copolymer composed of a backbone of poly-L-lysine, with chains of poly-DL-alanine attached to the amino groups of the polylysine, and elongated with short chains of L-tyrosine and L-glutamic acid, was shown to be immunogenic, leading to the production of specific antibodies in a variety of experimental animals. This first synthetic antigen paved the road to the elucidation of the molecular basis of immune phenomena, to the discovery of the genetic control of the immune response, as well as to the definition of sequential and conformational antigenic determinants (reviewed in [1]). Furthermore, a direct consequence of this approach is the development of synthetic vaccines against infectious diseases and of immunomodulators for the treatment of autoimmune diseases, as will be described in the following.

Peptide Drug Discovery and Development: Translational Research in Academia and Industry, First Edition.
Edited by Miguel Castanho and Nuno C. Santos.
© 2011 WILEY-VCH Verlag GmbH & Co. KGaA, Weinheim.
Published 2011 by WILEY-VCH Verlag GmbH & Co. KGaA

15.2
Peptides as Antigens and Vaccines

The antigenic properties of proteins are defined by two types of antigenic sites or epitopes: The B cell epitopes which are recognized by the receptors on B lymphocytes, as well as by antibodies, and the T-cell epitopes, recognized by T-cell receptors. Peptides or polypeptides corresponding to such epitopes are able to induce an immune response with similar specificity. Indeed, the investigation of peptides and polymers of amino acids led to a series of synthetic antigens capable of provoking antibodies reacting with native proteins. For example, the polymer of the tripeptide ProGlyPro led to antibodies cross-reacting with collagen [2], whereas a synthetic "loop" peptide, analogous to a loop in the sequence of hen egg-white lysozyme, in which a disulfide bridge was still intact, led – after attachment to a synthetic amino acid polymer carrier – to antibodies reacting with native lysozyme [3, 4]. These data proved the concept that it is possible to prepare synthetic peptide molecules which successfully mimic native proteins, while being much simpler and better defined.

The next step in the progress towards synthetic peptide vaccines was the success in preparing a peptide analogous to a fragment of the coat protein of bacteriophage MS2, and demonstrating that it inhibited the binding of anti-phage antibodies to the phage. Moreover, when this peptide was attached to multichain polyalanine, the resulting antigen led to antibodies capable of efficiently inactivating the bacteriophage [5]. While the bacteriophage as such is not a target for vaccination, these findings established the basis for anti-viral peptide vaccines.

A more relevant example is influenza virus, for which a synthetic peptide stemming from the viral hemaglutin demonstrated a capacity to induce anti-viral immunity, leading to protection against infection [6]. The case of influenza is of special interest, in view of the frequent and unpredictable changes in its surface proteins. Such changes, denoted shifts and drifts, result in serological differences among different strains of the virus and the demand for a new seasonal vaccine each year. Focus on conserved regions in the viral proteins resulted in several epitopes, eliciting B-cell, T-helper, as well as cytotoxic T-cell (CTL) immunity, and led to efficient long-term immunity and cross-strain protection in mice [7]. Taking this approach somewhat further, and identification of epitopes from several influenza proteins that are recognized by the human HLA [8], is the basis for the efforts of several laboratories and companies toward the development of a universal influenza vaccine [9]. A similar approach could be applicable in the case of human immunodeficiency virus (HIV), which causes AIDS, and for which no efficient vaccine is available as yet.

Synthetic peptides as vaccines were also shown to be effective in the domain of cancer. Thus, early studies demonstrated that antibodies to a synthetic undecapeptide analogous to the amino terminal segment of carcinoembryonic antigen (CEA), characteristic of several kinds of cancer tissues, reacted with the intact protein and with the relevant human sera [10]. Many studies since then have indicated the potential of synthetic peptides representing various epitopes of tumor-associated antigens (TAA), that can indeed induce an anti-cancer response. A few examples for such tumor-specific antigens are the melanoma proteins MAGE [11], the breast cancer-related Her2/neu [12], as well as the mucin MUC-1 [13], but there are many others. Cumulative data related to such antigens led to many cancer vaccine trials in the last decade that have raised hopes, but also led to disappointments. Nevertheless, advances in the engineering of peptides and in our understanding of the molecular mechanisms underlying an effective immune response against tumors have renewed the enthusiasm for peptide-based anti-cancer vaccines, as reviewed recently [14].

15.3
Peptides as Immunomodulators

In addition to their efficacy as immunogens, peptides are also endowed with the capability to modulate the immune response. In this context their effect could be either stimulatory or suppressive, and both types could be advantageous to human health. The immunostimulating peptides, or immune adjuvants, can restore the immune response in immunocompromized conditions, and thus can be of benefit and/or act in concert with chemotherapy in cancer treatment or other extreme situations. Both natural and synthetic peptides have been identified as immuno-modulators, including the naturally occurring cell wall-derived muramyl dipetide (MDP) and its synthetic analogues [15], as well as the IgG-derived tetrapeptide Tuftsin [16] and others. These immunopromoting peptides have been in clinical use for quite a while.

The other facet of peptide activity as immunomodulators is their capacity to reduce the immune response, an activity that is of importance both in immu-nosuppression for prevention of transplant rejection, and in the alleviation of autoimmune disorders. In this context as well, various peptides and polypeptides, natural and synthetic, have been explored. The most prominent among them are the fungal Cyclosporin A [17], and the immunosuppressive peptide FK-506 iso-lated from Streptomyces [18], both indispensible in the clinic for prevention of graft rejection after organ transplantation. Their proven efficacy prompted the preparation of many synthetic analogs, either modified or by substitution of different amino acid residues, in order to improve activity, with the ultimate goal of suppressing the humoral and cellular immune response to the trans-planted organ.

In the case of autoimmune disorders, the goal of immunomodulatory treatment is to dampen the immune response rather than to abrogate it altogether. Among the many agents that are being applied for this purpose, there are a number of regulatory peptides, proteins and glycoproteins (15–30 kDa), known as "soluble factors" cytokines/interleukins that affect the immune system. These include the interferons, and indeed, several recombinant products of IFN-β are approved as drugs for the treatment of multiple sclerosis [19]. Furthermore, they are presently under evaluation for a possible effect in other autoimmune diseases with shared immunological features. Antibodies, both polyclonal human IgG (IVIG) and monoclonal, specific towards various targets associated with the immune response, are also included in the arsenal of possible treatments for the immunomodulation of autoimmune disorders. The development of such monoclonal antibodies is at present a rapidly developing direction of many start-up companies, as well as established pharma, but is beyond the scope of this chapter.

In our laboratory we have developed a unique, synthetic polymer of amino acids denoted Copolymer 1 (Cop 1), or glatiramer acetate (GA), known commercially as Copaxone, which is an approved drug for the treatment of multiple sclerosis, and was shown to exert its activity via immunomodulation. The process of its development and its mode of action are detailed below.

15.4
Development of Copolymer 1 – a Polypeptide Immunomodulator Drug for the Treatment of Multiple Sclerosis

Multiple sclerosis (MS) is a chronic inflammatory demyelinating disease of the central nervous system, in which infiltrating lymphocytes, predominantly T-cells and macrophages, lead to the destruction of the myelin sheath and the formation of demyelinated lesions in the white matter which are the hallmark of this disease [20]. In addition, widespread neuronal pathology with substantial neurodegeneration and diffuse abnormalities in normal-appearing brain tissue are currently recognized as central components of MS pathology. Important data on MS has been obtained by using the animal model – experimental autoimmune encephalomyelitis (EAE) – that can be induced by immunization with myelin antigens such as myelin basic protein (MBP), myelin oligodendrocyte glycoprotein (MOG), or myelin proteolipid protein (PLP) [21]. EAE induction by the different encephalitogenic antigens, or their peptides, in susceptible animal strains leads to the development of various disease forms (acute, relapsing–remitting, or progressive) that mimics the different patterns of MS. Hence, in spite of certain discrepancies, the EAE model is an essential tool for testing novel therapies as well as for the elucidation of their mechanism of action.

In view of the immunological nature of MS and EAE, attempts have been made in several laboratories, since early on, to suppress the disease in animals challenged with MBP by desensitization procedures using the specific antigens relevant to the system. Thus, it has been shown that MBP, if given in high doses in incomplete Freund's adjuvant (IFA), is highly effective in preventing EAE in guinea pigs when administered before sensitization, or in suppressing EAE if given after sensitization. Furthermore, not only the whole encephalitogenic protein was effective in such treatment, but other non-encephalitogenic related substances, including degradation products or synthetic fragments of MBP, had a similar protective effect. On the other hand, several peptides with encephalitogenic activity were incapable of suppressing EAE [22]. This represented corroborating evidence for the assumption that the immunomodulating activity is not necessarily correlated with the encephalitogenicity, and paved the way for the development of synthetic polypeptide immunomodulators.

To this end, we synthesized in our laboratory several random basic copolymers, of amino acid composition approaching to a certain extent that of the natural encephalitogen MBP, and tested their activity in either inducing or suppressing EAE. Whereas none of these synthetic materials possessed any encephalitogenic activity, some of them showed high efficacy in suppressing the disease [23–25]. The most effective among them was copolymer 1 (Cop 1), composed of L-alanine, L-glutamic acid, L-lysine, and L-tyrosine in a molar ratio 6.0/1.9/4.7/1.0, which did not exert any encephalitogenic activity, but had a marked suppressive effect on EAE when injected either in adjuvant or even in aqueous solution [24]. In contrast to the diversity in the response among susceptible species to different determinants, and consequently their restricted susceptibility to specific encephalitogens, the suppressive effect of Cop 1 in EAE was not restricted and could be demonstrated in various species, such as guinea pig, rabbit, mouse as well as in two species of primate – rhesus monkeys and baboons [24, 26–30]. Cop 1 was also found effective in suppressing and preventing chronic relapsing EAE (CR-EAE) in guinea pigs induced by whole spinal cord homogenate [28]. In mice Cop 1 ameliorated acute EAE induced by MBP peptides 1–11 and 84–102, relapsing remitting EAE induced by PLP peptides 139–151 and 178–191, as well as chronic EAE induced by the MOG peptide 35–55 [26, 27]. These combined models simulate the various clinical and pathological features of human MS. The experiments in primates may be considered more relevant to demyelinating diseases in man, not only because of the closer phylogenetic relationship, but also due to the closer resemblance between manifestation of EAE in primates and the human disease. Hence, the significance of the finding that, in both the rhesus monkey and baboon, Cop1 suppresses EAE, even when administered to the animals after the onset of clinical symptoms, leading to a reversal of the disease state with full recovery [29]. Furthermore, the diseased baboons had histological damage typical of EAE, but in those fully recovered from the disease, almost no histopathological lesions were detected [30]. These results have prompted the investigation of Cop 1 in clinical trials for its effect on MS.

15.4.1
Clinical Studies with Cop 1 in MS Patients

Preliminary clinical studies using Cop 1 in MS patients were first conducted by Abramsky [31], and later by Bornstein [32]. These early studies were begun after toxicity studies in experimental animals showed that Cop 1 was non-toxic in both acute and subchronic administration in mice, rats, rabbits, and beagle dogs, and showed no significant uptake by any of the animals' organs. The first clinical application of Cop 1 involved 4 patients in the "terminal" stages of MS, two of whom showed some improvement in vision and speech, but more importantly, no side effects were noted [31]. The subsequent open study with Cop 1 examined its ability to alter the course of MS in 12 chronic-progressive and 4 exacerbating-remitting patients. Again, no undesirable side reactions were noted during their more than 2-year use of Cop 1, and in 3 of the chronic-progressive and 2 of the exacerbating-remitting patients, the disease was arrested and the patients improved [32]. These early trials were followed by a Phase II, double blind controlled trial involving 50 relapsing–remitting MS patients [33]. The patients were selected and pair-matched for age (20–35), disability (Kurtzke DSS 0–6) and exacerbation frequency. They were injected daily, for 24 months with either placebo or 20 mg Cop 1 (the optimal dose as determined in the previous trial). At the end of the 2 years, the results showed that 14 of 25 Cop 1-treated patients were exacerbation-free, compared to only six of 23 in the placebo group. Average exacerbations over 2 years were 2.7 for placebo and 0.6 for Cop 1 patients and the cumulative number of exacerbations showed a dramatic difference between the two groups (Figure 15.1a). Disability status changes were also favored – worsening by 0.75 units in the placebo compared to an improvement of 0.1 unit with Cop 1. All these differences, which showed statistical significance, were more pronounced in the less involved patients of disability score 0–2, than in the more severe patients. Finally, and of the utmost importance, adverse side effects were minimal.

The results of this trial secured the involvement of a pharmaceutical company that conducted a phase III multi-center double-blind trial with Cop 1, on 251 patients, which took place in 11 centers in the United States. This trial demonstrated a 32% decrease in relapse rate ($p = 0.002$) after 2.5 years and improvement in EDSS score ($p = 0.001$) in Cop 1 treated patients versus the placebo group [34, 35]. Additionally, the percentage of patients who improved was higher in the Cop 1 treated group. The treatment was well tolerated and the most common adverse experience was an injection-site reaction, with a very rare self-limited short-lasting systematic reaction [35]. An extension of this trial up to 35 months reconfirmed the clinical benefit as well as the excellent tolerability and safety profile of Cop 1 [36]. MRI studies have also indicated that Cop 1 reduces the frequency of new enhancing lesions and lesion load compared to baseline pre-treatment measure [37, 38].

As a consequence of these clinical trials, and considering the high safety profile of this synthetic polypeptide, Copolymer 1 was approved in 1996 by the FDA as a first line treatment for relapsing–remitting multiple sclerosis, under the commercial name Copaxone, and the generic name glatiramer acetate (GA). Since then, it has been approved in many other countries and is marketed worldwide. To date, over one million years of patient exposure have been accumulated. A follow up for 15 years of patients receiving Cop 1 as a sole disease-modifying therapy demonstrated a sustained persisting beneficial effect, with a 10-fold reduction of average annual rate of exacerbation, and a decrease in both disability progression and transition to progressive disease [39] (Figure 15.1b).

15.4.2
Immunological Mechanisms Involved in the Mitigation of Disease by Cop 1

The mechanism by which Cop 1 induces its beneficial effect in animals and patients was extensively investigated over the years by us and others. These studies

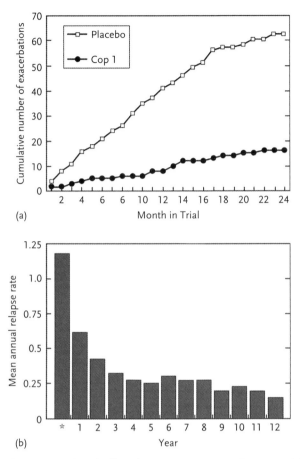

(a)

(b)

Figure 15.1 Clinical effect of Cop 1 treatment in MS Patients. (a) Cumulative number of exacerbations reported by Cop 1-treated in comparison to placebo-treated patients during two years of Phase II double blind controlled trial involving 50 relapsing–remitting MS patients. (b) Annual relapse rate – 12 years follow up of patients receiving Cop 1 as a sole disease-modifying therapy.* Annual relapse rate in the 2 years before starting Cop 1 treatment.

demonstrated that Cop 1 exerts its therapeutic activity by immunomodulating various levels of the immune response, which differ in their degree of specificity. The prerequisite step is the binding of Cop 1 to MHC class II molecules. Cop 1 was demonstrated to exhibit a very rapid, high, and efficient binding to various MHC class II molecules on murine and human antigen-presenting cells (APC), and it even displaced peptides from the MHC-binding site [40]. This competition for binding to the MHC prevents the presentation of other antigens to their specific T-cell receptors and can consequently lead to inhibition of various pathological effector functions. One example of this aspect in the mode of action of Cop 1 is its ability to modulate the immune response raised towards grafted tissue. As a consequence, Cop 1 was found effective in the prevention of graft rejection, either graft against host (GVH) response in bone marrow transplantation [41], or even the rejection of a grafted organ [42]. In both cases, Cop 1 did not react as a general immunosuppressive drug, but rather by diminishing the graft rejection. Combination of Cop 1 with one of the immunosuppressive drugs (Cyclosporin A or FK506) resulted in a synergistic effect [43].

In this process the treatment with Cop 1 inhibited the secretion of Th1 cytokines while inducing Th2 cells, thus emphasizing its role as an immunomodulator. It should be noted that this modulation, on the level of antigen-presenting cells, is the least specific step and can be beneficial for the modulation of detrimental immune responses to various antigens. However, in MS and EAE, the process is more specific and, in addition to the MHC blocking, Cop 1 was shown to inhibit the response to the immunodominant epitope of MBP peptide 82–100 in a strictly antigen-specific manner by acting as a T-cell receptor antagonist [44], indicative of the involvement of T-cells in the effect of Cop 1.

In our earlier studies we have already demonstrated that Cop 1-treated animals (either by subcutaneous injections or oral administration) develop Cop 1-specific T-cells in the peripheral immune system. These cells can adoptively transfer protection against EAE [45]. Furthermore, T-cell lines and hybridomas could be isolated from spleens of animals rendered unresponsive to EAE by Cop 1 [46]. Both cell types act as modulatory suppressor cells, as they inhibited *in vitro* the response of MBP-specific effector cells and inhibited *in vivo* EAE induced by different CNS antigens. The Cop 1-induced cells were indeed characterized as T-helper (Th) cells of the Th2/3 subtype, secreting high amounts of anti-inflammatory cytokines such as IL-4, IL-10, and transforming growth factor (TGF)-β, but not Th1 pro-inflammatory cytokines, in response to both Cop 1 and MBP [47]. Other myelin antigens such as PLP and MOG could not activate the Cop 1-induced cells to secrete Th2 cytokines. However, the disease induced by PLP and MOG could be suppressed by Cop 1 as well as by Cop 1-induced cells, probably by "bystander mechanisms" [48]. Furthermore, a shift from a pro-inflammatory Th1-biased cytokine profile toward an anti-inflammatory Th2-biased profile was observed also in Copaxone-treated MS patients [49–51], indicating that such Cop 1-specific cells are indeed involved in the therapeutic effect of this drug in MS. It is noteworthy that recent findings demonstrate that Cop 1 treatment is associated with a broader immunomodulatory effect on cells of both the innate and adoptive immune system. Hence, in addition to CD4$^+$ T-cells, Cop 1-mediated modulation of APCs, such as monocytes and dendritic cells, CD8$^+$ T-cells, Foxp3 regulatory T-cells (Tregs) and B-cells has been reported [52, 53].

15.4.3
Immunomodulation by Cop 1 in the CNS

Until several years ago, Cop 1-induced cells were demonstrated only in the periphery (spleens and lymph nodes of experimental animals, or peripheral blood mononuclear cells in humans) but not in the organ in which the pathological processes of EAE and MS occur. There was no information indicating whether they can reach the CNS and whether they actually function as suppressor cells *in situ*. More recent findings in our laboratory demonstrating the immunomodulatory activity of Cop 1 in the target organ of MS/EAE, namely the CNS, are of utmost relevance to the mode of action of Cop 1 in MS.

The existence in the CNS of Cop 1-specific T-cells, induced in the periphery either by parenteral or by oral treatment, was demonstrated by their actual isolation from brains of actively sensitized mice, as well as by their localization in the brain following passive transfer to the periphery. Thus, specific *ex vivo* reactivity to Cop 1, manifested by cell proliferation and by Th2 cytokine secretion, was found in whole lymphocyte populations isolated from brains of EAE-induced mice that had been treated by Cop 1 injection [54] or feeding [55]. Moreover, highly reactive Cop 1-specific T-cell lines, that secrete *in vitro* IL-4, IL-5, IL-10, and TGF-β in response to Cop 1, and cross-react with MBP at the level of Th2 cytokine secretion, were obtained from both brains and spinal cords of Cop 1-treated mice [54, 55]. The ability of the Cop 1-induced cells to cross the blood–brain barrier (BBB) and accumulate in the CNS was confirmed by the adoptive transfer (intraperitoneally) of fluorescently labeled Cop 1-specific T-cells and their subsequent detection in the brain. There is currently a consensus that the brain is not an immune privileged site and that activated T-cells, regardless of their specificity, cross the BBB [56]. However, T-cells specific to unrelated antigens subsequently migrate back or die, whereas T-cells specific to CNS antigens can be stimulated *in situ* and persist. The accumulation of Cop 1-specific cells in the brain can be attributed to their cross-reactivity with MBP [25, 46, 47]. While this cross-reactivity may not be essential for the Cop 1-specific cells to reach the brain, it may still enable their *in situ* activation.

Indeed, in the CNS, Cop 1-specific cells manifested intense *in situ* expression of the two potent regulatory anti-inflammatory cytokines IL-10 and TGF-β, but no trace of the detrimental inflammatory cytokine IFN-γ [57]. Of special interest is the finding that IL-10 and TGF-β were expressed not only by the Cop 1-specific T-cells but also by other cells in their vicinity, such as astrocytes. In contrast, the overall expression of IFN-γ in the brain tissue was drastically reduced. Recently, we demonstrated that Cop 1 treatment also induces drastic reduction in the occurrence of the pro-inflammatory Th-17 cells with parallel elevation of Tregs in the CNS of mice with either chronic (MOG-induced) or relapsing–remitting (PLP-induced) EAE [58], (Figure 15.2). These results indicated that Cop 1 treatment induces a bystander immunomodulatory effect on the CNS resident cells themselves and generates a Th1 to Th2/3 cytokine shift *in situ*, thus restraining the inflammatory pathological disease progression. However, the effect of Cop 1 is not restricted to anti-inflammation, and, as demonstrated in the following, it involves genuine neuroprotective processes.

15.4.4
Neuroprotection and Augmentation of Neurotropic Factors in the Brain

An essential challenge for MS therapy is to target not only the inflammatory aspect of the disease but also its neuronal pathology, aiming towards neuroprotective

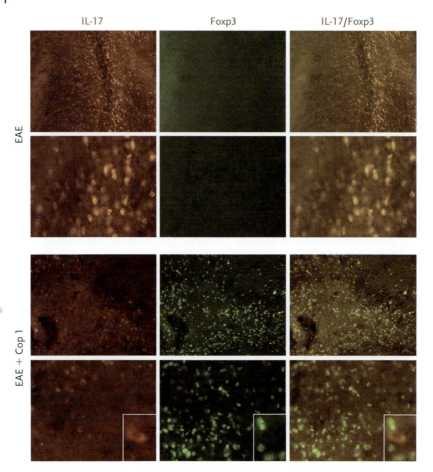

Figure 15.2 The effect of Cop 1 treatment on Th-17 cells and T-regulatory cells in the CNS of EAE-induced mice. Staining of brain sections from MOG-induced mice with antibodies to the pro-inflammatory cytokine IL-17 (orange) and to the T-regulatory marker Foxp3 (green), in the white matter area of the cortex. In brains of EAE untreated mice cellular infiltrations contain numerous IL-17[+] and minimal Foxp3[+] expressing cells, whereas in brains of Cop 1-treated mice, even when treatment started after disease manifestation (suppression regimen), rare IL-17[+] and many Foxp3[+] cells are found.

outcomes. By broad definition, neuroprotection is an effect that results in salvage, recovery, or regeneration of the nervous system, its cells, structure, and function [59].

During recent years accumulated findings revealed that Cop 1 treatment indeed generates neuroprotective consequences in the CNS. The initial indication for such effect was the ability of Cop 1-induced cells to secrete not only anti-inflammatory cytokines, but also the potent brain derived neurotrophic factor (BDNF). This was demonstrated for mouse Cop 1-specific T-cells originating from the periphery or the CNS, as well as for human T-cell lines, at both the protein and the mRNA levels [57, 59–63]. Furthermore, Cop 1-specific T-cells demonstrated extensive BDNF expression in the brain of EAE mice, in contrast to the low expression in the corresponding brain regions of EAE untreated mice [57]. In addition to the Cop 1-specific Th2/3 T-cells that penetrated the CNS, most of the BDNF positive cells were neurons and astrocytes. Namely, the CNS resident cells themselves. BDNF was also elevated in brains of mice that were injected daily (subcutaneously) with Cop 1 as such, parallel to the practice used in the treatment of MS patients. A similar phenomenon was found in brains of Cop 1-treated mice for two additional neurotrophic factors – NT3 and NT4 [63].

Members of the neurotrophin (NT) family, such as BDNF, NT-3, and NT-4, are important regulators of neuronal function and survival [64, 65]. Besides their well-established role in neuronal development, process growth and regulation of synaptic plasticity, they have the capacity to protect neurons against various pathological insults. BDNF, in particular, was shown to rescue degenerating neurons, promote axonal outgrowth, remyelination, and regeneration [65]. The elevation of these factors in the diseased organ may thus be of functional relevance and promote neuroprotective consequences. Of special significance is the finding that Cop 1 elevated the neurotrophic factors level, even when treatment started late – in the chronic disease phase, which is regarded as the stage in which exhausted self-compensating neuroprotection fails, and extensive neurodegeneration takes place [66, 67]. Reduced levels of BDNF in the serum and the cerebral spinal fluid of MS patients, and its reversal by Cop 1 treatment, have also been reported [68], suggestive of the relevance of this effect to human therapy.

The neuroprotective effect of Cop 1, as demonstrated by the augmentation of neurotrophins in the brain, was accompanied by considerable lowering of the neurological damage. This was manifested by preservation of the retinal ganglion cells in EAE-induced rats [69], as well as by the reduced amount and size of lesions in various brain regions of EAE-induced mice [70]. The beneficial effect of Cop 1 was also evident even when treatment was initiated long after the appearance of disease – in the chronic disease phase, thus suggesting induction of genuine repair mechanisms.

15.4.5
Myelin Repair and Neurogenesis

Repair processes, namely remyelination and neurogenesis, are major goals for MS therapy, involving a very active field of research, and hence they comprise a crucial aspect in the effect of immunomodulating treatments. The central elements of the CNS – the myelinating oligodendrocytes as well as the neurons – are terminally differentiated cells with a limited capacity to respond to injury. They depend for renewal on the availability of their precursors – the oligodendrocyte progenitor cells (OPCs) and the neuronal progenitor cells (NPCs), which need to undergo proliferation, migration and differentiation into the defined progeny. Moreover, to be effective in neuroprotection and repair they must survive in the hostile conditions within the inflamed lesions.

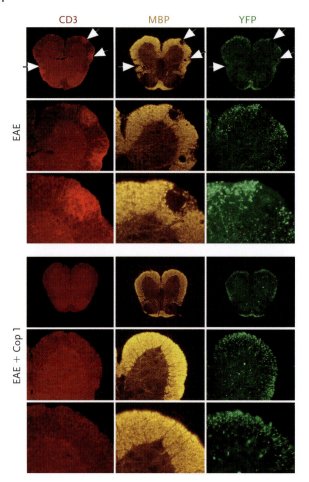

Figure 15.3 Immunohistochemical characterization of spinal cords from EAE mice and the effect of Cop 1 treatment. Corresponding coronal spinal cord sections from MOG-induced EAE mice revealing inflammation/T-cell infiltration (CD3 cells are stained in red), multiple demyelination sites (MBP is stained in yellow), accompanied by fiber deterioration (all neuronal fibers express YFP in green) in EAE untreated mouse (indicated by arrows), in contrast to the negligible damage detected in Cop 1-treated mouse.

During recent years, several studies have demonstrated that Cop 1 treatment led to neuroprotective outcome on the primary target of the EAE/MS pathological process – the myelin [71, 72]. Using scanning electron microscopy and immunohistochemistry, we found that Cop 1 prevented the typical EAE demyelination (Figure 15.3). Hence, treatment at the early disease stages prevented demyelination altogether. Moreover, even when treatment was initiated in the chronic disease phase, when substantial demyelination was already manifested, it resulted in a significant decrease in myelin damage. The mode of action of Cop 1 in this system was attributed to increased proliferation, and survival of oligodendrocyte

(a)   (b)   (c)

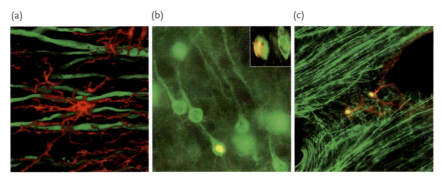

Figure 15.4 Neuroprotection *in situ* – progenitor cells in the CNS of EAE-induced mice treated by Cop 1. (a) Oligodendrocyte progenitor cell (stained for NG2 in red), extending multiple processes, intertwines several transected nerve fibers within a spinal cord lesion of transgenic mouse expressing YFP on its neuronal population (green). (b) Fate tracing of neuronal progenitor cells. A pyramidal neuron in the cortex, born during the concurrent injections of the proliferation marker BrdU and Cop 1, to an EAE-induced transgenic mouse, that selectively express YFP on its neuronal population. One month after treatment, neurons co-expressing BrdU (yelow) and YFP (green) with apical dendrites and axons are seen, indicative of mature functional neurons. Insert, BrdU positive cell (yellow) co-expressing the mature neuronal marker NeuN (green). (c) Penetration of neuronal progenitors into injury sites. Neuroprogenitor cells born during the concurrent injections of BrdU and Cop 1, co-expressing BrdU (yellow) and DCX (orange) are depicted inside a lesion in the frontal cortex (layer 5/6), accompanied by axonal sprouting and extension of YFP-expressing neuronal fibers (green) into the lesion.

progenitor cells (OPCs) along the oligodendroglial maturation cascade, and their recruitment into injury sites, thus enhancing repair processes *in situ*. Furthermore, Cop 1 treatment induced a morphological transformation of OPCs from the earlier bipolar progenitor to the more mature pre-oligodendrocyte multiprocessed form, suggesting its effect on the differentiation along the oligodendroglial maturation cascade (Figure 15.4).

Concerning the functional cells in the CNS – the neurons – current opinion claims that stem cells with potential to give rise to new neurons reside in different regions of the mammalian brain and may contribute to repair and recovery after injury [73]. In our own studies we investigated whether Cop 1 treatment can augment neurogenesis [70]. EAE induction as such triggered increased neuroprogenitor proliferation in the neuroproliferative zones, but this effect was of short duration and subsequently declined to levels below that of the naïve control mice. In contrast, Cop 1 treatment, applied at various disease stages, augmented neuronal proliferation to a higher level than that observed in EAE mice, and this effect persisted for a prolonged duration. Furthermore, neuronal progenitors diverged from the classic migratory streams and spread to adjacent atypical brain regions that do not normally undergo neurogenesis. After one month, neurons born during Cop 1 treatment that express mature neuronal markers and display mature morphology were found in the cortex of the treated mice (Figure 15.4). These newly formed neurons could constitute a pool for the replacement of dead or dysfunctional cells and/or induce a growth-promoting environment that supports neuroprotection and axonal growth. The latter activity was evidenced by BDNF expression of the new neurons. It can thus be concluded that an immunomodulatory treatment can essentially promote neurogenesis and the formation of new neurons in sites of injury, thus counteracting the neurodegenerative course of disease.

These neuroprotective effects induced by Cop 1, in particular its ability to induce a growth-promoting environment, in addition to its previously demonstrated ability to reduce inflammatory and immune rejection processes, supported its application for the improvement of stem/progenitor cell engraftment in the CNS. Indeed, we recently demonstrated that in EAE mice inoculated intra-ventricularly with muscle progenitor cells, Cop 1 treatment improved the incorporation and differentiation of the transplanted cells towards the neuronal pathway [74].

Findings from human studies support the notion that Cop 1 confers neuro-protection in MS patients as well, since treatment with Cop 1 reduced the formation of permanent T1 hypointense lesions that evolved into "black holes" which have been associated with irreversible neurological disability [75]. By quantitative MRI analysis, it was also shown that Cop 1 treatment for 1 year led to a significant increase in neurological markers compared to pre treatment values, suggestive of axonal metabolic recovery and protection from sub-lethal axonal injury [76]. Altogether, these findings may explain the long term beneficial effect of Cop 1 in patients followed up for 15 years and more [39].

15.4.6
The Effect of Cop 1 on Another Autoimmune Disease – Inflammatory Bowel Disease

Based on the immunomodulatory mode of action manifested by Cop 1, as well as its high safety profile, its application for an additional immune-mediated pathology, namely inflammatory bowel disease, has been explored. Inflammatory bowel disease (IBD), in particular Crohn's disease (CD), are severe gastrointestinal disorders characterized by detrimental immune reactivity in the gut, mainly $CD4^+$ Th1 cells and an imbalance between pro-inflammatory and anti-inflammatory cytokines [77]. In view of the immunopathological "autoimmune-like" nature of IBD, we tested the effect of Cop 1 in several IBD animal models and found that Cop 1 treatment ameliorated the various pathological manifestations in all these models, including trinitrobenzene sulfonic acid (TNBS)-induced colitis, dextran sulfate sodium (DSS)-induced colitis of different severity levels, as well as a spontaneous IBD model in transgenic mice [78, 79]. The beneficial effect of Cop 1 was manifested in significant abrogation of the weight loss, intestinal bleeding, diarrhea, and macroscopic colon damage that are characteristic to this disease, as well as in conserving glandular colon architecture, thus resulting in improved long-term survival. In all these models the detrimental proinflammatory response manifested by cell proliferation, as well as TNF-α and IFN-γ expression, was significantly decreased following Cop 1 treatment, whereas the regulatory anti-inflammatory TGF-β and IL-10 response was elevated. Furthermore, these beneficial effects could be achieved not only by Cop 1 treatment but also by adoptive transfer of specific T-cells originating in mice immunized with Cop 1 [80]. Similarly to their migratory pattern in EAE, upon transfer to DSS-induced mice, the Cop 1-specific cells localized in the diseased organ – in this case inner layers of the colon – and secreted *in situ* the anti-inflammatory regulatory cytokine TGF-β, thus inducing immunomodulation at the site in which the pathological process occurs. In view of the therapeutic consequence of Cop 1 in the various IBD models, its therapeutic effect is currently being tested in a clinical trial.

15.5
Additional Immunomodulatory Peptides as Drug Candidates

Additional peptide candidates as drugs against autoimmune diseases may be mentioned here. Three examples will be given: against autoimmune type 1 diabetes, against myasthenia gravis, and against lupus erythematosus. In all these cases, like in the case of Copaxone in multiple sclerosis, the drugs may be considered therapeutic vaccines.

15.5.1
Peptide Therapy for Type 1 Diabetes

Type 1 (insulin-dependent) diabetes mellitus is caused by an autoimmune process that leads to inappropriate inflammation directed at the pancreatic islets. The inflammation selectively causes the functional inactivation and ultimately the death of the insulin-producing beta cells. Irun Cohen and his colleagues have investigated several heat-shock proteins (HSP), and shown that mammalian HSP60 was the true target of autoimmunity in mice. They then identified a 24 amino acid peptide containing a major T-cell epitope: residues 437–460 in the sequence of human HSP60, and named the peptide p277. Its injection in incomplete Freund's adjuvant to NOD mice inhibited the development of spontaneous diabetes [81]. Moving to humans, a randomized, double-blind, phase II trial has been reported [82]. It showed preservation of beta-cell function associated with a specific Th2 shift, indicating the immunomodulatory effect of the peptide. In the improved p277 peptide the cysteine residues were replaced with valine residues. The DiaPep277 used in the trial is peptide p277 in vegetable oil with a mannitol filler, and it is presently in phase III trial.

Therapeutic vaccination with p277 can arrest the spontaneous diabetogenic process both in NOD mice and in humans, associated with a Th1 to Th2 cytokine shift specific for the autoimmune T-cells. P277 can directly signal human T-cells also via innate toll-like receptor (TLR)-2, leading to up-regulation of integrin-mediated adhesion to fibronectin, and inhibition of chemotaxis to the chemokine SDF-1a *in vivo* [83]. Thus, T-cells do respond innately to p277, and signaling by soluble p277 through TLR-2- could contribute to the treatment of type 1 diabetes. P277 may stop the destruction of beta cells by signaling in concert both innate and adaptive receptors on T-cells.

15.5.2
Myasthenia Gravis (MG)

The attack of specific antibodies on the acetylcholine receptor (AChR) is the accepted cause of disease in MG. Weakness and fatigability of voluntary muscles characterize both MG and experimental autoimmune MG (EAMG). Although the symptoms of MG are caused by autoantibodies produced by B-cells, there is ample evidence that T-cells have a key role in the etiopathology of the disease in humans and animals. Because the a-subunit of the AChR was shown to be predominant for T-cells epitopes, use was made of the peptides representing different sequences of the human AChR subunit. Two sequences of the latter, namely, peptides p195-212 and p259-271, were able to stimulate peripheral blood lymphocytes (PBL) of patients with MG. Furthermore, PBL of seronegative MG patients responded by either proliferation or IL-2 secretion to these peptides, emphasizing the importance of AChR-specific T-cells in MG. Peptides p195-212 and p259-271 were further shown to be immunodominant T-cell epitopes in SJL and BALB/c mice, respectively.

Ideally, the goal of therapy in MG should be the elimination of autoimmune responses to the AChR specifically, without interfering with immune responses to other antigens. To this end, altered myasthenia peptides, which are single amino acid-substituted analogs of peptide p195-212 (207Ala) and p259-271 (262Lys), as well as a dual-altered peptide ligand (APL), composed of the randomly arranged two single peptide analogs (262Lys-207Ala), were synthesized and shown to inhibit the pro-liferative responses of both p195-212 and p259-271-specific T-cell lines *in vitro* [84].

It was also shown that oral administration of the dual APL to BALB/c mice afflicted with EAMG induced by the pathogenic p259-271-specific T-cell line reversed EAMG manifestations in the treated mice. Furthermore, it also affects beneficially EAMG manifestations induced in rats.

The dual analog vaccine candidate acts by specifically and actively suppressing myasthenogenic T-cell responses. This active suppression is mediated by the upregulation of transforming growth factor-β (TGF-β) secretion and down-regulation of IFN-γ and IL-2 (Th1-type cytokines). A state of nonresponsiveness is induced by the dual analog, which, at least partially, causes the cells to undergo anergy. Thus, the dual analog can definitely be considered a candidate for a therapeutic vaccine. More recently, experiments were performed that clearly show that the dual APL downregulates myasthenogenic T-cell responses by upregulat-ing CD25$^+$ and CTLA-4 expressing T-cells [85], as well as CD8$^+$ CD28$^+$ regulating cells [86], indicating its effect as an immunomodulator.

Furthermore, the cumulative result of all of the cell populations and stages affected by the dual APL is the amelioration of an established EAMG.

15.5.3
A Novel Tolerogenic Peptide for the Specific Treatment of Systemic Lupus Erythematosus

Systemic lupus erythematosus (SLE) is a complex disease characterized by the generation of autoantibodies and clinical involvement of multiple organs. T- and

B-cells play a role in the development of SLE. Current therapies for SLE are mainly based on the use of non-specific immunosuppressive drugs and have serious side effects. As a potential candidate for the specific treatment of SLE patients, a tolerogenic peptide, designated hCDR1, that is based on the sequence of the heavy chain complementarity determining region (CDR)1 of a human monoclonal anti-DNA, has been designed and synthesized [87]. hCDR1 was tested for its ability to ameliorate SLE manifestations in spontaneous and induced models of SLE in mice. Administration of hCDR1 subcutaneously, once a week for 10 weeks, resulted in a significant amelioration of the serological manifestations that developed either in the spontaneously SLE-prone (NZB × NZW)F1 mice, or in several experimentally induced animal models of SLE. Furthermore, tolerogenic administration of low doses of hCDR1 ameliorated the serological, renal, and neurological manifestations of SLE in murine models [88].

In view of the various immunomodulatory effects of hCDR1 in the murine models of lupus, it was of interest to determine the effects of the peptide on SLE patients. *In vitro* studies with the patients' PBMC showed that hCDR1 downregulated significantly their IL-1β, IFN-γ, and IL-10 gene expression. Moreover, it upregulated the expression of the anti-apoptotic molecule Bcl-xL and downregulated the pro-apoptotic caspase-3, resulting in reduced rates of apoptosis. HCDR1 also increased the expression of the immunosuppressive cytokine TGF-β and of the regulatory master gene FoxP3 [89]. The elevated gene expression of FoxP3 was due to hCDR1-induced upregulation of TGF-β, resulting in an increase in CD4$^+$CD25$^+$FoxP3$^+$ functional, regulatory cells. These results showed that hCDR1 immunomodulated PBMC' of SLE patients via mechanisms similar to those observed in murine lupus models, suggesting that hCDR1 might have beneficial effects in SLE patients. Indeed, a study in which 9 SLE patients participated showed that treatment with hCDR1 downregulated significantly, both on the mRNA level and *in vivo*, the gene expression of pathogenic cytokines, apoptosis, as well as other SLE-related genes, and upregulated immunosuppressive molecules, restoring the global immune dysregulation of lupus patients. Due to the limited number of patients the clinical results should be interpreted with caution. However, the effects of hCDR1 on the gene expression were associated with clinical amelioration [90]. Hence, taking into consideration the safety of treatment with hCDR1 and the fact that its effects are specific to SLE-associated responses, the results suggest a potential role for hCDR1 in the treatment of lupus.

15.6
Summary and Concluding Remarks

This chapter illustrates the multifaceted role played by peptides and polypeptides in modulating the immune response. This modulation may result, on the one hand, in stimulation of the immune response, which may lead, in turn, to peptide-based vaccines, both prophylactic and therapeutic, either against infectious diseases, or for the treatment of autoimmune diseases. On the other hand, peptides can mitigate the immune response, which can lead to immunosuppression, thus giving rise to most powerful drugs for the prevention of graft rejection after organ transplantation. However, less drastic and more controlled suppression of the immune response can also be mediated by peptides and polypeptides which serve as immunomodulators for the amelioration of quite a few autoimmune diseases. One example is the synthetic amino acid copolymer Cop 1, an effective approved drug (Copaxone®) for the treatment of multiple sclerosis, which may prove effective in the case of other autoimmune diseases as well. All these peptide immunomodulators have a specific effect on the cells involved in the immune response and the cytokines they secrete, allowing, on the one hand, the *in vitro* assessment of the immunomodulatory activity, and, on the other hand, the determination of the *in situ* expression of these cytokines in the damaged organ affected by the autoimmune process. In such cases a correlation between the immunomodulating activity and the amelioration of the autoimmune process can be drawn, thus providing the rationale for their therapeutic efficacy. Finally, different synthetic peptides based on the relevant antigenic specificity are demonstrated as disease-specific immunomodulators which may provide a novel therapeutic approach for the treatment of various autoimmune diseases.

References

1 Sela, M. (1969) Antigenicity: some molecular aspects. *Science*, **166**, 1365–1374.

2 Maoz, A., Fuchs, S., and Sela, M. (1973) On immunological cross-reactions between the synthetic ordered polypeptide (L-Pro-Gly-L-Pro)n and several collagens. *Biochemistry*, 4246–4252.

3 Arnon, R. and Sela, M. (1969) Antibodies to a unique region in lysozyme provoked by a synthetic antigen conjugate. *Proc. Natl. Acad. Sci. USA.*, **62**, 163–170.

4 Arnon, R., Maron, E., Sela, M., and Anfinsen, C.B. (1971) Antibodies reactive with native lysozyme elicited by a completely synthetic antigen. *Proc. Natl. Acad. Sci. USA.*, **68**, 1950–1955.

5 Langbeheim, H., Arnon, R., and Sela, M. (1976) Antiviral effect on MS-2 coliphage obtained with a synthetic antigen. *Proc. Natl. Acad. Sci. USA.*, **73**, 4636–4640.

6 Muller, G.M., Shapira, M., and Arnon, R. (1982) Anti-influenza response achieved by immunization with a

synthetic antigen. *Proc. Natl. Acad. Sci. USA.*, **79**, 569–573.

7 Levi, R. and Arnon, R. (1996) Synthetic recombinant influenza vaccine induces efficient long-term immunity and cross-strain protection. *Vaccine*, **14** (1), 85–92.

8 Ben-Yedidia, T., Marcus, H., Reisner, Y., and Arnon, R. (1999) Intranasal administration of peptide vaccine protects human/mouse radiation chimera from influenza infection. *Int. J. Immunol.*, **11** (7), 1043–1051.

9 Cassone, A. and Rappuoli, R. (2010) Universal vaccines: Shifting to one for many. *mBio*, **1**, e00042–10.

10 Arnon, R., Bustin, M., Calif, E., Chaitchik, S., Haimovich, J., Novik, N., and Sela, M. (1976) Immunological cross-reactivity of antibodies to a synthetic undecapeptide analogous to the amino terminal segment of carcinoembryonic antigen, with the intact protein and with human sera. *Proc. Natl. Acad. Sci. USA.*, **73**, 2123–2127.

11 Coulie, P.G., Karanikas, V., Lurquin, C., Colau, D., Hanagiri, T., Van Pel, A.,

Lucas, S., Godelaine, D., Lonchay, C., Marchand, M., Van Baren, N, and Boon, T. (2002) Cytolytic T-cell responses of cancer patients vaccinated with a MAGE antigen. *Immunol. Rev.*, **188**, 33–42.

12 Disis, M.L., Gralow, J.R., Bernhard, H., Hand, S.L., Rubin, W.D., and Cheever, M.A. (1996) Peptide-based, not whole protein, vaccines elicit immunity to HER-2/neu, oncogenic self-protein. *J. Immunol.*, **156** (9), 3151–3158.

13 Moyal-Amsellem, N. and Arnon, R. (2010) *Therapeutic Muc1-Based Vaccine Expressed in Flagella – Efficacy in Aggressive Model of Breast cancer*, submitted for publication.

14 Khazaie, K., Bonertz, A., and Beckhove, P. (2009) Current developments with peptide-based human tumor vaccines. *Curr Opin Oncol.*, **6**, 524–530.

15 Chedid, L. and Lederer, E. (1978) Past, present and future of the synthetic immunoadjuvant MDP and its analogs. *Biochem Pharmacol.*, **27**, 2183–2186.

16 Najjar, V.A. and Nishioka, K. (1970) Tuftsin: a natural phagocytic stimulating peptide. *Nature*, **228**, 672–673.

17 Borel, J.F, Feurer, C., Gubler, H.U, and Stähelin, H. (1976) Biological effects of cyclosporin A: a new anti lymphocytic agent. *Agents Actions*, **6**, 468–475.

18 Kino, T., Hatanaka, H., Hashimoto, M., Nishiyama, M., Goto, T., Okuhara, M., Kohasaka, M., Aoki, H., and Imanaka, H. (1987) FK-506, a novel immunosuppressant isolated from a Streptomyces. I. Fermentation, isolation, and physico-chemical and biological characteristics. *J. Antibiot.*, **40**, 1249–1255.

19 Jacobs, L. and Johnson, K.P. (1994) A brief history of the use of interferons as treatment for multiple sclerosis. *Arch. Neurol.*, **51**, 1245–1252.

20 Lassmann, H., Bruck, W., and Lucchinetti, F. (2007) The immunopathology of MS: an overview. *Brain Pathol.*, **17**, 210–218.

21 Furlan, R., Cuomo, C., and Martino, G. (2009) Animal models of multiple sclerosis. *Methods Mol. Biol.*, **549**, 157–173.

22 Arnon, R. (1981) Experimental allergic encephalomyelitis-susceptibility and suppression. *Immunol. Rev.*, **55**, 5–30.

23 Teitelbaum, D., Meshorer, A., Hirshfeld, T., Arnon, R., and Sela, M. (1971) Suppression of experimental allergic encephalomyelitis by a synthetic basic copolymer. *Eur. J. Immunol.*, **1**, 242–248.

24 Teitelbaum, D., Webb, C., Meshorer, A., Arnon, R., and Sela, M. (1973). Suppression by several synthetic polypeptides of experimental allergic encephalomyelitis induced in guinea pigs and rabbits with bovine and human basic encephalitogen. *Eur. J. Immunol.*, **3**, 273–279.

25 Webb, C., Teitelbaum, D., Hertz, A., Arnon, R., and Sela, M. (1976) Molecular requirements involved in suppression of EAE by synthetic basic copolymers of amino acids. *Immunochemistry*, **13**, 333–337.

26 Teitelbaum, D., Fridkis-Hareli, M., Arnon, R., and Sela, M. (1996) Copolymer 1 inhibits the onset of chronic relapsing experimental autoimmune encephalomyelitis and interferes with T-cell responses to encephalitogenic peptides of myelin proteolipid protein. *J. Neuroimmunol.*, **64**, 209–217.

27 Ben-Nun, A., Mendel, I., Bakimer, R., Fridkis-Hareli, M., Teitelbaum, D., Arnon, R., and Sela, M. (1966). The autoimmune reactivity to myelin oligodendrocyte glycoprotein (MOG) in multiple sclerosis is potentially pathogenic: effect of copolymer-1 on MOG induced disease. *J. Neurol.*, **243**, S14–S22.

28 Keith, A.B., Arnon, R., Teitelbaum, D., Caspary, E.A., and Wisniewski, H.M. (1979) The effect of Cop 1, a synthetic polypeptide, on chronic relapsing experimental allergic encephalomyelitis in guinea pigs. *J. Neurol. Sci.*, **42**, 267–274.

29 Teitelbaum, D., Webb, C., Bree, M., Meshorer, A., Arnon, R., and Sela, M. (1974) Suppression of experimental allergic encephalomyelitis in rhesus monkeys by a synthetic basic copolymer. *Clin. Immunol. Immunopathol.*, **3**, 256–262.

30 Teitelbaum, D., Meshorer, A., and Arnon, R. (1977) Suppression of experimental allergic encephalomyelitis in baboons by cop 1. *Israel J. Med. Sci.*, **13**, 1038.

31 Abramsky, O., Teitelbaum, D., and Arnon, R. (1977) Effect of a synthetic polypeptide (Cop 1) on patients with multiple sclerosis and with acute disseminated encephalomyelitis. *J. Neurol. Sci.*, **31**, 433–438.

32 Bornstein, M.B., Miller, A.J., Teitelbaum, D., Arnon, R., and Sela, M. (1982). Multiple sclerosis: trial of a synthetic polypeptide. *Ann. Neurol.*, **11**, 327–319.

33 Bornstein, M.B., Miller, A., Slagle, S., Weitzman, M., Crystal, H., Drexler, E., Keilson, M., Merriam, A., Wassertheil-Smoller, S., Spada, V., Weiss, W., Arnon, R., Jacobsohn, I., Teitelbaum, D., and Sela, M. (1987). A pilot trial of Cop 1 in exacerbating-remitting multiple sclerosis. *N. Engl. J. Med.*, **317**, 408–414.

34 Johnson, K.P., Brooks, B.R., Cohen, J.A., Ford, C.C., Goldstein, J., Lisak, R.P., Myers, L.W, Panitch, H.S., Rose, J.W, Schiffer, R.B., Vollmer, T., Weiner, L.P., and Wolinsky, J.C (1995). Copolymer reduces relapse rate and improves disability in relapsing-remitting multiple sclerosis. Results of a phase III multicenter double blind, placebo-controlled trial. *Neurology*, **1**, 65–70.

35 Johnson, K.P. and The Copolymer I Multiple Sclerosis Study Group (1996). Extended report of the positive multicenter III phase III trial of copolymer 1 for the treatment of relapsing remitting multiple sclerosis. *Neurology*, **46**, A406.

36 Johnson, K.P., Brooks, B.R., Cohen, J.A., Ford, C.C., Goldstein, J., Lisak, R.P., Myers, L.W., Panitch, H.S., Rose, J.W, Schiffer, R.B., Vollmer, T., Weiner, L.P. *et al.* (1998). Extended use of glatiramer acetate (Copaxone) is well tolerated and maintains its clinical effect on multiple sclerosis relapse rate and degree of disability. Copolymer 1 Multiple Sclerosis study Group. *Neurology*, **50**, 701–708.

37 Mancardi, G.L., Sardanelli, F., Parodi, R. C., Capello, E., Ingles, M. *et al.* (1988) Effect of copolymer-1 on serial

gadolinium enhanced MRI in relapsing remitting multiple sclerosis. *Neurology*, **50** (4), 1127–1133.

38 Comi, G., Filippi, M., and Wolinsky, J.S. (2001) European/Canadian multicenter, double-blind, randomized, placebo controlled study of the effects of glatiramer acetate on magnetic resonance imaging-measured disease activity and burden in patients with relapsing multiple sclerosis. European/Canadian Glatiramer Acetate Study Group. *Ann. Neurol.*, **49**, 290–297.

39 Ford, C., Goodman, A.D., Johnson, K., Kachuk, N., Linsey, J.W., Lisak, R., Luzzio, C., Meyers, L, Panitch, H., Preiningerova, J., Pruitt, A., Rose, J., Rus, H., and Wolinsky, J. (2010). Continuous long-term immunomodulatory therapy in relapsing multiple sclerosis: results from the 15 year analysis of the US prospective open-label study of glatiramer acetate. *Multiple Sclerosis*, 1–9.

40 Fridkis-Hareli, M., Teitelbaum, D., Gurevich E., Pecht I., Brautbar, C., Oh Joong, K., Brenner, T., Arnon, R., and Sela, M. (1994). Direct binding of myelin basic protein and synthetic copolymer 1 to class II major histocompatibility complex molecules on living antigen presenting cells-specificity and promiscuity. *Proc .Natl. Acad. Sci. USA.*, **91**, 4872–4876.

41 Schlegel, P., Aharoni, R., Chen, J. Teitelbaum, D., Arnon, R., Sela, M., and Chao, N.J. (1996). A synthetic random basic copolymer with promiscuous binding to class II major histocompatibility complex molecules inhibits T-cell proliferative responses to major and minor histocompatibility antigens *in vitro* and confers the capacity to prevent murine graft-versus-host disease *in vivo*. *Proc. Natl. Acad. Sci. USA.*, **93**, 5061–5066.

42 Aharoni, R., Teitelbaum, D., and Sela, M. (2001). Copolymer 1 inhibits manifestations of graft rejection. *Transplantation*, **72** (4), 598–605.

43 Aharoni, R., Yussim, A., Sela, M., and Arnon. R. (2005). Combined treatment of Glatiramer Acetate and low doses of

immunosuppressive drugs is effective in the prevention of graft rejection. *Int. Immunopharm.*, **5**, 23–32.

44 Aharoni, R., Teitelbaum, D., Arnon, R., and Sela. M. (1999) Copolymer 1 acts against the immunodominant epitope 82–100 of myelin basic protein by T-cell receptor antagonism in addition to major histocompatibility complex blocking. *Proc. Natl. Acad. Sci. USA.*, **96**, 634–639.

45 Lando, Z., Teitelbaum, T., and Arnon, R. (1979) Effect of cyclophosphamide on suppressor cell activity in mice unresponsive to EAE. *J. Immunol.*, **123**, 2156–2160.

46 Aharoni, R., Teitelbaum, D., and Arnon, R. (1993). T-suppressor hybridomas and IL-2 dependent lines induced by copolymer 1 or by spinal cord homogenate down regulate experimental allergic encephalomyelitis. *Eur. J. Immunol.*, **23**, 17–25.

47 Aharoni, R., Teitelbaum, D., Sela, M., and Arnon, R. (1997) Copolymer 1 induces suppressor T-cells of the Th2 type that cross react with myelin basic protein and suppress experimental autoimmune encephalomyelitis. *Proc. Natl. Acad. Sci. USA.*, **94**, 10821–10826.

48 Aharoni, R., Teitelbaum, D., Sela, M., and Arnon, R. (1998) Bystander suppression of experimental autoimmune encephalomyelitis by T-cell lines and clones of the Th2 type induced by Copolymer 1. *J. Neuroimmunol.*, **91**, 135–146.

49 Miller, A., Shapiro, S., Gershtein, R., Kinarty, A., Rawashdeh, H., Honigman, S., and Lahat, N. (1998). Treatment of multiple sclerosis with copolymer-1 (Copaxone): implicating mechanisms of Th1 to Th2/Th3 immune-deviation. *J. Neuroimmunol.*, **92**, 113–121.

50 Neuhaus, O., Farina, C., Yassouridis, A., Wiendl, H., Then Bergh, F., Dose, T., Wekerle, H., and Hohlfeld, R. (2000). Multiple sclerosis: comparison to copolymer-1-reactive T-cell lines from treated and untreated subjects reveals cytokine shift from T helper 1 to T helper 2 cells. *Proc. Natl. Acad. Sci. USA.*, **97** (13), 7452–7457.

51 Duda, P.W., Schmied, M.C., Cook, S.L., Krieger, J.I., and Hafler, D.A. (2000) Glatiramer acetate (Copaxone) induces degenerate, TH2-polarized immune responses in patients with multiple sclerosis. *J. Clin. Invest.*, **105**, 967–976.

52 Weber, M.S, Prod'homme, T., Youssef, S. *et al.* (2007) Type II monocytes modulate T-cell-mediated central nervous system autoimmune disease. *Nature Med.*, **13** (8), 935–943.

53 Ziemssen, T. and Schrempf, W. (2007) Glatiramer acetate: mechanisms of action in multiple sclerosis. *Int. Rev. Neurobiol.*, **9**, 537–570.

54 Aharoni, R., Teitelbaum, D., Leitner, O., Meshorer, A., Sela, M., and Arnon, R. (2000) Specific Th2 cells accumulate in the central nervous system of mice protected against EAE by copolymer. *Proc. Natl. Acad. Science USA.*, **97**, 11472–11477.

55 Aharoni, R., Meshorer, A., Sela, M., and Arnon, R. (2002) Oral treatment of mice with Copolymer 1 results in the accumulation of specific Th2 cells in the central nervous system. *J. Neuroimmunol.*, **126**, 58–68.

56 Skundric, D.S., Kim, C., Tse, H.Y., and Raine, C.S. (1993) Homing of T-cells to the central nervous system throughout the course of relapsing experimental autoimmune encephalomyelitis in Thy-1 congenic mice. *J. Neuroimmunol*, **46** (1–2), 113–121.

57 Aharoni, R., Kayhan, B., Eilam, R., Sela, M., and Arnon, R. (2003) Glatiramer acetate specific T-cells in the brain express TH2/3 cytokines and brain-derived neurotrophic factor *in situ*. *Proc. Natl. Acad. Sci. USA.*, **100** (24), 14157–14162.

58 Aharoni, R., Eilam, R., Stock, A., Vainshtein, A., Shezen, E., Gal, H., Friedman, N., and Arnon, R. (2010) Glatiramer acetate reduces Th-17 inflammation and induces regulatory T-cells in the CNS of mice with relapsing-remitting or chronic EAE. *J. Neuroimmunol.*, **225**, 100–111.

59 Aharoni, R. and Arnon, R. (2009) Linkage between immunomodulation, neuroprotection and neurogenesis. *Drugs News Prospect.*, **22** (6), 301–312.

60 Kipnis, J., Yoles, E., Porat, Z., Cohen, A., Mor, F., Sela, M., Cohen, I.R., and Schwartz, M. (2000) T-cell immunity to copolymer 1 confers neuroprotection on the damaged optic nerve: possible therapy for optic neuropathies. *Proc. Natl. Acad. Sci. USA.*, **97**, 7446–7451.

61 Ziemssen, T., Kumpfel, T., Kinkert, W. E.F., Neuhaus, O., and Hohlfeld, R. (2002) Glatiramer acetate-specific T-helper 1- and 2-type cell lines produce BDNF: implications for multiple sclerosis therapy. Brain-derived neurotrophic factor. *Brain*, **125**, 2381–2391.

62 Chen, M., Valenzuela, R.M., and Dhib-Jalbut, S. (2003) Glatiramer acetate-reactive T-cells produce brain derived neurotrophic factor. *J. Neurol. Sci.*, **215**, 37–44.

63 Aharoni, R., Eylam, R., Domev, H., Labunsky, G., Sela, M., and Arnon, R. (2005) The immunomodulator glatiramer acetate augments the expression of neurotrophic factors in brains of experimental autoimmune encephalomyelitis mice. *Proc. Natl. Acad. Sci. USA.*, **102** (52), 19045–19050.

64 Lessman, V., Gottmann, K., and Malcangio, M. (2003) Neurotrophin secretion: current facts and future prospect. *Prog. Neurobiol.*, **69**, 341–374.

65 Riley, C.P., Cope, T.C., and Buck, C.R. (2004) CNS neurotrophins are biologically active and expressed by multiple cell types. *J. Mol. Histol.*, **35**, 771–783.

66 Bjartmar, C., Wujek, J.R., and Trapp, B. D. (2003) Axonal loss in the pathology of MS: consequences for understanding the progressive phase of the disease. *J. Neurol. Sci.*, **15**, 165–171.

67 Hobom, M., Storch, M.K., Weissert, R., Maier, K., Radhakrishnan, A., Kramer, B., Bahr, M., and Diem, R. (2004) Mechanisms and time course of neuronal degeneration experimental autoimmune encephalomyelitis. *Brain Pathol.*, **14**, 148–157.

68 Azoulay, D., Vachapova, V., Shihman, B., Miler, A., and Karni, A. (2005) Lower brain-derived neurotrophic factor in serum of relapsing remitting MS: reversal by glatiramer acetate. *J. Neuroimmunol.*, **167**, 215–218.

69 Maier, K., Kuhnert, A.V., Taheri, N., Sättler, M.B., Storch, M.K., Williams, S. K., Bähr, M., and Diem, R. (2006) Effects of glatiramer acetate and interferon-beta on neurodegeneration in a model of multiple sclerosis: a comparative study. *Am. J. Pathol.*, **169** (4), 1353–1364.

70 Aharoni, R., Arnon, R., and Eilam, R. (2005) Neurogenesis and neuroprotection induced by peripheral immunomodulatory treatment of experimental autoimmune encephalomyelitis. *J. Neurosci.*, **25** (36), 8228–8217.

71 Gilgun-Sherki, Y., Panet, H., Holdengreber, V., Mosberg-Galili, R., and Offen, D. (2003) Axonal damage is reduced following glatiramer acetate treatment in C57/bl mice with chronic-induced experimental autoimmune encephalomyelitis. *Neurosci. Res.*, **47**, 201–207.

72 Aharoni, R., Herschkovitz, A., Eilam, R., Blumberg-Hazan, M., Sela, M., Bruck, W., and Arnon, R. (2008) Demyelination arrest and remyelination induced by glatiramer acetate treatment of experimental autoimmune encephalomyelitis. *Proc. Natl. Acad. Sci. USA.*, **32**, 11358–11363.

73 Magavi, S.S., Leavitt, B.R., and Macklis, J.D. (2000) Induction of neurogenesis in the neocortex of adult mice. *Nature*, **405**, 951–955.

74 Aharoni, R., Aizman, E., Fuchs, O., Arnon, R., Yaffe, D., and Sarig, R. (2010) Transplanted myogenic progenitor cells express neuronal markers in the CNS and ameliorate disease in experimental autoimmune encephalomyelits. *J. Neuroimmunol.*, **225** (1–2), 100–111.

75 Filippi, M., Rovaris, M., Rocca, M.A., and the European/Canadian Glatiramer Acetate Study Group (2001) Glatiramer acetate reduces the proportion of new MS lesions evolving into "black holes". *Neurology*, **57**, 731–733.

76 Khan, O., Shen, Y., Caon, C. et al. (2005) Axonal metabolic recovery and potential neuroprotective effect of glatiramer acetate in relapsing-remitting multiple sclerosis. *Multiple Sclerosis*, **11**, 646–651.

77 Shanahan, F. (2001) Immunodiagnostics in immunotherapeutics and ectotherapeutics. *Gastroenterology*, **120**, 622–635.

78 Aharoni, R., Kayhan, B., and Arnon, R. (2005) Theraputic effect of the immunomodulator glatiramer acetate on trinitrobenzene sulfonic acid-induced experimental colitis. *Inflam. Bowel Dis.*, **11**, 106–115.

79 Aharoni, R., Kayhan, B., Brenner, O., Domev, H., Lubanskay, G., and Arnon, R. (2006) Immunomodulatory therapeutic effect of glatiramer acetate on several murine models of inflammatory bowel disease. *J. Pharmacol. Exp. Ther.*, **318**, 68–78.

80 Aharoni, R., Sonego, H., Brenner, O., Eilam, R., and Arnon, R. (2007) The therapeutic effect of glatiramer acetate in murine model of inflammatory bowel disease is mediated by anti-inflammatory T-cells. *Immunol. Lett.*, **112**, 110–119.

81 Elias, D., Birk, O.S., Van Der Zee, R., Walker, M.D., and Cohen, I.R. (1991) Vaccination against autoimmune mouse diabetes with a T-cell epitope of the human 60 kDa heat shock protein. *Proc. Natl. Acad. Sci. USA*, **88**, 3088–3091.

82 Raz, I., Elias, D., Avron, A., and Tamir, M. (2001) Beta-cell function on a new-onset type 1 diabetes and immunomodulation with a heat-shock protein peptide (DiaPep277): a randomized, double-blind, phase II trial. *Lancet*, **358**, 1749–1753.

83 Nussbaum, G., Zanin-Zhorov, A., Quintana, F., Lider, O., and Cohen, I.R. (2001) Peptide p277 of HSP60 signals T-cells: inhibition of flammatory chemotaxis. *Int. Immunol*, **18**, 1413–1419.

84 Sela, M. and Mozes, E. (2004) Therapeutic vaccines in autoimmunity. *Proc. Natl. Acad. Sci. USA.*, **101** (Supp. 2), 14586–14592.

85 Aruna, B.V., Sela, M., and Mozes, E. (2005) Suppression of myasthenogenic responses of a T-cell line by a dual altered peptide ligand by induction of CD4⁺ CD25- regulatory cells. *Proc. Natl. Acad. Sci. USA.*, **102**, 10285–10290.

86 Ben-David, H., Sharabi, A., Dayan, M., Sela, M., and Mozes, E. (2007) The role of CD8⁺ CD28- regulatory cells in suppressing myasthenia gravis-associated responses by a dual altered peptide ligand. *Proc. Natl. Acad. Sci. USA.*, **104**, 17459–17464.

87 Mozes, E. and Sharabi, A. (2010) A novel tolerogenic peptide for the specific treatment of systemic lupus erythematosus. *Autoimmun. Rev.*, **10**, 22–26.

88 Luger, D., Dayan, M., Zinger, H., Liu, J.-P., and Mozes, E. (2004) A peptide based on the complimentarity determining region 1 of a human monoclonal autoantibody ameliorates spontaneous and induced lupus manifestations in correlation with cytokine immunomodulation. *J. Clin. Immunol.*, **24**, 579–590.

89 Shtoeger, Z. M., Sharabi, A., Dayan, M., Zinger, H., Asher, I., Sela, U., and Mozes, E. (2009) The tolerogenic peptide, hCDR1, down-regulates pathogenic cytokines and apoptosis and up-regulates immunosuppressive molecules and regulatory T-cells in peripheral blood mononuclear cells of lupus patients. *Human Immunol.*, **70**, 139–145.

90 Shtoeger, Z.M., Sharabi, A., Molad, Y., Asher, I., Zinger, H., Dayan, M., and Mozes, E. (2009) Treatment of lupus patients with a tolerogenic peptide hCDR1 (Edratide): immunomodulation of gene expression. *J. Autoimmun.*, **33**, 77–82.

16
Development of Antibody Fragments for Therapeutic Applications

Sofia Côrte-Real, Frederico Aires da Silva, and João Gonçalves

16.1
Antibodies

Throughout the development of therapeutic antibodies over the past 30 years, many obstacles have been overcome and, today, therapeutic antibodies have entered a new era. Mouse hybridomas were the first therapeutic antibodies approved by the Food and Drug Administration (FDA). However, early studies on the use of murine mAbs determined that they had properties which could limit their clinical utility [1]. First, the human immune system recognizes murine mAbs as foreign material, producing human anti-mouse antibodies (HAMAs) leading to their clearance from the body, thereby limiting their therapeutic benefit. Second, murine mAbs were shown to have short serum half-lives and an inability to trigger human effector functions [1–3]. In an attempt to increase efficacy and reduce the immunogenicity of murine antibodies in humans, chimeric antibodies with mouse variable regions and human constant regions were developed by recombinant DNA technology [4, 5]. However, even though chimeric antibodies were less immunogenic than murine antibodies, human anti-chimeric antibody (HACAs) responses were still observed. Therefore, to further minimize the mouse component of antibodies, "humanized" antibodies were developed by protein engineering. Patients with Crohn's disease treated with infliximab develop human anti-chimeric antibodies (HACAs) in 8–61% of patients. These HACAs can bind to the therapeutic antibody, limiting its half-life and clinical effectiveness, as well as causing infusion-related anaphylaxis in some patients. The incidence of HACA development can be attenuated by co-administration of immunosuppressive agents in patients with Crohn's disease or with rheumatoid arthritis. The advent of humanization protocols and development of human antibodies have minimized this immunogenicity. However, patients treated with humanized or human antibodies still develop human anti-human antibodies (HAHAs). Adalimumab, a phage-derived human antibody, has an incidence of 12% neutralizing HAHAs in patients with rheumatoid arthritis receiving monotherapy, that is decreased

Peptide Drug Discovery and Development: Translational Research in Academia and Industry, First Edition.
Edited by Miguel Castanho and Nuno C. Santos.
© 2011 WILEY-VCH Verlag GmbH & Co. KGaA, Weinheim.
Published 2011 by WILEY-VCH Verlag GmbH & Co. KGaA

to ~1% in patients also treated with the immunosuppressant methotrexate. In such "humanized" antibodies, only the complementarity determining regions (CDRs) that are responsible for the antigen binding are grafted into the human variable-domain framework (FR) [6]. This ability to manipulate antibodies into more human variants finally made antibodies clinically useful [7–9]. There are currently 23 monoclonal antibodies in the market approved by the FDA as therapeutic agents in a wide range of indications, including transplant rejection, rheumatoid arthritis, cancer, Crohn's disease, and antiviral prophylaxis (Table 16.1). With more than 150 candidates in late-phase clinical trials, it is clear that monoclonal antibodies are becoming the most rapidly growing class of human therapeutics and the second largest class of biodrugs after vaccines. The introduction of humanization protocols, phage display technologies, the use of genetically modified mice expressing human immunoglobulins, and the application of PEGylation to increase the half-life of the antibody fragment have partially solved one of the historic obstacles of antibodies – immunogenicity.

As antibodies are such versatile and highly specific molecules, fine tuned by millions of years of evolution to be optimal agents for targeted disease elimination, their development for various indications has evolved greatly.

In antibody-based therapies, the goal is to eliminate or neutralize the pathogenic infection or the disease target, for example, bacterial, viral, or tumor targets. Therapeutic antibodies can function by three principal modes of action: by blocking the action of specific molecules, by targeting specific cells, or by functioning as signaling molecules. In other scenarios, effective treatment requires a more general immune response, and antibodies must boost effector functions such as antibody-dependent cellular cytotoxicity (ADCC) and/or complement-dependent cytotoxicity (CDC) [9]. In ADCC responses, antibodies bind to antigens on target cells and the antibody Fc domains engage Fc receptors (FcγRs) on the surface of effector cells such as macrophages and natural killer cells. These cells, in turn, trigger phagocytosis or lyse the targeted cell. In CDC, antibodies kill the targeted cells by triggering the complement cascade at the cell surface. These effector functions contribute to the therapeutic efficacy of several antibodies in clinical settings in which the destruction of target cells is desired, such as the removal of tumor cells or virally infected cells. A strong evidence for an Fc-mediated contribution to antibody efficacy in patients is the Rituximab (Genentech) monoclonal antibody [10]. Rituximab is a chimeric IgG1 that specifically targets the CD20 surface antigen expressed on normal and neoplastic B-lymphoid cells. Rituximab is currently indicated in both follicular and aggressive B-cell non-Hodgkin's lymphomas (NHL) and its impact on clinical treatment is clearly evidenced by its high effectiveness in triggering both ADCC and CDC responses [10–14].

16.1.1
Antibody Structure

Antibodies (or immunoglobins, Ig) have a basic structure consisting of two antigen-binding fragments (Fabs), which are linked via a flexible region (the hinge) to a constant (Fc) region, generally involved in interaction with effector systems such

Table 16.1 FDA approved therapeutic monoclonal antibodies in the United States.

Trade Name	Antibody Type	Antigen	Therapeutic use	Company	Approval year
OKT3	Murine IgG2a	CD3	Allograft rejection	Ortho Biotech	1986
ReoPro	Chimeric Fab	GPIIb/IIIa	Cardiovascular disease	Centocor	1994
Rituxan	Chimeric IgG1	CD20	Non-Hodgkin's lymphoma	Genentech	1997
Zenapax	Humanized IgG1	CD25	Transplant rejection	Roche	1997
Simulect	Chimeric IgG1	CD25	Transplant rejection	Novartis	1998
Synagis	Humanized IgG1	RSV	RSV propylaxis	MedImmune	1998
Remicade	Chimeric IgG1	TNF-α	Crohn's disease	Centocor	1998
Herceptin	Humanized IgG1	Her2	Metastatic breast cancer	Genentech	1998
Mylotarg	Humanized IgG4	CD33	Acute myeloid leukemia	Wyeth	2000
Campath	Humanized IgG1	CD52	Chronic myeloid leukemia	Genzyme	2001
Zevalin	Murine IgG1	CD20	Non-Hodgkin's lymphoma	Biogen Idec	2002
Humira	Human IgG1	TNFα	Crohn's disease	Abbott	2002
Xolair	Humanized IgG1	IgE	Asthma	Genentech	2003
Bexxar	Murine IgG2a	CD20	Non-Hodgkin's lymphoma	GlaxoSmithKline	2003
Raptiva	Humanized IgG1	CD11a	Psoriasis	Genentech	2003
Erbitux	Chimeric IgG1	EGFR	Colorectal cancer	Imclone Systems	2004
Avastin	Humanized IgG1	VEGF	Colorectal cancer	Genentech	2004
Tysabri	Humanized IgG4	α4-integrin	Multiple sclerosis	Biogen Idec	2004
Lucentis	Humanized Fab	VEGF	Wet macular degeneration	Genentech	2006
Panitumumab	Human IgG2	EGFR	Colorectal cancer	Amgen	2006
Eculizumab	Humanized IgG1	C5	Inflammatory diseases	Alexion Pharmaceuticals	2007
Certolizumab pegol	PEGylated Humanized Fab	TNF	Crohn's disease	UCB	2008
Golimumab	PEGylated Humanized Fab	TNF	RA, psoriathic arthritis and AS	Centocor	2009

RSV, respiratory syncytial virus; VEGF, vascular endothelial growth factor; EGFR, epidermal growth factor receptor; TNF, tumor necrosis factor; RA, Rheumatoid arthritis.

as complement, as well as molecules that determine the bio-distribution of the antibody (Figure 16.1).

The identical pair of heavy (H) chain polypeptides and a pair of identical light (L) chain polypeptides are held together by disulfide bridges and noncovalent bonds [15, 16]. Each of the heavy chains is encoded by: variable (V_H), diversity (D), joining (J_H), and constant (C_H) genetic segments; while each of the light chains is encoded by V_L, J_L, and C_L segments. The DNA and the amino acid sequences of the C region are relatively conserved within a given species while those of the V region are antigen dependent.

Pairing of the heavy V–D–J regions and light chain V–J regions creates an antigen-binding site (paratope) which recognizes a single antigenic determinant (epitope) [17]. The intervening strands of more rigid anti-parallel β-sheet are termed framework regions and are highly conserved. The hypervariable loops of a pair of VH and VL domains (H1, H2, and H3 and L1, L2, and L3) together form the antigen binding site. These loops, which vary in length and in sequence, are also known as complementarity-determining regions (CDRs) due to their dominant role in determining the shape of the binding site and its specificity. Each V region consists of an alternating framework (FR) and three complementarity-determining regions. The first 2 CDRs are encoded by the V segment while the third CDR is

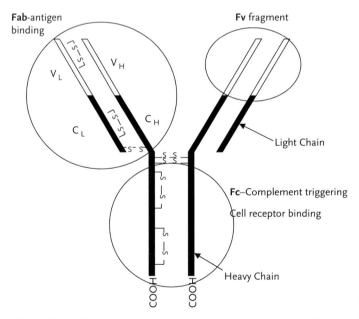

Figure 16.1 Schematic representation of the four chain structure of IgG emphasizing the relationship between structure and function. Disulfide bridges (⌒S⌒S⌒) link the two H chains and also the L and H chains. A regular arrangement of intrachain disulfide bonds is also found.

the product of the junction of the V–D–J for the heavy chain or V–J for the light chain. Analysis of the relationship between the sequence and three-dimensional structure of the combining sites revealed that, except for H3, the other loops have one of a small number of main-chain conformations or canonical structures. So, most of the binding specificity of an antibody is determined by the V_H domain, specifically by its CDR H3. The canonical structure formed in a particular loop is determined by its size and the presence of certain residues at key sites in the loop and in framework regions.

16.1.2
Antibody Fragments

Most marketed antibodies are comprised of a full-length IgG molecule that provides long half-life and effector functions. However, there is a range of therapeutic applications in which other antibody formats may be more desirable [18]. For instance, in some conditions a long antibody serum half-life results in poor contrast in imaging applications, and inappropriate activation of Fc receptor-expressing cells may lead to massive cytokine release and associated toxic effects. In addition, due to their high molecular weight ($\sim$150 kDa), IgG antibodies are known to diffuse poorly into solid tumors and clear slowly from the body. Therefore, to avoid Fc-associated effects in some clinical settings and to address the size limitations of IgGs, smaller antibody molecules such as the antigen-binding fragment (Fab) or the variable fragment (Fv) may be produced and become more attractive as therapeutic agents [18–25].

Cleavage of the IgG molecule with papain or recombinant technology can be used to yield Fab and Fv fragments (Figure 16.1). Both these fragments are stable, small molecular entities that exhibit most of the same properties as when they are part of the whole antibody molecule. The smaller Fv fragment (fragment variable) is composed of the V_H and V_L regions only. The recombinant version of the Fv fragment is termed the single-chain variable fragment (scFv) and the two variable regions are joined artificially by a flexible peptide linker, to produce scFv with improved antibody folding and stability (Figure 16.2a). Linkers of different compositions may result in different levels of oligomerization and may also alter the interface of the V_H and V_L regions (Figure 16.2). Single-chain fragments in which the light and heavy-chain variable regions are connected with a short peptide linker tend to form dimers, called bivalent diabodies, whereas scFvs with long linkers tend to be monomers. Bivalent diabodies can have the advantage of binding with higher avidity to their antigen, but the use of a short linker can also lead to selection of unwanted low-affinity binders.

The Fab fragment of an antibody is a structurally independent unit that contains the antigen-binding site; its stability is not influenced by the Fc part, as it is separated by the hinge region. The four domains of the Fab fragment (V_H, C_H1, V_L, C_L) interact through a large interface between the chains (V_H/V_L and C_H1/ C_L) and a small one between the variable and constant domains (V_H/ C_H1 and V_L/ C_L) of each chain (Figure 16.2).

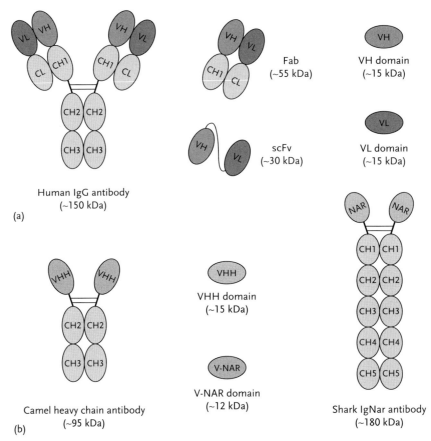

(a)

Human IgG antibody
(~150 kDa)

Fab
(~55 kDa)

scFv
(~30 kDa)

VH domain
(~15 kDa)

VL domain
(~15 kDa)

(b)

Camel heavy chain antibody
(~95 kDa)

VHH domain
(~15 kDa)

V-NAR domain
(~12 kDa)

Shark IgNar antibody
(~180 kDa)

Figure 16.2 Schematic representation of antibody constructs of biotechnological and clinical interest. (a) The engineering of antibody fragments that can be generated from an intact conventional IgG: antigen-binding fragment (Fab), single-chain Fv fragment (scFv) and heavy and light chains only (V domains). (b) Camelid and shark immunoglobulins are constituted only by heavy chains. They present no light chain and the displayed V domains of both species bind their target independently. Camelid heavy chain antibodies comprise a homodimer of one variable domain (VHH) and two C-like constant domains (CH). Shark IgNARs comprise a homodimer of one variable domain (V-NAR) and five C-like constant domains (CH). [26].

At this time, three non-IgG antibody molecules have been approved for human therapy. Abciximab (Centocor), the first one to be approved, is a chimeric Fab with mouse variable and human constant domains that inhibit platelet activation by blocking platelet glycoptotein IIb/IIIa receptor [27, 28]. Another antibody fragment is Ranibizumab, (Genentech), a humanized VEGF-specific Fab that is efficacious for treating neovascular age-related macular degeneration [29]. The most recently approved antibody fragment is Cimzia from UCB, a PEGylated Fab against TNF-alpha. In addition, many others are already in clinical trials. Examples include

Pexelizumab (Alexion Pharmaceuticals), a humanized scFv that is in Phase II/III testing for reducing mortality and myocardial infarction in patients undergoing graft surgery for coronary artery bypass [30]. Trubion Pharmaceuticals together with Pfizer was also developing TRU-015, a small modular immunopharmaceutical (SMIP™) drug candidate designed to target and deplete B-cells using a balance of effector functions optimized for inflammatory disease. *In vitro* and *in vivo* studies on TRU-015 demonstrate B-cell CD20 binding, ADCC and apoptosis activity, together with reduced CDC activity. Pfizer has presently discontinued TRU-015 but is completing a Phase II study with SBI-087, a humanized, subcutaneous CD20 RA product candidate in rheumatoid arthritis patients with active disease.[31] (see Table 16.2).

16.1.3
Single-Domain Antibodies

Fv and single-chain Fv (scFv) fragments are usually viewed as the smallest antibody units, which form complete antigen binding sites. However, early observations in the late 1960s indicated that sometimes VH domains alone retain a significant part of the original binding activity [32–34]. Based on this concept, in 1989 Greg Winter's group at the Medical Research Council, Cambridge,UK, isolated heavy chain variable domains with antigen affinity against lysozyme derived from an immunized murine VH library [35]. Despite such promising results, the efficient expression of VH fragments is usually confronted with folding problems, low solubility, and a high tendency for aggregation caused by the exposure of the hydrophobic VH/VL interface upon removal of the VL domain. Nevertheless, these problems seem to have been overcome, or at least greatly reduced for some mouse and rabbit VH domains by the identification and design of mutations that minimize the hydrophobic interface, and by direct selection of highly stable single-domains from phage display libraries [36–45]. In contrast, another promising alternative is the naturally heavy chain antibodies devoid of light chain that were recently discovered in two types of organisms, the camelids (camels and llamas) [46] and cartilaginous fish (wobbegong and nurse shark) [47–49] (Figure 16.2B). These heavy-chain antibodies recognize the antigen by one single variable domain and can be obtained from either immunized or non-immunized animals. In camelids, the variable heavy chains are referred to VHH ($\sim$ 15 kDa) and consist of four framework regions and three CDRs [50]. On the other hand, shark variable heavy chain are called IgNAR and contain only two CDR loops due to the deletion of a large portion of CDR2, which make them the smallest natural antigen binding site ($\sim$ 12 kDa) [47]. In VHH and IgNAR the third antigen-binding loop (CDR3) is often stabilized by disulfide bonds and is, on average, longer than a human or mouse VH-CDR3 loop. These smaller antibody molecules might, therefore, reach targets not easily recognized by currently marketed mAbs therapies, such as enzyme active sites and canyons in viral and infectious disease biomarkers [45, 51]. Further advantages include ease of manufacture, high stability, improved tumor tissue penetration, and rapid blood clearance [52–55]. As a result, it is clear that

Table 16.2 Protein and antibody scaffolds.

Trade name	Scaffold or format	Developer or licensee	Parent protein structure	Clinical trial phase	Target
Excallantide (Kalbitor/DX88)	Kunitz domain	Dyax	Human lipoprotein-associated coagulation inhibitor (LACI)	FDA approved (December 2009)	Kallikrein inhibitor
SBI-087	SMIP	Trubion/Pfizer	humanized, subcutaneous CD20 RA product candidate	Phase II	CD20
Dom-0200/ART621	Domain Antibody	Domantis (GSK)/Cephalon	V_H or V_L antibody domain; 100–130 amino acids	Phase II	TNF
MT103	BiTE	Micromet	scFv-scFv; 200–260 aa	Phase II	CD19 and CD3
Angiocept	Adnectin	Adnexus (Bristol Myers Squibb)	10th FN3 domain of fibronectin; 94 aminoacids	Phase II	VEGFR2
ALX-0018 and ALX-0681	Nanobody	Ablynx	VHH; 100 aa	Phase II	vWf
ALX-0141	Nanobody	Ablynx	VHH; 100 aa	Phase I	RANKL
ATN-103 and ALX-0061	Nanobody	Ablynx	VHH; 100 aa	Phase II	TNF and IL6R
ESBA105	scFv	ESBAtech/Alcon (Novartis)	scFv with hyperstable properties	Phase II	TNF
MT110	BiTE	Micromet	scFv-scFv; ~500aa	Phase I	EPCAM and CD3
ABY-002	Affibody	Affibody	Z domain of protein A from *Staphylococcus aureus*; 58 amino acids	Phase I	HER2
MP0112	DARPin	Molecular Partners	Ankyrin repeat proteins; 67 amino acids plus a repeating motif of 33 amino acids	Phase I	VEGF
PRS-050 (Angiocal)	Anticalin	Pieris	Lipocalin; 160–180 aa	Phase I	VEGF

ACS, acute coronary syndrome; ALL, acute lymphoblastic lymphoma; BiTE, bispecific T-cell engager; DARPin, designed ankyrin repeat protein; EPCAM, epithelial cell adhesion molecule; FDA, United States Food and Drug Administration; HER2, human epidermal growth factor receptor 2; IL, interleukin; LDL, low-density lipoprotein; NHL, non Hodgkin's lymphoma; NSCLC, non-small-cell lung carcinoma; R, receptor; scFv: single-chain variable domain antibody fragment; SMIP, small modular immunopharmaceutical; TNF, tumor necrosis factor; TTP, thrombotic thrombocytopenic purpura; VEGF, vascular endothelial growth factor; V_H, heavy chain variable domain; VHH, heavy chain variable domain (in camelids); V_L, light chain variable domain; vWF, von Willebrand factor.

single-domain antibodies will quickly become one of the most promising new generations of therapeutic mAbs. Indeed, there are currently three biotech companies focused only on single-domain antibodies as therapeutic agents. Domantis is one of these companies that was launched in the end of 2000 by Sir Gregory Winter and Dr Ian Tomlinson at the Medical Research Council, Cambridge, UK, with the aim to build up a series of large and highly functional libraries of fully human V_H and V_L domains. Today, Domantis has more than a dozen proprietary human single-domain antibody therapeutic programs in the fields of inflammation and oncology [45]. The other biopharmaceutical company is Ablynx, founded in Belgium in 2002 and engaged in the development of camelid single-domain antibodies [18]. The power of Ablynx's discovery platform has resulted so far in two VHH single-domains in pre-clinical trials for treatment of rheumatoid arthritis and inflammatory bowel disease and other mAbs for prevention of thrombosis associated with arterial stenosis. The third company is Technophage, a Portuguese biopharmaceutical company engaged in the research and development of therapeutics and diagnostics in three main R&D programs, managed by different Business Units, one of them being TechnoAntibodies that is developing single domain antibody fragments (sdAbs), using proprietary IP, against targets for inflammatory diseases, tumor antigens and cardiology. TechnoAntibodies is expected to finish preclinical studies and file an IND application in 2011 for inflammation therapeutics [56].

16.1.4
Engineering Multivalent, Bispecific, and Bifunctional Fragments

Converting whole IgG antibodies into Fab, scFv, or even single-domains fragments is usually associated with decrease in the antigen binding activity due to the loss of avidity. Nevertheless, this loss in binding activity can be compensated by engineering multivalent antibody fragments. Indeed, several antibody conjugates have already been constructed through the use of either chemical or genetic cross-links. These molecules span a molecular weight range of 60–150 kDa, and valences from two to four binding sites. For example, Fab fragments have been chemically cross-linked into di- and tri-valent multimers, leading to an increase in functional affinity [57–59]. On the other hand, several strategies have been devised to create multimeric scFvs genetically, however, the most successful design has been the simple reduction of the scFv linker length from 15–20 amino acids to 5 or less amino acids [18, 20]. While fragments with a 5 amino acid linker generally result in the formation of dimeric molecules (diabodies, ~60 kDa) with two binding sites, further reduction often leads to the assembly of trimers (triabodies, ~90 kDa) or tetramers (tetrabodies, ~120 kDa). An alternative format is the arrangement of two single-chain antibody fragments (scFv) connected by a flexible polypeptide linker on a single polypeptide chain.

In general, all multivalent antibody fragments are generated as being mono-specific. Nevertheless, some of the above strategies have also been applied to generate bispecific multimers. These bispecific antibodies have two different binding specificities fused together in a single molecule. Due to the dual specificity they can bind to two adjacent epitopes on a single antigen, thereby improving avidity. Alternatively, bispecific antibodies can cross-link two different antigens and be powerful therapeutic agents in some clinical settings [24]. The first approach to construct and produce bispecific antibodies was the quadroma technology that is based on the somatic fusion of two different hybridoma cell lines expressing murine monoclonal antibodies with the desired specificities of the bispecific antibody [60–62]. However, this technique is complex and time-consuming, and it produces unwanted pairing of the heavy and light chains. Far more effective methods incorporate chemical conjugation or genetic conjugation to couple two different Fab modules or smaller antibody fragments together [24, 63, 64]. Among the first bispecific antibodies were constructs designed to redirect T-cells against cancer target cells [65, 66]. Target cells were killed when cytotoxic T lymphocytes were tethered to tumor cells and simultaneously triggered by one arm of the bispecific antibody that interacted with the T-cell receptor (TCR)-CD3 complex. The use of the monomorphic CD3 complex for triggering T-cells circumvented the restrictions of clonotypic T-cell specificity, and enabled a polyclonal cytotoxic T lymphocyte response against target cells bearing the antigen recognized by the second arm of the bispecific antibody. Another development is bispecific antibodies that simultaneously bind tumor cells and an activating Fcγ receptor, for example, CD64/FcγRI on monocytes [67, 68]. Their binding to Fcγ receptors can elicit effector cell activation, without being competed by simultaneously binding normal IgG.

Antibody engineering has also been applied to build up bifunctional antibodies. In contrast to bispecific antibody fragments, bifunctional molecules combine the antigen binding site of an antibody with a biological function encoded by a linked or fused partner [24]. These include radionuclides, cytokines, toxins, enzymes, peptides, and proteins. Currently, Zevalin (Biogen Idedc Inc.), Bexxar (GlaxoSmithKline), and Mylotarg (Wyeth) are three examples of FDA approved bifunctional antibodies designed to specifically deliver cytotoxic drugs into cancer cells. Zevalin [69] and Bexxar [70] are both mouse anti-CD20 antibodies attached to yttrium-90 and Iodine-131 radioisotopes, respectively. Due to their bifunctional properties they can target the surface of mature B-cells and B-cell tumors, and induce cellular damage in the target and neighboring cells. In contrast, Mylotarg is a humanized monoclonal antibody that is linked to the anti-tumor agent calicheamicin, a bacterial toxin [71]. The antibody is targeted to CD33, which is expressed in about 90% of all acute myelogenic leukemia (AML) cases, and has been approved for administration to patients who have relapsed AML. Recently, bifunctional antibodies have also been developed to improve antibody pharmacokinetics. The small size of antibody fragments and single-domains improves their ability to penetrate tumors, and leads to rapid clearance from the circulation through the kidney. In some therapeutic applications, the rapid clearance is beneficial; however, in other cases it is desirable to increase the half-life of the antibody. This can be achieved by linking the antibody fragment or single-domain by chemical conjugation to a biocompatible polymer (PEG, polyethylene glycol) or peptides that bind to albumin or fibronectin, thus extending the half-life. PEGy-lation is clinically proven with PEGylated products worth over $8 bn pa currently being used by patients. PEGylation is particularly appropriate in decreasing the immunogenic response that is often experienced by patients [72, 73]. To date, one pEGylated antibody Fab fragment, Cimzia from UCB, as mentioned before, is already in the market. It has a circulating half-life prolonged to 14 days by site-specific PEGylation in the hinge region [74]. Cimzia has demonstrated that PEGylation can be used to extend the half-life of a Fab antibody fragment for use as a TNF-alpha inhibitor. Half-lives of each of the TNF-specific antibodies also define dosing schedules and modes of delivery. Infliximab has the shortest half-life ($\sim$8–10 days) among the TNF-specific antibodies and is administered intrave-nously every 4–8 weeks. By contrast, adalimumab and golimumab, both with half-lives of $\sim$2 weeks, are administered subcutaneously every 2–4 weeks, respectively. Subcutaneous administration is more convenient for patients, particularly those with chronic diseases requiring long-term therapy, as intravenous administration requires visits to physicians' offices or infusion centers.

16.1.5
Intracellular Antibodies (Intrabodies)

Intracellular antibodies, termed intrabodies, represent a new family of molecules that can be expressed within the context of a cell to define or mediate function(s) of a particular gene product [75]. When fused to well-characterized intracellular protein localization/trafficking signal peptides, antibodies can be expressed in different subcellular compartments, depending on the trafficking signals that are used. They are directed within a particular cellular compartment by the intracel-lular localization signals genetically fused to the N- or C-terminus of the antibody. When genetically fused to an intrabody, these short polypeptide "signals" (e.g., PKKKRKV derived from the large T antigen of SV40) can direct the intrabody to a specific subcellular localization (e.g., the nucleus) of its target antigen [76]. In principle, upon interaction with its target, an intrabody can modulate target pro-tein function or achieve functional knockout by one of the following mechanisms:

- Modulate protein enzymatic activities by inhibiting an activity directly, by sequestering substrate, or by maintaining the catalytic site in an active or inactive conformation.
- Disrupt the signaling pathway of a target protein through interference with its protein–protein, protein–DNA, or protein–RNA interactions.
- Divert a target protein from its normal site of action such as sequestering nuclear localized proteins in the cytosol, targeting of cytosolic proteins to the nucleus, and retention of secreted or cell surface-expressed proteins in the endoplasmic reticulum (ER).
- Accelerate degradation of target protein.

Besides specificity, other important criteria for choosing an intrabody would be the high antigen-binding affinity of the scFv binding site [77]. However, when expressed inside a cell, the behavior of scFvs is often unpredictable, and does not always correlate with their *in vitro* binding affinities. Several studies have shown that the intracellular stability of an intrabody, not affinity, is highly critical for its efficacy. The main factors contributing to scFvs stability are disulfide bond formation and correct protein folding. The primary amino acid sequence of an scFv also contributes directly to its stability. In its natural environment, an antibody is directed to the secretory pathway, where it is synthesized and processed to allow correct folding and disulfide formation [78, 79]. Once released outside a cell, an antibody maintains its correct conformation and thus is stable in the oxidized extracellular environment. However, in the reducing environment of the cytosol, formation of intrachain disulfide bonds does not occur, and maintenance of correct folding is inefficient, which would result in protein aggregation [80]. This is why scFvs which do not have disulfide bonds are used as intrabodies, and not Fabs which have a higher affinity, but cannot fold efficiently in the reducing environment of a cell. Gene therapy application of intrabodies in animal studies, or eventually as therapeutic agents in human diseases, needs to overcome other problems that are common for gene therapy, such as development of efficient gene transfer vehicles and high level gene expression that is not only long-term, but also regulatable. These advances combined with the recent improvements in viral and non-viral vectors that are safer, less immunogenic and capable of achieving tissue-specific gene transfer through cell surface targeting should enable intrabody technology to prosper [80].

16.1.5.1 Immunogenicity of Engineered Antibodies

Antibody therapeutics continues to demonstrate clinical efficacy in an ever-wider array of indications. Murine monoclonal antibodies have proved to be tremendously useful in diagnostics. However, when used in the treatment of patients with various ailments, their effect is not always sustained. This is often due to the development of HAMA, leading to clearance of the murine mAb and adverse events that are sometimes fatal. HAMA has been the impetus for efforts over the last 20 years to reduce the murine content of therapeutic mAb. Chimeric antibodies, constructed by linking murine variable and human constant regions [5], were an important first step in Ab immunogenicity reduction. Although they possess greatly reduced immunogenicity relative to murine versions, chimerics still pose a significant risk of eliciting an immune response [81]. The development of CDR grafting [7], whereby CDRs from a murine donor Ab are grafted onto human variable regions acceptor FRs, was a subsequent advancement. The variety of humanization methods based on this technique [82] has produced antibodies that are more homologous to human sequences than the original chimeric mAbs, often resulting, but not always, in a reduction in the Ab imunogenicity to clinically acceptable levels [81]. The main goal of CDR-grafting based humanization methods is the maximization of identity between a single donor and a single acceptor sequence. The underlying assumption is that higher global sequence identity of a humanized sequence to the human acceptor results in a lower risk of immunogenicity. Nevertheless, with respect to molecular immunology, the global identity is just a fraction of the immunogenic potential. The immunogenicity of a recombinant antibody agent depends on its ability to trigger either a cellular or a humoral immune response. In the first case, the T-cells recognize small peptides resulting from proteolytic processing of the agent displayed on the binding groove of the MHC molecule of the antigen-presenting cells. In the second case, the B-cells recognize the biotherapeutic agent as strange and produce antibodies against it. In contrast to foreign proteins, the native human Ab repertoire is non-immunogenic because the corresponding peptides either fail to bind to MHC-II, or are not recognized by reactive T-cells. Hence, an administered protein will be non-immunogenic to the extent that its corresponding peptide sequences lack MHC and/or T-cell reactivity. Therefore, the identification and removal of MHC-II and T-cell reactive epitopes have become key strategies to reduce the immunogenicity of therapeutic proteins. This molecular understanding of immune reaction and tolerance highlights the limitations of humanization methods that employ CDR grafting. Standard protocols based on CDR grafting are poor engineering tools for addressing these other properties. CDR grafting typically leads to structural incompatibilities between CDRs and FRs, as well as across the VH/VL interface, resulting in substantial reductions in antigen affinity. These problems are often partially resolved by back-mutating crucial FR residues to the original murine amino acids, creating additional non-human sequences and thereby potentially restoring or generating new immunogenic potential. Because CDRs are often treated as inviolable, grafting of foreign donor CDRs onto a human acceptor framework leaves many non-human agretopes, including not only those within the foreign CDRs, but also those generated at the FR/CDR boundaries. CDR grafting generally maximizes the donor–acceptor identity of the frameworks at the expense of linear sequence epitopes within the CDRs and at the FR/CDR boundaries [83]. This may, in part, be responsible for the lack of robustness in immune evasion observed for humanized antibodies. In fact, several humanized antibodies elicit a significant immune response when administered clinically [81], and response incidences as high as 63% have been reported [84].

16.1.5.2 Engineering New Protein Scaffolds

Recent advances in novel methods of combinatorial protein engineering have made it possible to develop antibody-based and other protein scaffolds that can potentially substitute most of the antibody functions. It is conceivable that many different natural human protein backbones are suitable to be used as structural templates for engineering: antibody-derived scaffolds, novel proteins with a single binding interface, protein domains that offer a rigid core structure appropriate for grafting loops or, instead, protein scaffolds tolerating the fusion of variable loops in suitable configuration. Nevertheless, only a few have yielded the necessary properties to be translated into novel therapeutic proteins. The most important of these are potential broad specificities towards any potential target, high yield production, reduced size, good tolerability, and low immunogenicity. Circumventing antibody-associated patents is often a major if not primary goal of developing these new protein scaffolds. Nevertheless, to translate scaffold discovery into successful therapeutic protein candidates they have to show clear advantages compared to whole antibodies.

While many protein scaffolds have been proposed during the past years, the technology shows a trend toward consolidation, with a smaller set of systems that are being applied against multiple targets and in different settings, with emphasis on the development of drug candidates for therapy or *in vivo* diagnostics: Adnectins, Affibodies, Anticalins, DARPins, and engineered Kunitz-type inhibitors, among others. These new small protein scaffolds are currently being tested as alternatives to antibodies. They may be cheaper to produce and have advantages associated with smaller size, such as deeper tumor penetration. Such small protein-based drugs can have highly specific binding properties derived usually from human proteins. Some of them are described in Table 16.2 and more than 10 protein scaffolds have entered clinical trials. More recently ecallantide (Kalbitor/DX-88; Dyax) which is a Kunitz domain-based scaffold that targets human plasma kallikrein, was approved in December 2009 by the FDA for the treatment of attacks of hereditary angioedema. [85–87] Once again, one of the main disadvantages of these new drugs is their potential immunogenicity and safety profile, however, it is encouraging that none of them elicited severe adverse reactions or anti-drug antibody responses during Phase I clinical trials.

Only few data from early clinical studies are available yet, but many more are likely to come in the near future, thus providing a growing basis for assessing the therapeutic potential – but possibly also some limitations – of this exciting new class of protein drugs.

16.2
Conclusions

Enormous strides have been made in the past decade toward the discovery, optimization and therapeutic application of antibodies to a wide variety of pathologies. The Kohler and Milstein endeavor of mAbs as elegantly sensitive therapeutics has finally been fulfilled. The examples presented above indicate that this class of drugs can be highly effective as therapeutic agents. From a stalled start, mAbs now represent around 30% of the novel biological entities entering clinical trials, indicating that the biotechnology community at large has finally recognized the speed and efficiency of the antibody platform.

As a proven maturity of the field, the latest advances in antibody design and scaffold engineering are poised to contribute to more innovative and extensive applications in the field of biodrugs. It has been demonstrated that V-like domains provide alternative and efficient scaffolds for the presentation of paratopes capable of reaching buried epitopes and targeting, therefore, refractory antigens. Due to the recent advances in scaffold design, repertoire construction and selection strategies there is currently rapid progress in the generation of specific, high affinity mAb fragments against virtually any antigen. After intensive engineering and preclinical/clinical testing, antibody fragments are now set to join mAb as powerful therapeutic and diagnostic agents.

Overall, it is also becoming clear (and ironic) that the classical mAbs may yet become the commercial savior of the high-tech proteomics and genomics revolutions. Increasingly, antibody fragments are also being applied to proteomic discovery of new cancer biomarkers, and exploitation at the level of robust and sensitive immunosensors.

References

1 Khazaeli, M.B., Conry, R.M., and LoBuglio, A.F. (1994) Human immune response to monoclonal antibodies. *J. Immunother.*, **15** (1), 42–52.

2 Köhler, G. and Milstein, C. (1975) Continuous cultures of fused cells secreting antibody of predefined specificity. *Nature*, **256** (5517), 495–497.

3 Hwang, W.Y. and Foote, J. (2005) Immunogenicity of engineered antibodies. *Methods*, **36** (1), 3–10.

4 Presta, L.G. (2006) Engineering of therapeutic antibodies to minimize immunogenicity and optimize function. *Adv. Drug Deliv. Rev.*, **58** (5), 640–656.

5 Morrison, S.L., Johnson, M.J., Herzenberg, L.A. *et al.* (1984) Chimeric human antibody molecules: mouse antigen-binding domains with human constant region domains. *Proc. Natl. Acad. Sci. U. S. A.*, **81** (21), 6851–6855.

6 Jones, P.T., Dear, P.H., Foote, J. *et al.* (1986) Replacing the complementarity-determining regions in a human antibody with those from a mouse. *Nature*, **321** (6069), 522–525.

7 Brekke, O.H. and Sandlie, I. (2003) Therapeutic antibodies for human diseases at the dawn of the twenty-first century. *Nat. Rev. Drug Discov.*, **2** (1), 52–62.

8 Reichert, J.M., Rosensweig, C.J., Faden, L.B. *et al.* (2005) Monoclonal antibody successes in the clinic. *Nat. Biotechnol.*, **23** (9), 1073–1078.

9 Carter, P.J. (2006) Potent antibody therapeutics by design. *Nat. Rev. Immunol.*, **6** (5), 343–57.

10 Reff, M.E., Carner, K., Chambers, K.S. *et al.* (1994), Depletion of B cells *in vivo* by a chimeric mouse human monoclonal antibody to CD20. *Blood*, **83** (2), 435–445.

11 Cartron, G., Watier, H., Golay, J. *et al.* (2004) From the bench to the bedside: ways to improve rituximab efficacy. *Blood*, **104** (9), 2635–2642.

12 Flieger, D., Renoth, S., Beier, I. *et al.* (2000) Mechanism of cytotoxicity induced by chimeric mouse human monoclonal antibody IDEC-C2B8 in CD20-expressing lymphoma cell lines. *Cell Immunol.*, **204** (1), 55–63.

13 Harjunpaa, A., Junnikkala, S., and Meri, S. (2000) Rituximab (anti-CD20) therapy of B-cell lymphomas: direct complement killing is superior to cellular effector mechanisms. *Scand. J. Immunol.*, **51** (6), 634–641.

14 Golay, J., Lazzari, M., Facchinetti, V. *et al.* (2001) CD20 levels determine the *in vitro* susceptibility to rituximab and complement of B-cell chronic lymphocytic leukemia: further regulation by CD55 and CD59. *Blood*, **98** (12), 3383–3389.

15 Harlow, E. and Lane, D. (1988) *Antibodies: A Laboratory Manual*, New York, Cold Spring Harbor Laboratory.

16 Barbas, C.F. III, Burton, R., Scott, J.K., and Silverman, G.J. (2001) *Phage Display, A Laboratory Manual* Cold Spring Harbor Laboratory.

17 Azzazy, H.M. and Highsmith, W.E. Jr (2002) Phage display technology: clinical applications and recent innovations. *Clin. Biochem.*, **35** (6), 425–445.

18 Holliger, P. and Hudson, P.J. (2005) Engineered antibody fragments and the rise of single domains. *Nat. Biotechnol.*, **23** (9), 1126–1136.

19 Huston, J.S., McCartney, J., Tai, M.S. *et al.* (1993) Medical applications of single-chain antibodies. *Int. Rev. Immunol.*, **10** (2), 195–217.

20 Hudson, P.J. (1998) Recombinant antibody fragments. *Curr. Opin. Biotechnol.*, **9** (4), 395–402.

21 Dall'Acqua, W. and Carter, P. (1998) Antibody engineering. *Curr. Opin. Struct. Biol.*, **8** (4), 443–450.

22 Hudson, P.J. (1999) Recombinant antibody constructs in cancer therapy. *Curr. Opin. Immunol.*, **11** (5), 548–557.

23 Presta, L. (2003) Antibody engineering for therapeutics. *Curr. Opin. Struct. Biol.*, **13** (4), 519–525.

24 Hudson, P.J. and Souriau, C. (2003) Engineered antibodies. *Nat. Med.*, **9** (1), 129–134.

25 Kipriyanov, S.M. (2003) Generation of antibody molecules through antibody engineering. *Methods Mol. Biol.*, **207**, 3–25.

26 Aires da Silva, F., Corte-Real, S., and Goncalves, J. (2008) Recombinant antibodies as therapeutic agents. *Biodrugs*, **22** (5), 301–314.

27 Reverter, J.C., Beguin, S., Kessels, H. *et al.* (1996) Inhibition of platelet-mediated, tissue factor-induced thrombin generation by the mouse/human chimeric 7E3 antibody. Potential implications for the effect of c7E3 Fab treatment on acute thrombosis and "clinical restenosis". *J. Clin. Invest.*, **98** (3), 863–874.

28 Coller, B.S. (1997) GPIIb/IIIa antagonists: pathophysiologic and therapeutic insights from studies of c7E3 Fab. *Thromb. Haemost.*, **78** (1), 730–735.

29 Kaiser, P.K. and Do, D.V. (2007) Ranibizumab for the treatment of neovascular AMD. *Int. J. Clin. Pract.*, **61** (3), 501–509.

30 Haverich, A., Shernan, S.K., Levy, J.H. *et al.* (2006) Pexelizumab reduces death and myocardial infarction in higher risk cardiac surgical patients. *Ann. Thorac. Surg.*, **82** (2), 486–492.

31 Available on http://www.trubion.com

32 Haber, E. and Richards, F.F. (1966) The specificity of antigenic recognition of antibody heavy chain. *Proc. R. Soc. London, Ser. B Biol. Sci.*, **166** (3), 176–187.

33 Rockey, J.H. (1967) Equine antihapten antibody. The subunits and fragments of

34 Jaton, J.C., Klinman, N.R., Givol, D. *et al.* (1968) Recovery of antibody activity upon reoxidation of completely reduced polyalanyl heavy chain and its Fd fragment derived from anti-2,4-dinitrophenyl antibody. *Biochemistry*, **7** (12), 4185–4195.

35 Ward, E.S., Gussow, D., Griffiths, A.D. *et al.* (1989) Binding activities of a repertoire of single immunoglobulin variable domains secreted from *Escherichia coli*. *Nature*, **341** (6242), 544–546.

36 Cai, X. and Garen, A. (1996) A melanoma-specific V_H antibody cloned from a fusion phage library of a vaccinated melanoma patient. *Proc. Natl. Acad. Sci. U.S.A.*, **93** (13), 6280–6285.

37 Davies, J. and Riechmann, L. (1994) 'Camelising' human antibody fragments: NMR studies on V_H domains. *FEBS Lett.*, **339** (3), 285–290.

38 Davies, J. and Riechmann, L. (1996) Single antibody domains as small recognition units: design and *in vitro* antigen selection of camelized, human V_H domains with improved protein stability. *Protein Eng.*, **9** (6), 531–537.

39 Tanha, J., Xu, P., Chen, Z. *et al.* (2001) Optimal design features of camelized human single-domain antibody libraries. *J. Biol. Chem.*, **276** (27), 24774–24780.

40 Aires da Silva, F., Santa-Marta, M., Freitas-Vieira, A. *et al.* (2004) Camelized rabbit-derived VH single-domain intrabodies against Vif strongly neutralize HIV-1 infectivity. *J. Mol. Biol.*, **340** (3), 525–542.

41 Dottorini, T., Vaughan, C.K., Walsh, M.A. *et al.* (2004) Crystal structure of a human VH: requirements for maintaining a monomeric fragment. *Biochemistry*, **43** (3), 622–628.

42 Jespers, L., Schon, O., James, L.C. *et al.* (2004) Crystal structure of HEL4, a soluble, refoldable human V(H) single domain with a germ-line scaffold. *J. Mol. Biol.*, **337** (4), 893–903.

43 Jespers, L., Schon, O., Famm, K. *et al.* (2004) Aggregation-resistant domain antibodies selected on phage by heat

denaturation. *Nat. Biotechnol.*, **22** (9), 1161–1165.

44 Tanha, J., Nguyen, T.D., Ng, A. *et al.* (2006) Improving solubility and refolding efficiency of human V(H)s by a novel mutational approach. *Protein Eng. Des. Sel.*, **19** (11), 503–509.

45 Holt, L.J., Herring, C., Jespers, L.S. *et al.* (2003) Domain antibodies: proteins for therapy. *Trends Biotechnol.*, **21** (11), 484–490.

46 Hamers-Casterman, C., Atarhouch, T., Muyldermans, S. *et al.* (1993) Naturally occurring antibodies devoid of light chains. *Nature*, **363** (6428), 446–448.

47 Greenberg, A.S., Avila, D., Hughes, M. *et al.* (1995) A new antigen receptor gene family that undergoes rearrangement and extensive somatic diversification in sharks. *Nature*, **374** (6518), 168–173.

48 Nuttall, S.D., Krishnan, U.V., Hattarki, M. *et al.* (2001) Isolation of the new antigen receptor from wobbegong sharks, and use as a scaffold for the display of protein loop libraries. *Mol. Immunol.*, **38** (4), 313–326.

49 Roux, K.H., Greenberg, A.S., Greene, L. *et al.* (1998) Structural analysis of the nurse shark (new) antigen receptor (NAR): molecular convergence of NAR and unusual mammalian immunoglobulins. *Proc. Natl. Acad. Sci. U.S.A.*, **95** (20), 11804–12089.

50 Muyldermans, S. (2001) Single domain camel antibodies: current status. *J. Biotechnol.*, **74** (4), 277–302.

51 Desmyter, A., Decanniere, K., Muyldermans, S. *et al.* (2001) Antigen specificity and high affinity binding provided by one single loop of a camel single-domain antibody. *J. Biol. Chem.*, **276** (28), 26285–26290.

52 Cortez-Retamozo, V., Lauwereys, M., Hassanzadeh, Gh.G. *et al.* (2002) Efficient tumour targeting by single-domain antibody fragments of camels. *Int. J. Cancer*, **98** (3), 456–462.

53 Cortez-Retamozo, V., Backmann, N., Senter, P.D. *et al.* (2004) Efficient cancer therapy with a nanobody-based conjugate. *Cancer Res.*, **64** (8), 2853–2857.

54 van der Linden, R.H., Frenken, L.G., De Geus, B. *et al.* (1999) Comparison of physical chemical properties of llama VHH antibody fragments and mouse monoclonal antibodies. *Biochim. Biophys. Acta*, **1431** (1), 37–46.

55 Frenken, L.G., van der Linden, R.H., Hermans, P.W. *et al.* (2000) Isolation of antigen specific llama VHH antibody fragments and their high level secretion by Saccharomyces cerevisiae. *J. Biotechnol.*, **78** (1), 11–21.

56 Available on http://www.technophage.pt.

57 Casey, J.L., Napier, M.P., King, D.J. *et al.* (2002) Tumour targeting of humanised cross-linked divalent-Fab' antibody fragments: a clinical phase I/II study. *Br. J. Cancer*, **86** (9), 1401–1410.

58 Weir, A.N., Nesbitt, A., Chapman, A.P. *et al.* (2002) Formatting antibody fragments to mediate specific therapeutic functions. *Biochem. Soc. Trans.*, **30** (4), 512–516.

59 Casey, J.L., King, D.J., Chaplin, L.C. *et al.* (1996) Preparation, characterisation and tumour targeting of cross-linked divalent and trivalent anti-tumour Fab' fragments. *Br. J. Cancer*, **74** (9), 1397–405.

60 Milstein, C. and Cuello, A.C. (1983) Hybrid hybridomas and their use in immunohistochemistry. *Nature*, **305** (5934), 537–540.

61 Staerz, U.D. and Bevan, M.J. (1986) Hybrid hybridoma producing a bispecific monoclonal antibody that can focus effector T-cell activity. *Proc. Natl. Acad. Sci. U. S. A.*, **83** (5), 1453–1457.

62 Suresh, M.R., Cuello, A.C., and Milstein, C. (1986) Bispecific monoclonal antibodies from hybrid hybridomas. *Methods Enzymol.*, **121**, 210–228.

63 Holliger, P., Prospero, T., Winter, G. *et al.* (1993) Diabodies: small bivalent and bispecific antibody fragments. *Proc. Natl. Acad. Sci. U.S.A.*, **90** (14), 6444–6448.

64 Kipriyanov, S.M., Moldenauer, G., Schuhmacher, J. *et al.* (1999) Bispecific tandem diabody for tumor therapy with improved antigen binding and

pharmacokinetics. *J. Mol. Biol.*, **293** (1), 41–56.

65 Staerz, U.D., Kanagawa, O. and Bevan, M.J. (1985) Hybrid antibodies can target sites for attack by T cells. *Nature*, **314** (6012), 628–631.

66 Loffler, A., Gruen, M., Wuchter, C. *et al.* (2003) Efficient elimination of chronic lymphocytic leukaemia B cells by autologous T cells with a bispecific anti-CD19/anti-CD3 single-chain antibody construct. *Leukemia*, **17** (5), 900–909.

67 Karpovsky, B., Titus, J.A., Stephany, D.A. *et al.* (1984) Production of target-specific effector cells using hetero-cross-linked aggregates containing anti-target cell and anti-Fc gamma receptor antibodies. *J. Exp. Med.*, **160** (6), 1686–1701.

68 De Jonge, J. Heirman, C., De Veerman, M. *et al.* (1998) *In vivo* retargeting of T cell effector function by recombinant bispecific single chain Fv (anti-CD3 x anti-idiotype) induces long-term survival in the murine BCL1 lymphoma model. *J. Immunol.*, **161** (3), 1454–1461.

69 Vose, J.M., Bierman, P.J., Loberiza, F.R. Jr *et al.* (2007) Phase I trial of (90)Y-ibritumomab tiuxetan in patients with relapsed B-cell non-Hodgkin's lymphoma following high-dose chemotherapy and autologous stem cell transplantation. *Leuk. Lymphoma*, **48** (4), 683–690.

70 Macklis, R.M. (2006) Iodine-131 tositumomab (Bexxar) in a radiation oncology environment. *Int. J. Radiat. Oncol. Biol. Phys.*, **66** (Suppl. 2), S30–S34.

71 Larson, R.A., Boogaerts, M., Estey, E. *et al.* (2002) Antibody-targeted chemotherapy of older patients with acute myeloid leukemia in first relapse using Mylotarg (gemtuzumab ozogamicin). *Leukemia*, **16** (9), 1627–1636.

72 Chapman, A.P. (2002) PEGylated antibodies and antibody fragments for improved therapy: a review. *Adv. Drug Deliv. Rev.*, **54** (4), 531–545.

73 Chapman, A.P., Antoniw, P., Spitali, M., West, S., Stephens, S., and King, D.J. (1999) Therapeutic antibody fragments with prolonged *in vivo* half-lives. *Nat. Biotechnol.*, **17** (8), 780–783.

74 Choy, E.H., Hazleman, B., Smith, M. *et al.* (2002) Efficacy of a novel PEGylated humanized anti-TNF fragment (CDP870) in patients with rheumatoid arthritis: a phase II double-blinded, randomized, dose-escalating trial. *Rheumatology (Oxford).*, **41** (10), 1133–1137.

75 Marasco, W.A. (1998) *Intrabodies – Basic Research and Clinical Gene Therapy Applications*, in (ed. W.A. Marasco), Springer, New York, pp. 1–22.

76 Bradbury, A. (1997) Recombinant antibodies for ectopic expression, in (eds A. Cattaneo and S. Biocca), *Intracellular Antibodies: Development and Applications.* New York, Springer-Verlags and Landes Biosciences, pp. 15–40.

77 Zhu, Q. and Marasco, W.A. (2003) Intracellular targeting of antibodies in mammalian cells, in (ed. S.C. Makrides), *Gene Transfer and Expression in Mammalian Cells.* Elsevier Science B.V.

78 Worn, A. and Pluckthun, A. (1998) An intrinsically stable antibody scFv fragment can tolerate the loss of both disulfide bonds and fold correctly. *FEBS Lett.*, **427** (3), 357–361.

79 Osbourn, J., Jermutus, L., and Duncan, A. (2003) Current methods for the generation of human antibodies for the treatment of autoimmune diseases. *Drug Discovery Today*, **8**, 845–851.

80 Rondon, I.J. and Marasco, W.A. (1997) Intracellular antibodies (Intrabodies) for gene therapy of infectious diseases. *Annu. Rev. Microbiol.*, **51**, 257–283.

81 Hwang, W.Y., Almagro, J.C., Buss, T.N. *et al.* (2005) Use of human germline genes in a CDR homology-based approach to antibody humanization. *Methods*, **36** (1), 35–42.

82 Tsurushita, N. and Vasquez, M. (2003) Humanization of monoclonal antibodies, in (eds T. Honjo, F. Alt, and M. Neuberger), *Molecular Biology of B Cells*, Academic Press, San Diego, 533–545.

83 Clark, M. (2000) Antibody humanization: a case of the 'Emperor's new clothes'?. *Immunol. Today*, **21** (8), 397–402.

84 Ritter, G., Cohen, L.S., and Williams, C. Jr *et al.* (2001) Serological analysis of human anti-human antibody responses in colon cancer patients treated with repeated doses of humanized monoclonal antibody A33. *Cancer Res.*, **61** (18), 6851–6859.

85 Wurch, T. *et al.* (2008) Development of novel protein scaffolds as alternatives to whole antibodies for imaging and

therapy: status on discovery research and clinical validation. *Curr. Pharm. Biotechnol.*, **9**, 502–509.

86 Gebauer, M. and Skerra, A. (2009) Engineered protein scaffolds as next generation antibody therapeutics. *Curr. Opin. Chem. Biol.*, **13**, 245–255.

87 Hughes, B. (2010) 2009 FDA drug approvals. *Nature Rev. Drug Discov.*, **9**, 89–92.

Index

Peptide Drug Discovery and Development: Translational Research in Academia and Industry, First Edition.
Edited by Miguel Castanho and Nuno C. Santos.
© 2011 WILEY-VCH Verlag GmbH & Co. KGaA, Weinheim.
Published 2011 by WILEY-VCH Verlag GmbH & Co. KGaA